www.harcourt-international.com

Bringing you products from all Harcourt Health Sciences companies including Baillière Tindall, Churchill Livingstone, Mosby and W.B. Saunders

- ▶ **Browse** for latest information on new books, journals and electronic products

- ▶ **Search** for information on over 20 000 published titles with full product information including tables of contents and sample chapters

- ▶ **Keep up to date** with our extensive publishing programme in your field by registering with eAlert or requesting postal updates

- ▶ **Secure online ordering** with prompt delivery, as well as full contact details to order by phone, fax or post

- ▶ **News** of special features and promotions

If you are based in the following countries, please visit the country-specific site to receive full details of product availability and local ordering information

USA: www.harcourthealth.com

Canada: www.harcourtcanada.com

Australia: www.harcourt.com.au

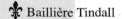 Baillière Tindall 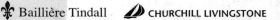 CHURCHILL LIVINGSTONE Mosby 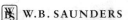 W.B. SAUNDERS

Respiratory Nursing

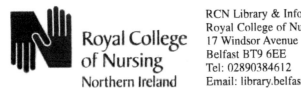
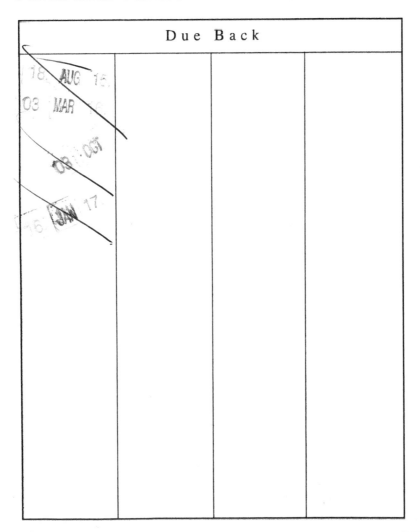

For Baillière Tindall:

Senior Commissioning Editor: Ninette Premdas
Project Manager: Gail Murray
Project Development Manager: Mairi McCubbin
Designer: George Ajayi

Respiratory Nursing

Edited by

Glenda Esmond BSc(Hons) Dip Nursing RGN
Lecturer Practitioner, City University, St Bartholomew School
of Nursing and Midwifery and London Chest Hospital,
London, UK

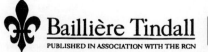 Baillière Tindall
PUBLISHED IN ASSOCIATION WITH THE RCN

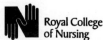 Royal College
of Nursing

EDINBURGH LONDON NEW YORK PHILADELPHIA ST LOUIS SYDNEY TORONTO 2001

BAILLIÈRE TINDALL

An imprint of Harcourt Publishers Limited
© Harcourt Publishers Limited 2001

 is a registered trademark of Harcourt Publishers Limited

The right of Glenda Esmond to be identified as editor of this
work has been asserted by her in accordance with the Copyright,
Designs and Patents Act 1988

First published 2001

ISBN 0 7020 2427 9

British Library Cataloguing in Publication Data
A catalogue record for this book is available from the British
Library

Library of Congress Cataloging in Publication Data
A catalog record for this book is available from the Library of
Congress

Note
Medical knowledge is constantly changing. As new information
becomes available, changes in treatment, procedures, equipment
and the use of drugs become necessary. The editor, contributors
and the publishers have taken care to ensure that the information
given in this text is accurate and up to date. However, readers are
strongly advised to confirm that the information, especially with
regard to drug usage, complies with the latest legislation and
standards of practice.

The
Publisher's
policy is to use
paper manufactured
from sustainable forests

Printed in China

Contents

Contributors

Cecilia Connolly RGN
Welfare Advisor Assistant (Women's Section),
Royal British Legion, London, UK

Carol Lynn Cox BSc(Hons) MSc MAEd PhD PEDipEd RN
MSc Programme Leader, City University,
St Bartholomew School of Nursing and
Midwifery, London, UK

Liz Dunn BSc(Hons) RGN
Clinical Nurse Manager, Lane Fox Unit, Guy's
and St Thomas' Hospital Trust, London, UK

Glenda Esmond BSc(Hons) Dip Nursing RGN
Lecturer Practitioner, City University,
St Bartholomew School of Nursing and
Midwifery and London Chest Hospital,
London, UK

Paul Hateley BSc Dip Counselling DMS RGN RMN
Head of Nursing, Pathologies and Patient
Services, St Bartholomew's Hospital, London, UK

Linda M Mackay BSc MSc RGN Higher Dip HV
Formerly Teamleader, Respiratory Nursing
Services, Riverside Community Health Care
NHS Trust, London, UK

Susan Madge MSc SRN RSCN
Clinical Nurse Specialist, Respiratory Unit,
Great Ormond Street Hospital, London, UK

Carl Margereson BSc(Hons) MSc DipN(Lond) RGN
RMN RNT
Senior Lecturer, Thames Valley University,
Faculty of Health and Human Sciences,
London, UK

Christine Mikelsons BSc(Hons) MCSP
Superintendent Physiotherapist,
Physiotherapy Department, London Chest
Hospital, London, UK

Sadhna Murphy BPharm(Hons) MPharmS
Principal Pharmacist, London Chest Hospital,
London, UK

Tracy Parker BSc(Hons) PGDip Dietetics SRD Accredited
Sport Dietitian
Senior Dietitian, Dietetic Department,
London Chest Hospital, London, UK

Jennifer Percival RGN RM RHV Dip Counselling FETC
Training Consultant/Personal Development
Counsellor, London, UK

Sharon Rudkin
Nurse Manager, Airliquide Healthcare New
Zealand Ltd, Auckland, New Zealand

Preface

The development of specialties within medicine during the last century is, in the main, a success story in that it has resulted in a number of exciting scientific discoveries and a revolution in the way that some diseases are now treated.

The success of the specialization within respiratory medicine, however, has not been without cost. Different sub-specialties within respiratory medicine may at times detract from an appreciation of the wider public health impact of respiratory disease generally. Someone obtaining a copy of any national or local public health report, apart from the inclusion of asthma, lung cancer and more recently tuberculosis, could be excused for thinking that respiratory illness is not really a major health issue. Nothing could be further from the truth!

Chronic obstructive pulmonary disease (COPD) is very common in the United Kingdom. In general practice the consultation rates per 10 000 population rise from 417 at age 45–64 to 886 at age 65–74 and 1032 at age 75–84, and these values are 2–4 times the equivalent rates for angina (British Thoracic Society 1997). With only one in four cases being recognized, the quality of life of people with COPD is among the worst of all chronic illness groups. In the past health professionals have had low expectations when caring for patients with COPD but now there is renewed interest with the realization that much can be done to improve quality of life.

Asthma continues to cause great concern and, despite effective treatments being available, morbidity continues to be high with between 5% and 10% of adults suffering in the United Kingdom. Moreover, 1600 people die annually as a result of asthma and most of these deaths are avoidable. It is estimated that asthma prescriptions alone cost the National Health Service (NHS) over £381 million annually, accounting for 10% of the total NHS spending on drugs (British Lung Foundation 1996).

It is now beyond dispute that smoking is a major cause of lung cancer, yet, without effective government policies, respiratory healthcare professionals will be kept busy well into the next decade. Indeed, in some parts of the United Kingdom lung cancer has overtaken breast cancer as the most common cause of death among women. The British Lung Foundation estimates that the annual cost of treating all lung cancers is more than £130 million. Despite the huge numbers dying as a consequence of smoking-related disorders, the tobacco industry remains successful in recruiting replacement smokers, particularly amongst the young. The poor prognosis for people with lung cancer means that the incidence of 40 000 each year in the United Kingdom is almost the same as the mortality, which is 38 000 each year (Muers 1995).

Interstitial lung disease (ILD) includes more than 200 disease entities, although they are classified together because of common clinical, radiographic, physiological and pathological features (Borous et al 1997). Very little is known about the epidemiology of ILD, although these diseases are not rare, with mortality from cryptogenic fibrosing alveolitis increasing substantially over the last two decades (Hubbard et al 1996). Bronchiectasis is another respiratory disorder which affects a smaller but nevertheless significant group.

Cystic fibrosis is the most common genetic disorder and, although it is a disease which affects a number of organs, most patients experience deteriorating respiratory function. However, there have been real improvements as a result of effective treatment of lung infection and improved nutrition. It has moved from being a childhood disease to one that affects equal numbers of children and adults.

Those with impaired immune responses, particularly the elderly, have an increased susceptibility to respiratory infection and it is estimated that around 50 000 people in the United Kingdom are admitted into hospital with pneumonia annually. Many developed countries, including the United Kingdom, have seen a 20% rise in tuberculosis (TB) within recent years (Davis 1995) and because tuberculosis is responsible for over 3 million deaths worldwide each year, the World Health Organization has declared tuberculosis a global crisis. The resurgence of tuberculosis is a chilling reminder of the dangers of complacency and the need to address not only treatment issues but also socio-economic factors. The overall burden as a result of lower respiratory tract infections is great and, with the emergence of more multi-resistant organisms, effective strategies in prevention and treatment are required.

Respiratory illness is responsible for a great deal of acute and chronic ill health in the United Kingdom. More people consult their GPs for respiratory problems than for any other group of diseases and the cost in terms of medical intervention, days off work, and to the employment prospects of the next generation as a consequence of time lost from school is correspondingly large (British Lung Foundation 1996). It is likely that the psychological and economic costs as a result of respiratory illness will continue, and indeed will most likely escalate in the future.

London 2001   Glenda Esmond

REFERENCES

Borous D, Psathakis K, Siafakas N M 1997 Quality of life in interstitial lung disease. European Respiratory Review 7(42): 66–70

British Lung Foundation 1996 The lung report. Lung disease: a shadow over the nation's health. British Lung Foundation, London

British Thoracic Society 1997 Guidelines for the management of chronic obstructive pulmonary disease. Thorax 52(suppl 5): S1–S28

Davis P D O 1995 Tuberculosis. Medicine 23(8): 318–321

Hubbard R, Johnson I, Coultas D B, Britton J 1996 Mortality rates from cryptogenic fibrosing alveolitis in 7 countries. Thorax 51(7): 711–716

Muers M 1995 Lung cancer. Medicine 4(4): 361–369

1

Anatomy and physiology

Carl Margereson

PULMONARY FUNCTION

Oxygen must be available to cells for aerobic metabolism so that adenosine triphosphate (ATP) in the mitochondria may be produced. ATP supplies energy which is needed for a myriad of different chemical and mechanical processes. When glucose is broken down in the presence of oxygen then far more ATP is released than in anaerobic (without oxygen) conditions. The utilization of oxygen in the mitochondria to form ATP is called oxidative phosphorylation because adenosine diphosphate (ADP) is converted to energy packed ATP by adding phosphate (Nunn 1993). For this process of oxidative phosphorylation the body requires approximately 250 ml of oxygen per minute at rest (oxygen demand).

Oxygen demand will vary enormously of course depending on the metabolic needs of the body and, more specifically, of different organs. Carbon dioxide is a waste product of cellular metabolism estimated to be approximately 200 ml per minute. As a result of respiratory disease hypoxaemia (a low PaO_2) may develop and if severe may lead to hypoxia (low cellular PO_2). This will result in anaerobic metabolism with the formation of lactic acid as a waste product and this form of metabolism is very inefficient. It is through effective ventilation of the lungs that the partial pressures of arterial oxygen (PaO_2) and carbon dioxide ($PaCO_2$) are kept within acceptable limits, thus facilitating effective oxidative phosphorylation.

1

Although the main function of the respiratory system is the maintenance of PaO_2 and $PaCO_2$ within acceptable limits, the following list illustrates just how complex this system is.

Functions of the respiratory system:

- phonation
- acid–base balance
- defence against pathogens/foreign matter
- oxidative phosphorylation
- synthesis and metabolism of various chemical mediators
- angiotensin converting enzyme converts angiotensin I to angiotensin II
- produces cytokines
- nitric oxide (NO) released from airway epithelium – epithelium derived relaxing factor (EpDRF).

ANATOMY OF THE RESPIRATORY SYSTEM AND LUNG VOLUMES

Figure 1.1 illustrates the anatomical features of the respiratory system. During inspiration air is warmed, filtered and moistened by the nose before passing down a number of air passages which branch repeatedly before finally ending as respiratory bronchioles, alveolar ducts and sacs. There are approximately 300 million air sacs in the lung and with a corresponding pulmonary capillary network there is a huge surface area for gaseous exchange.

The trachea divides at the fifth thoracic vertebra into the right and left primary bronchi and thereafter there are three secondary bronchi from the right bronchus and two secondary bronchi from the left bronchus. In total there are about 23

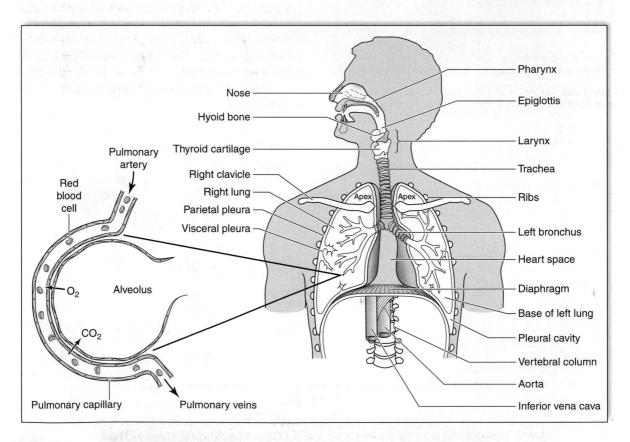

Figure 1.1 Anatomy of the respiratory system. A single alveolus is shown demonstrating the alveolar capillary membrane (0.5 microns thick) where gaseous exchange occurs (i.e. external respiration).

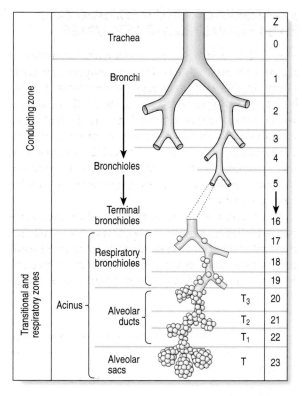

Figure 1.2 Diagram of airway branching in the human lung. Reproduced with permission from Weibel 1963.

generations. The bronchi are lined with ciliated columnar epithelium and the walls are supported with cartilage. Cartilage helps to maintain patency of the airway lumen but small bronchioles do not have this cartilage and pathological processes may reduce lumen size significantly.

The trachea, bronchi, bronchioles and terminal bronchioles (0–16 generations) are conducting passages only (Fig. 1.2). The air in these sections is not available for exchange and this is referred to as anatomical dead space. Ventilated areas of the lungs with poor perfusion increase the overall dead space further and this is called physiological dead space. In the apices of the lung, for example, ventilation is normally greater than perfusion at rest, increasing dead space. Exercise will reduce this dead space by improving pulmonary perfusion as a result of increased cardiac output.

From the 17th generation respiratory bronchioles, alveolar ducts and alveolar sacs comprise the acini which contain air which is available for gaseous exchange. The name terminal bronchiole is somewhat confusing as these are not the final anatomical structures at all but are part of the conducting zone.

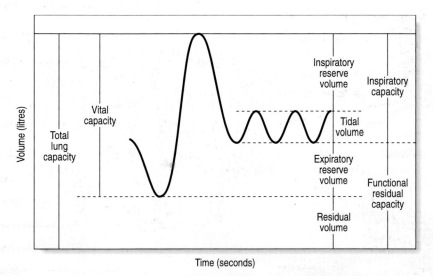

Figure 1.3 Normal lung volumes and capacities. Tidal volume = volume of air in or out per breath. Vital capacity = sum of the tidal volume, inspiratory and expiratory reserve volumes. Functional residual capacity = volume remaining in the lungs at the end of a normal tidal expiration (about 3 L in a healthy adult). Reproduced with permission from Cherniack 1992.

Normal ventilation (inspiration and expiration) ensures that enough air is available in the lungs for gaseous exchange. Minute volume (V_E), or pulmonary ventilation, is the air breathed in each minute and at rest is approximately 6–8 L. This may increase greatly during exercise, of course. Minute volume is calculated by multiplying the volume of air in one breath (tidal volume = V_T) by the breathing frequency (f) per minute, which at rest is approximately 6 L:

$$500 \text{ ml } (V_T) \times 12 \text{ (f)} = 6000 \text{ ml (MV or } V_E)$$

However, not all this air making up the minute volume is available for gaseous exchange because some of it remains in the anatomical dead space. The volume of air in the anatomical dead space is equivalent to 150 ml in an adult although this will vary with body size.

Because minute volume includes dead space air, it is more useful to consider the alveolar volume. This is the air which has entered the acini over one minute and is therefore available for gaseous exchange. Alveolar dead space is calculated by first subtracting the anatomical dead space from the tidal volume and then multiplying by the frequency, e.g.

$$360 \text{ ml } (500 \, V_T - 150 \, V_D) \times 12 = 4000 \text{ ml } (V_A)$$

Alveolar ventilation is important as this determines PaO_2 and $PaCO_2$ levels. When tidal volumes fall or breathing becomes very rapid then dead space air makes up a larger proportion of the tidal volume (Fig. 1.3 illustrates the various lung volumes). As a result, a falling alveolar volume may result in hypoxaemia and a rise in $PaCO_2$ (hypercapnia or hypercarbia). Patients with respiratory disease may not be able to generate adequate alveolar volumes and ventilatory failure may ensue.

GASES IN RESPIRATORY PHYSIOLOGY

Before considering the mechanism of breathing it may be useful to outline some basic principles regarding the pressures of different gases. Atmospheric air is made up of a number of gases among which are:

- Oxygen (O_2) 20.98%
- Carbon dioxide (CO_2) 0.04%
- Nitrogen (N_2) 76%.

Each gas in the atmosphere exerts a pressure of its own (partial pressure = P) and the sum total of these partial pressures is called atmospheric or barometric pressure (P_B). This property of gases is called Dalton's law. At sea level atmospheric pressure is 101 kPa, therefore the partial pressure of oxygen is:

$$\frac{20.98}{100} \times 101 = 21.18 \text{ kPa}$$

Knowing the atmospheric pressure therefore enables us to work out the partial pressure of each gas. Atmospheric pressure decreases with altitude (halves every 18 000 feet) therefore the PO_2 falls. Mountain climbers may run into problems, therefore, when the air becomes 'thinner', resulting in a

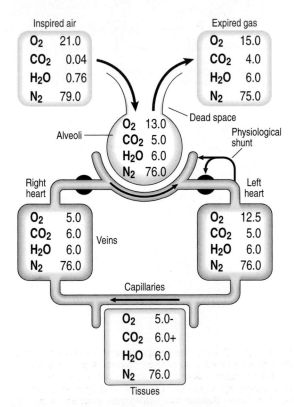

Figure 1.4 Partial pressure of gases (kPa) in various parts of the respiratory system and in the circulatory system. Reproduced with permission from Ganong 1993.

fall in PaO$_2$ and oxygen saturation with the development of altitude sickness. On inspiration by the time the air reaches the alveoli it is fully saturated with water (water vapour exerts a partial pressure of 6 kPa) and the concentration of oxygen is 14% and not 20.98%. Before calculating the partial pressure of oxygen the pressure exerted by water vapour is first subtracted from the atmospheric pressure. The composition of air in the alveoli remains relatively constant and the partial pressure of oxygen is:

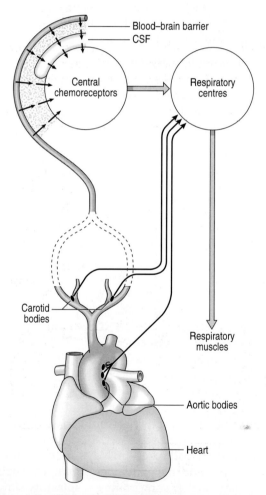

Carotid bodies
Central chemoreceptors
Blood–brain barrier
CSF
Respiratory centres
Respiratory muscles
Aortic bodies
Heart

Figure 1.5 The central and peripheral chemoreceptors. The carotid bodies are bilaterally situated, one at each carotid bifurcation, and their afferent fibres are in the glossopharyngeal nerves. The central chemoreceptors are found in the medulla oblongata and are supplied with cerebrospinal fluid and with materials that penetrate the blood–brain barrier. Reproduced with permission from Widdicombe & Davies 1983.

$$\frac{14}{100} \times 95 \,(101 - 6) = 13\ kPa$$

The amount of O$_2$ and CO$_2$ varies at different points in the respiratory cycle. Figure 1.4 illustrates the different partial pressures of gases at different sites. Note that gases move down a pressure gradient from a region of high pressure to a region of lower pressure. In health a concentration of 21% oxygen will maintain PaO$_2$ within the normal range to meet the demands of the body, but in respiratory illness the fractional inspired oxygen (FIO$_2$) may need to be increased above 21% to ensure adequate saturation of haemoglobin.

NORMAL BREATHING

Although breathing may be brought under voluntary control for a short period of time, fortunately for most of us breathing is something we don't have to think about as it takes so little effort. The normal stimulus to breathe is the rising level of CO$_2$ in the blood. In the brain this CO$_2$ diffuses over into the cerebrospinal fluid (CSF) where it hydrates to form carbonic acid (H$_2$CO$_3^-$). This dissociates into bicarbonate ions (HCO$_3^-$) and hydrogen ions (H$^+$) and it is these hydrogen ions which stimulate the central chemoreceptors in contact with the CSF and which stimulate respiratory neurones of the medulla oblongata (Fig. 1.5). The following reversible equation shows how these hydrogen ions are formed:

$$CO_2 + H_2O \Leftrightarrow H_2CO_3 \Leftrightarrow HCO_3^- + H^+$$

As a result of stimulation of the respiratory centre, neuronal discharge of motor impulses results in contraction of the respiratory muscles. The diaphragm is the main muscle of breathing at rest, although the intercostal and accessory muscles become important with increased respiratory effort. Muscular contraction is necessary to bring about the thoracic volume and pressure changes needed to move air into the lungs. Boyle's law states that if the temperature of a gas is kept constant then the volume occupied by the gas is inversely proportional to the gas pressure. Thus, when the volume of the thoracic cavity is increased during inspiration the pressure is decreased. When considering the pressure

Box 1.1   Events occuring during inspiration and expiration

The following sequence brings about the necessary pressure volume changes to move air in and out of the lungs. Normally there is no energy expenditure during expiration.

Inspiration (active process):

- $\uparrow CO_2$ in cerebrospinal fluid
- Respiratory centre stimulated
- Cervical/thoracic/phrenic nerves
- Diaphragm (+ ex intercostals)
- Thoracic volume $\uparrow$
- Pleural pressure $\downarrow$
- Alveoli expand
- Alveolar pressure $\downarrow$
- Air enters by bulk flow

Expiration (normally passive):

- Brain output ceases
- Inspiratory muscles relax
- Thoracic volume $\downarrow$
- Pleural pressure less negative
- Elastic recoil of alveoli
- Alveolar pressure $\uparrow$
- Air flows out of the lungs

changes that occur during breathing, in pulmonary physiology atmospheric pressure which is 101 kPa is referred to as 0. Box 1.1 outlines the events which take place during the normal breathing cycle.

As the thoracic cavity increases on inspiration, the alveoli must expand and the intrapulmonary pressure is reduced (i.e. more negative than atmospheric pressure). Air moves by bulk flow from the atmosphere into the lungs. On expiration, normally a passive process, the thoracic cavity decreases, the pressure increases relative to atmospheric pressure and air is moved out of the lungs.

The lungs lie on both sides of the mediastinum. The mediastinum and chest wall are lined by parietal pleura and the lungs are covered by visceral pleura. Normally there is no gas in the pleural cavity and only a small amount of pleural fluid. Thus, the pleural cavity is a potential space and is in the middle of two opposing forces:

- the tendency of the elastic alveolar walls to recoil inwards
- the tendency of the elastic chest wall to recoil outwards.

This creates a slight negative pressure in the pleural cavity, i.e. slightly lower than atmospheric pressure. Maintenance of this potential space and negative pressure is important in keeping the alveoli open and preventing collapse.

Distending pressure

To understand the pressure changes which occur during the breathing cycle it is useful to think about the state which exists at the end of expiration and before inspiration begins. The volume in the lungs at this time is called the functional residual capacity (FRC) and:

- no volume change occurs in alveoli
- alveolar pressure is the same as atmospheric
- intrapleural pressure is −0.5 kPa (relative to P_B)
- there is no airflow.

No muscles are contracting at FRC and there are the two opposing forces of the chest wall (outwards) and lung tissue (inwards). The chest wall is holding the alveoli open and the alveoli do not collapse. Many interventions employed in respiratory care by nurses and physiotherapists are aimed at increasing FRC. This not only facilitates effective gaseous exchange but also prevents closure of alveoli. Body position, for example, can affect lung volumes and recumbency is associated with a 30% fall in FRC compared with the upright position (Jenkins et al 1988).

There is a point below FRC volume at which small airways begin to collapse. In health this closing volume is usually at low lung volumes, i.e. below FRC. However, in the elderly and in some patients with chronic respiratory illness closing volume may occur at higher lung volumes. Collapse of airways results in a loss of surface area for gaseous exchange. In addition, reopening of collapsed airways requires much greater distending pressures. Changes during sleep may further compromise respiratory status. In COPD sleep may result in reduced FRC, shallow breathing, hypoventilation and alteration in $\dot{V}/\dot{Q}$ matching, all resulting in hypoxaemia (Douglas & Flenley 1990).

During inspiration and expiration intrapleural pressure is normally less negative than airway pressure. This transpulmonary pressure difference is important as it keeps the airways open. However, if a forced expiratory effort is made then intrapleural pressure becomes much more positive with respect to the airway lumen. As the transpulmonary pressure difference is reduced this can cause dynamic airway collapse (West 1992). Coughing against a closed glottis may cause this, and techniques such as 'huff' coughing against an open glottis will generate less pressure. This technique is also more effective in moving secretions from the distal air passages.

The work of breathing

Although for most of us breathing involves very little effort, energy must nevertheless be expended to overcome several opposing forces during a normal breathing cycle. This work of breathing may be greatly increased in patients with respiratory disease. Energy is needed for the following work during breathing:

- distending the elastic tissues of the chest wall and lungs (compliance work)
- moving inelastic tissues (tissue resistance work)
- moving air through the respiratory passages (airway resistance work).

The oxygen cost of normal quiet breathing is normally less than 5% of total body oxygen uptake and this may increase to 30% and more during exercise and in respiratory disease (Levitzky et al 1990). This may be problematic for patients with respiratory illness who have poor energy reserves anyway. Fatigued muscles may eventually result in ventilatory (pump) failure.

Compliance work

One major portion of the work of breathing is to overcome the elastic recoil of the lungs and chest wall (65% of the work). Compliance refers to the change in lung volume per unit change in airway pressure and is the distensibility (compliance) of

the lung and chest wall. Compliance is the opposite of elastic recoil and is the ease with which something can be stretched. Healthy lungs have good compliance and very little pressure needs to be generated to move air in. Usually only a small pressure change is needed for a normal tidal volume of 500 ml. Try blowing 500 ml of air into a balloon. Which is less compliant (stiffer), the balloon or your lungs? Hopefully, your lungs are more compliant than a balloon which has poor distensibility but good elastic recoil.

In conditions such as pulmonary fibrosis, pulmonary oedema and pneumothorax the lungs become 'stiffer' and compliance is therefore reduced. Obesity and muscular disorders will also result in low compliance. In all these disorders greater pressures must be generated during inspiration to move the same volume of air into the lungs. Breathing will become much more of an effort and the sensation of breathlessness increased.

In emphysema compliance is increased. Here, the lungs have no problem stretching out but elastic recoil is reduced, therefore air trapping occurs. Once again, patients may generate greater pressures to exhale, increasing the risk of airway collapse.

Surface tension in the alveoli

Surface tension is generated at an air/liquid interface and this occurs on the alveolar surface where gas molecules come into contact with liquid molecules. Molecules on the surface of the liquid generate a cohesive force inwards and this surface tension contributes to their collapse. Therefore, to reduce this surface tension Type II epithelial cells in the alveolar wall release surfactant. This is produced in the lung, particularly during inspiration, and reduces the surface tension thereby increasing compliance and reducing the work of breathing.

High surface tension also tends to draw fluid from the interstitial space, therefore surfactant also helps to keep the alveoli relatively 'dry'. Surfactant is a detergent-like substance consisting of lipids (90%) and proteins (10%) and is first detectable in the fetal lung just over halfway through gestation (Gibson 1997). Premature babies may therefore develop respiratory distress syndrome (RDS) due to surfactant deficiency. Surfactant production may be reduced in smokers and in patients whose breathing is monotonous with absence of an occasional deep inspiratory effort (sigh).

Airway resistance

Air flow is influenced by the diameter of the airways and with greater diameters there is less chance of molecules colliding. If the length of a tube is increased by half, airway resistance doubles but if the radius is halved the resistance increases 16 times (Dettenmeier 1992). Airway resistance accounts for approximately 28% of the work of breathing. Most of this airway resistance is in the larger upper airways as although the small bronchioles are narrower, their total cross sectional area is greater. A number of factors may alter airway resistance in health and disease (Box 1.2).

Ventilation and perfusion

Another important factor in determining effective pulmonary gas exchange is matching of ventilation and perfusion and in an ideal state the two would match. However, even in health there are areas in the lungs where ventilation and perfusion do not match and this can be even greater in respiratory disease. Blood flow through the pulmonary circulation (perfusion) is dependent upon cardiac output and is abbreviated as $\dot{Q}$.

$$\frac{\text{Alveolar ventilation } (\dot{V}) \quad = 4\,L/min}{\text{Pulmonary perfusion } (\dot{Q}) \quad = 5\,L/min} = 0.8$$

The normal $\dot{V}/\dot{Q}$ ratio is 0.8 but the $\dot{V}/\dot{Q}$ relationship changes in various parts of the lung according to gravitational forces. In the upright position, due to gravity, ventilation is greater at the base of the lung than at the apex. At the beginning of inspiration intrapleural pressure is less negative at the bases, therefore apices are more expanded (but stiffer) and there may be more dead space (greater ventilation to perfusion). Further volume increases during inspiration are greater at the base where the lungs are less stiff. Perfusion is also greater at the base than at the apex. Because the change in blood flow from apex to base is greater than the relative change in ventilation, the following differences exist:

- base – low $\dot{V}/\dot{Q}$ ratio (perfusion is greater)
- apex – high $\dot{V}/\dot{Q}$ ratio (ventilation is greater).

Arterial oxygenation may be improved in unilateral lung disease when patients lie on their good lung. This improves perfusion in the dependent lung and drainage from the upper lung. In patients with adult respiratory distress syndrome (ARDS) the prone position has been found to improve PaO_2. This is thought to be due to better $\dot{V}/\dot{Q}$ matching and improved ventilation as a result of better diaphragmatic movement (Krayer et al 1989). Improved PaO_2 has also been demonstrated in acute respiratory failure on chronic respiratory insufficiency (Chatte et al 1997).

Pulmonary circulation

The pulmonary blood vessels accommodate a blood flow which is almost equal to that of all other organs in the body. The pulmonary vascular system can be described as a high volume/low pressure system. Resistance in the pulmonary circulation is mainly in the arterioles

---

Box 1.2 Factors affecting airway resistance

Many factors in health and disease may affect airway resistance, either increasing or decreasing the work of breathing.

Factors increasing and decreasing airway resistance:

- Cholinergic (vagal) activity ↑
- Irritant/cough receptors ↑
- Chemicals (e.g. histamine) ↑
- Nonadrenergic noncholinergic (NANC) nerves ↓
- Catecholamines (e.g. adrenaline) ↓
- Beta$_2$ agonists, e.g. salbutamol and ipratropium bromide ↓
- Radial traction of surrounding lung tissue ↓
- Sputum/pulmonary oedema ↑

(Widdicombe & Davies 1991)

and capillaries. Increasing the dilation of capillaries and recruiting those that are closed may reduce resistance further. If there are small units in the lungs that are poorly oxygenated then the capillaries supplying these will constrict, diverting blood to where there is a greater oxygen supply.

The pulmonary circulation has a remarkable ability to change in order to accommodate changes in blood flow. Pulmonary arterioles may also constrict in response to localized hypoxia and in chronic lung disease this may in the long term result in prolonged vasoconstriction, increased red cells and cardiac output resulting in right ventricular failure (cor pulmonale) and often death (Ferguson & Cherniack 1993). Local hypoxia in the lungs is therefore a normal compensatory response which, although adaptive, may cause further problems in chronic respiratory disease.

The right ventricular output is not the same as the left cardiac output because a portion of the bronchial venous blood drains into the pulmonary veins. Some of the coronary circulation arising from the aorta partly drains via the Thebesian veins into the left ventricle. A small proportion, therefore, of the pulmonary arterial blood flow (approximately 2%) is not available for oxygenation and this venous blood is returned to the left side of the heart creating a form of shunt. This small anatomical shunt is quite normal and it is only when a greater proportion of the flow remains deoxygenated that serious problems may develop. Such an increase in the shunt fraction may need to be treated as a matter of urgency if severe hypoxaemia and ultimately hypoxia are to be avoided. Increased shunting of this kind may occur in pneumonia and atelectasis and to a lesser degree in other disorders where ventilation is reduced. Venous admixture refers to all sources of 'wasted blood flow' which is not oxygenated (e.g. right to left shunts). This is regarded as a proportion of the cardiac output which has bypassed the lungs.

$\dot{V}/\dot{Q}$ differences therefore occur in health but changes may become more marked and clinically significant in various pathophysiological states (Fig. 1.6).

TRANSPORT OF GASES

As mentioned earlier, the partial pressure of oxygen in the alveoli (PaO_2) is approximately 13 kPa. Blood returning from the right side of the heart in the pulmonary artery (mixed venous blood) has a PO_2 of around 5.7 kPa. There is therefore a pressure gradient across the alveolar capillary membrane. The alveolar capillary membrane is quite complex, comprising alveolar epithelium, the interstitial space, capillary endothelium, plasma and erythrocyte cell membrane. Despite this complexity, however, the thickness is only about 0.5 microns and gas exchange by diffusion takes place quite easily. Because of the differences in partial pressures, O_2 diffuses from the alveolus into the pulmonary capillary blood and CO_2 diffuses in the opposite direction. Equilibrium

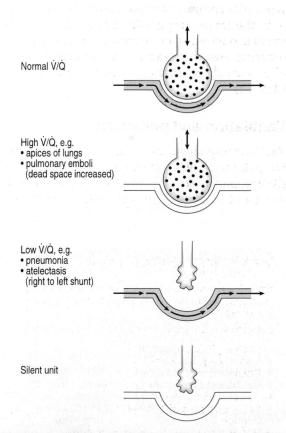

Figure 1.6   Different ventilation/perfusion relationships in the lungs. Ventilated units with poor perfusion will increase physiological dead space. Perfusion to poorly ventilated units will result in a right to left shunt.

between the pressures of O_2 and CO_2 takes place in around 0.25 seconds. It is useful here to consider Fick's law which governs the flow of gas per unit of time into a membrane-bound fluid phase. This is directly proportional to the:

- surface area – surface area is at least 70 m² in healthy adults (surface area will be reduced where are units poorly ventilated)
- pressure gradient of gases (adequate partial pressures in alveolar air will normally provide the pressure gradient required)
- solubility of gas (CO_2 is about 20 times more soluble than O_2 but O_2 diffuses readily because of its affinity for haemoglobin)

and inversely proportional to the:

- thickness of the membrane (Increased thickness of the alveolar capillary membrane is rarely a problem until the late stages in pulmonary disease. Most problems in respiratory disease are caused by $\dot{V}/\dot{Q}$ mismatch.)

Normal PaO_2 falls within a range of 10–13 kPa with the higher levels usual in healthy young adults. In the elderly and in patients with chronic respiratory illness a lower PaO_2 is to be expected. It is important to establish what is normal for each patient as it may be quite inappropriate to attempt to restore blood gases to unrealistic and often unachievable values. In some patients with chronic respiratory failure the 'normal' PaO_2 may be remarkably low (< 8 kPa) causing relatively few problems.

Once the oxygen has diffused across the alveolar capillary membrane it is carried in the blood in two ways. Around 3% is dissolved in the plasma with the remaining 97% carried in the red cells, bound to haemoglobin as oxyhaemoglobin. With a normal PaO_2 there is approximately 0.3 ml of oxygen dissolved in plasma. It is the partial pressure of plasma oxygen which is measured in arterial blood gas analysis.

Oxyhaemoglobin

Haemoglobin is a combination of iron (haem) and protein (globin). Oxygen readily combines with haemoglobin and this is a reversible equa-

tion. Hb is deoxyhaemoglobin which is often referred to as reduced haemoglobin. Each haemoglobin molecule has four sites each able to carry one molecule of oxygen as follows:

$$Hb_4 + 4O_2 \Leftrightarrow Hb_4O_8$$

Oxygen saturation gives the percentage of these sites which are loaded with O_2 (Fig. 1.7).

The proportion of haemoglobin combined with O_2 depends on PO_2, irrespective of the amount of Hb present. In anaemia, for example, patients may still have good saturations if PaO_2 is within the normal range. In heavy smokers carbon monoxide will be carried by some of the haemoglobin as carboxyhaemoglobin, but a pulse oximeter will read this as saturated haemoglobin regardless. In anaemia there may only be half the usual amount of haemoglobin and, despite an acceptable PaO_2 and saturation, cellular hypoxia may still occur! Saturation gives useful information about gas exchange but little about O_2 content (if haemoglobin is halved then so will be oxygen content). However, although not always accurate, using pulse oximetry is useful when initiating and evaluating oxygen therapy. Where PaO_2 is normal yet tissue hypoxia remains a possibility (e.g. low cardiac output, anaemia), mixed venous PO_2 ($P\overline{v}O_2$) measured in pulmonary arterial blood approximates to mean tissue PO_2 and reflects tissue oxygenation (Bateman & Leach 1998).

Oxygen capacity

Because saturation of haemoglobin alone does not guarantee effective oxygen delivery it is

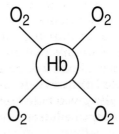

Figure 1.7   Oxyhaemoglobin (Hb_4O_8) showing full saturation (100%). Each molecule of haemoglobin has four sites for oxygen to combine. Saturation of these sites is determined by the partial pressure of oxygen.

important to be aware of other factors which contribute to oxygen delivery. When the haemoglobin is fully saturated (100%) each gram of haemoglobin can hold 1.39 ml of O_2 and this is called the oxygen capacity. With a haemoglobin of 15 g/100 ml the maximum amount of O_2 that can be combined with Hb in every 100 ml of blood will be:

$$15 \times 1.39 = 20 \text{ ml } O_2/100 \text{ ml blood}$$

Actually, the oxygen capacity is slightly lower than this at around 19.5 ml/100 ml. Nevertheless, it should be clear that capacity depends on the amount of haemoglobin and full saturation (and saturation depends on PaO_2).

Oxygen content

Not everyone, of course, has a haemoglobin count of 15 g/100 ml. To work out the actual amount of O_2 attached to haemoglobin and dissolved in the plasma (i.e. the oxygen content) we need to know the haemoglobin value for an individual together with the saturation. Remember that there are 0.3 ml of O_2 dissolved in every 100 ml of plasma. This small amount has been omitted in the following calculation for oxygen content:

$$\frac{\text{Sat of Hb}}{100} \times O_2 \text{ capacity of Hb (Hb}/100 \times 1.39)$$

$$\text{e.g. } \frac{98}{100} \times (12 \times 1.39) = 16.34 \text{ ml}/100 \text{ ml}$$

This oxygen content of arterial blood is abbreviated to CaO_2. Knowing the oxygen content it is then possible to work out the oxygen available each minute. Let us assume that the oxygen content is close to capacity at 19.5 ml/100 ml. For a cardiac output of around 5000 ml at rest the oxygen available per minute will be almost 1000 ml and this is called the oxygen delivery (DO_2). Values are usually given based on cardiac index or CI (cardiac output adjusted for body surface area) (Box 1.3).

Knowing the content of arterial and venous blood gives some indication regarding the consumption of oxygen by the cells. In health and at

Box 1.3 Oxygen delivery and consumption

Whole body O_2 delivery (DO_2)
$CI \times CaO_2 \times 10$
(Normal: 520–720 ml/min/m^2)

Whole body O_2 consumption (VO_2)
$CI \times (CaO_2 - CvO_2) \times 10$
(Normal: 100–180 ml/min/m^2)

rest, there will be an arterial oxygen content (CaO_2) of around 19.5 ml/100 ml and a venous oxygen content (CvO_2) of 14.5 ml/100 ml. Thus, at rest, only 5 ml of oxygen is extracted per 100 ml of blood. This is the oxygen consumption (VO_2) and over one minute is around 250 ml. Normally, therefore, the VO_2 is only approximately one quarter of the DO_2 (expressed as the O_2 extraction ratio or OER, normally 22–30%), leaving plenty in reserve for when demand increases. Monitoring these parameters is important in critical care settings where tissue hypoxia is always a threat and where early recognition is vital. Currently it is difficult to determine the oxygen demand of specific organs but severe hypoxia can occur in a single organ even in the presence of a normal PaO_2. Figure 1.8

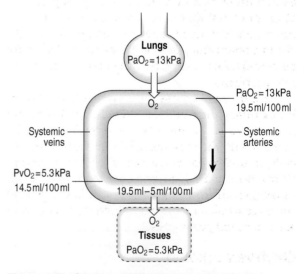

Figure 1.8 Oxygen partial pressure and content at different points. Note how under normal conditions only approximately 25% of the oxygen is removed per 100 ml of blood at tissue level.

shows how oxygen partial pressure and content change at different points.

OXYHAEMOGLOBIN DISSOCIATION CURVE

The relationship between the saturation of haemoglobin and PaO_2 is depicted graphically in the oxyhaemoglobin dissociation curve (Fig. 1.9). The curve shows how changes in the chemical environment will result in physiological changes in the transport of oxygen by the haemoglobin.

The oxyhaemoglobin dissociation curve is an S or sigmoid curve. Looking at the curve you can see that so long as the PaO_2 remains between 10 and 13 kPa, saturations on the flat portion of the curve remain high. Even with a PaO_2 of 8 kPa the saturation is around 90%. When singing, laughing and even talking there can be great fluctuations in PaO_2. However, saturations will remain high because of the physiological properties of the curve.

In order for the oxygen dissociation curve to be in its normal position temperature, pH (or H^+ ion concentration) and CO_2 must be within normal limits. When any one or more of these parameters changes, then the affinity for haemoglobin and oxygen also changes and oxygen delivery to the tissues may be compromised. During anaerobic glycolysis 2,3-diphosphoglycerate (2,3-DPG) within the red cell is produced and this will also affect the bond between oxygen and haemoglobin. Levels of 2,3-DPG are increased during hypoxia to facilitate unloading of oxygen to the tissues.

Shifts to the right (→)

When the curve shifts to the right there is less attraction between the haemoglobin and oxygen and the latter is readily offloaded. For a given PaO_2 therefore, less oxygen is combined with haemoglobin and saturation will be lower. A shift of the curve to the right facilitates the unloading of oxygen as the blood flows through the tissues.

Shifts to the left (←)

When the curve shifts to the left there is a greater attraction between the haemoglobin and oxygen. For a given PaO_2 the saturation is greater. The curve shifts to the left normally as blood flows through the lungs. This occurs when venous blood in the lung releases carbon dioxide, thereby decreasing the number of hydrogen ions. Although loading of oxygen in the lungs is beneficial, a shift to the left as the blood flows through the tissues will not favour unloading and cellular hypoxia may develop.

In summary, the following should all be considered where there are problems with oxygen transport possibly resulting in cellular hypoxia:

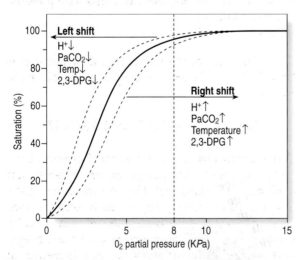

Figure 1.9   Oxyhaemoglobin dissociation curve. With a PaO_2 of 8 kPa and more, saturations will remain high (flat portion of curve). N.B. The middle dark line is the normal position of the curve.

> **Box 1.4**   Factors shifting the position of the oxyhaemoglobin dissociation curve
>
> O_2 dissociation curve shifts to the right with:
>
> - increase in temperature
> - increased H^+ (↓ pH)
> - increased CO_2
> - increased 2,3-DPG
>   (more O_2 released from Hb)
>
> O_2 dissociation curve shifts to the left with:
>
> - decrease in temperature
> - decrease in H^+ (↑ pH)
> - decrease in CO_2
> - decrease in 2,3-DPG
>   (less O_2 released from Hb)

- Is the PAO_2 and PaO_2 adequate?
- Is there adequate functional haemoglobin?
- Is cardiac output satisfactory?
- Is oxygen being unloaded normally?

Consider someone with chronic respiratory illness who normally copes quite well with a PaO_2 of little more than 8 kPa. Despite such a low PaO_2, saturations remain just over 90%. However, if this same person then develops a chest infection there will be an increase in temperature and an increase in CO_2. The CO_2 may be even more elevated if ventilation is poor and this will lead to an increase in hydrogen ions. The increased temperature, CO_2 and hydrogen ions will shift the oxygen dissociation curve to the right, which will place this individual on the steep portion where saturations fall rapidly. Although this may be advantageous at tissue level, this decreased affinity between haemoglobin and oxygen will be disadvantageous in the lungs where oxygen uptake will be reduced. The PaO_2 may well fall below 8 kPa with a further fall in saturations.

From the above example it should become clear that although oxygen administration may be useful in such circumstances, it is also important to address the factors which have shifted the position of the curve.

If PaO_2 falls below 8 kPa respiratory failure Type I is present. This is also called pulmonary failure and one of the commonest causes is $\dot{V}/\dot{Q}$ problems resulting in hypoxaemia. Uncorrected, arterial hypoxaemia may well result in cellular hypoxia. In chronically hypoxaemic patients, however, adequate delivery of oxygen to tissues is achieved by compensatory mechanisms including polycythaemia, a shift in the oxyhaemoglobin dissociation curve and an increase in the oxygen extraction ratio (Bateman & Leach 1998).

Hypoxaemia (low PaO_2 in arterial blood) may occur in:

1. Ventilation/perfusion mismatch (most common).
2. Low inspired O_2.
3. Anatomical right to left shunt.
4. Hypoventilation.

Effective ventilatory drive is necessary in order to 'blow off' CO_2 and maintain acceptable $PaCO_2$ levels. If ventilatory or pump failure occurs then $PaCO_2$ levels will rise and be accompanied by a hypoxaemia of less than 8 kPa. This picture of hypercapnia and hypoxaemia is called respiratory failure Type II. Some people with respiratory disease have this type of chronic respiratory failure and have developed effective compensatory mechanisms enabling them to cope with a low PaO_2 and elevated $PaCO_2$.

ACID–BASE BALANCE

Having considered the transport of oxygen we can now turn to the transport of carbon dioxide. A brief overview of acid–base balance relevant to respiratory disease will also be given in this section.

Like oxygen, carbon dioxide is also transported in the plasma and the red cells as follows:

- 70% is dissolved in plasma
- 30% enters the red cells.

As well as being dissolved in the plasma carbon dioxide is also in combined form as:

- carbonic acid (10%)
- carbamino haemoglobin and also with plasma proteins (20%)
- bicarbonate (70%).

The following equation introduced earlier shows how CO_2 is able to be transported in different forms:

$$CO_2 = H_2O \Leftrightarrow H_2CO_3 \Leftrightarrow HCO_3^- + H^+$$

An important homeostatic mechanism in the body is the maintenance of an appropriate acid–base environment. This is vital for effective enzyme functioning, important in many metabolic pathways. Acid–base status is measured by the hydrogen (H^+) concentration and an acceptable range is 35–45 nmol/L. An increase in hydrogen ions results in an increase in acidity. Acids produced in the body add hydrogen ions to the body's fluids.

Acids may be formed through the ingestion of dietary protein containing sulphur (sulphuric acid) and phosphorus (phosphoric acid) or as a result of diseases where acids accumulate, e.g. ketoacidosis (acetoacetic acid/hydroxybutyric acid), and during anaerobic metabolism (lactic acid). These acids may be described as fixed or non-volatile acids and must be excreted principally by the kidneys. An increase in these acids results in a metabolic acidosis.

Another important acid in the body is formed by the hydration of CO_2 which forms carbonic acid (H_2CO_3). Carbonic acid is a volatile acid and is removed by the lungs. It is the accumulation of carbonic acid which occurs in respiratory disorders where ventilation is compromised. A rising $PaCO_2$, for example, is indicative of a respiratory acidosis as the carbonic acid adds hydrogen ions to the body.

The body has a number of base compounds which are able to accept hydrogen ions and therefore maintain acid–base balance. An important base is bicarbonate (HCO_3^-).

Acid–base status depends on the ratio of the total dissolved CO_2 and HCO_3^- (which may be quantified as PCO_2 and bicarbonate (HCO_3^-)) as follows:

$$[H^+] + \frac{[HCO_3]}{[PCO_2]} = \frac{20}{1}$$

The ratio of HCO_3 to PCO_2 should be 20:1. In respiratory acid–base disorders it is the PCO_2 which is either too high (respiratory acidosis) or too low (respiratory alkalosis). Changes on the PCO_2 side therefore usually represent a respiratory problem and changes on the HCO_3 side a metabolic problem. Disorders resulting in these changes can be seen in Table 1.1. Where both are abnormal, one will be responsible for the change in acid–base status and the other will be compensating, either successfully or unsuccessfully. The body compensates for abnormalities by trying to return the base:acid ratio to 20:1. If the primary process is respiratory, the compensating mechanism is metabolic and vice versa.

When acid–base status is altered the body will attempt to maintain homeostasis in three ways:

Table 1.1 Acid–base abnormalities

Respiratory acid–base imbalance	Causes
$\uparrow$ PaCO$_2$ = acidosis Increase in hydrogen ions	• Chronic obstructive pulmonary disease • Depressed respiratory centre: – sedation – head injury – anaesthesia • Neuromuscular disorders • Acute respiratory infection
$\downarrow$ PaCO$_2$ = alkalosis Decrease in hydrogen ions	• Hyperventilation, e.g. extreme anxiety
Metabolic acid–base imbalance	**Causes**
$\downarrow$ HCO$_3$ = acidosis Increase in metabolic acids Loss of bicarbonate	• Ketoacidosis in diabetes • Anaerobic metabolism • Diarrhoea • Renal disease
$\uparrow$ HCO$_3$ = alkalosis Loss of acid	• Vomiting • Nasogastric aspiration • Excessive alkali intake

1. **Buffer system**. These substances are able to accept hydrogen ions; examples are bicarbonate, proteins and phosphates. This mechanism is activated almost immediately.

2. **Respiratory system**. Whether the primary disorder is respiratory or metabolic, the lungs will remove or retain CO_2. This mechanism soon follows the buffer response.

3. **Renal system**. The renal tubules are able to secrete or retain ions such as bicarbonate and hydrogen and although this response is delayed it is the most efficient.

In some patients with chronic respiratory disease there is often an elevated PCO_2. These patients retain bicarbonate as a compensatory mechanism and this is seen in the plasma bicarbonate, which is also elevated, and the base excess which is higher than normal. In chronic respiratory failure this retained bicarbonate may desensitize the central chemoreceptors. In this situation the peripheral chemoreceptors

Table 1.2 Normal values for arterial and venous blood

Normal values	Arterial blood	Venous blood
pH	7.35–7.45	7.31–7.41
Hydrogen ions	35–45 nmol/L	
PO_2	12–14 kPa	4.6–5.8 kPa
PCO_2	4.6–6.0 kPa	5.5–6.8 kPa
HCO_3	22–26 mmol/L	22–26 mmol/L
O_2 saturation	95% +	70–75%
Base excess/deficit	–2 to +2	–2 to +2

become important in stimulating breathing and this is referred to as hypoxic drive.

Where hyperventilation occurs, too much CO_2 is exhaled and the falling $PaCO_2$ will result in a respiratory alkalosis. This may result in dizziness, muscle tremor and spasm, palpitations, tachycardia, fatigue and weakness.

When determining whether or not an acid–base abnormality exists, arterial blood gas analysis should be carried out in a systematic way as follows:

1. Check H^+ concentration – is this normal or does it show acidosis or alkalosis?
2. Check the $PaCO_2$ (respiratory).
3. Check the HCO_3 (metabolic).
4. Determine the primary imbalance.
5. Determine any secondary compensation.
6. Check PaO_2 and saturation.

Table 1.2 gives the normal arterial and venous blood values.

AIRWAY EPITHELIUM AND NEUROHORMONAL CONTROL

Research into disorders such as bronchial asthma has increased our knowledge of pathophysiological mechanisms greatly, including the complex pathways involved in the control of human airways. Smooth muscle in the airways can be affected by hormones, various peptides and by neurotransmitters from nerve endings. For instance, the focus on neural mechanisms in asthma has helped towards our understanding of the complex interaction between neural control and the effect of mediators on neurotransmission (Fig. 1.10).

Research on the respiratory epithelium has identified a host of different factors possibly initiating and maintaining inflammatory processes in chronic respiratory disorders. Although there is agreement in some areas, there is controversy in others.

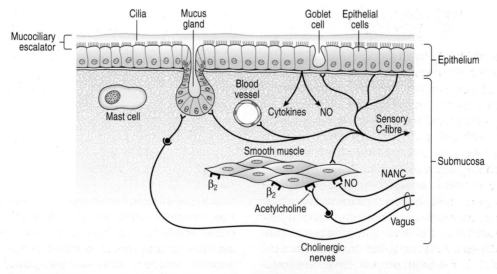

Figure 1.10 The airway epithelium. NO = nitric oxide, NANC = nonadrenergic noncholinergic nerves, β_2 = beta$_2$ adrenergic receptor. Bronchomotor tone is regulated by neurohormonal factors and influenced by many chemical mediators released from many different cells. The airways are dilated by NANC nerves releasing nitric oxide (NO). Note the presence of beta$_2$ receptors which are stimulated by beta$_2$ agonists such as salbutamol and terbutaline. Reproduced with permission from Barnes 1993.

One problem lies in the fact that many experimental studies are performed in vitro. With regard to neurotransmitters, for example, these studies usually concentrate on only one neurotransmitter and one target tissue, whilst the in vivo situation is far more complex, with possibly co-release of transmitters and secondary responses affecting the release of other agents (Widdicombe 1998). Despite the complexity of airway epithelium, this section will provide a brief overview of its many activities both in health and disease.

Neural control of airways

Control of airway tone is not as straightforward as once thought and a number of factors, including not only neural mechanisms but also a variety of hormones, vasoactive peptides and molecules, are released locally from other cells within the airways (Thompson et al 1996). It has been known for some time that autonomic nerves contribute to the regulation of many physiological and pathophysiological processes in the airways. These activities include smooth muscle tone, secretions, blood flow, microvascular permeability and the migration and release of inflammatory cells (Barnes 1990).

The autonomic nervous system is made up of two opposing branches, parasympathetic and sympathetic (Fig. 1.11). These nerves supply, in the main, smooth (involuntary) muscle, cardiac muscle and glandular tissue. An organ is usually supplied by the two branches, i.e. it has double innervation, where one branch is inhibitory and the other excitatory. Parasympathetic nerves to the airways are branches of the vagus nerve and the neurotransmitter is acetylcholine which results in smooth muscle contraction.

The acetylcholine released by these cholinergic nerves acts on muscarinic receptors and results in not only contraction of smooth muscle but also secretion of mucus. There are five subtypes of muscarinic receptors (M_1–M_5) but M_3 receptors are found on airway smooth muscle. Drugs are sometimes given which mimic acetylcholine; an example is metacholine which is used in bronchial challenge tests. Conversely, drugs such as atropine and ipratropium bromide may be given to block

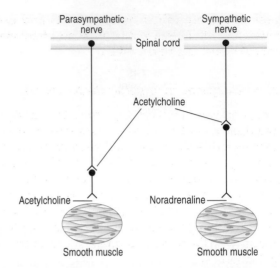

Figure 1.11   The divisions of the autonomic nervous system. Although airway smooth muscle has a parasympathetic supply (bronchoconstriction) it is adrenaline from the adrenal medulla which dilates through beta$_2$ stimulation.

the acetylcholine receptors and are called anticholinergic or antimuscarinic agents.

Sympathetic nerves supply a number of different target organs where the neurotransmitter released is noradrenaline. However, sympathetic effects are also mediated by adrenaline, released from the adrenal medulla. Noradrenaline and adrenaline are catecholamines and sympathetic nerves are described as adrenergic.

Although sympathetic nerves release noradrenaline, the effect which it has depends on the receptor (i.e. adrenoceptor) site on the target cell membrane. Bronchial smooth muscle cells have beta$_2$ receptors and when these are stimulated the muscle relaxes and there is bronchodilation. For many years it was believed that the main bronchodilator of human airways was via sympathetic nerves. However, studies have shown that sympathetic nerves are of no major importance in the lung and that adrenergic fibres do not control smooth muscle in human airways directly. However, it seems that circulating adrenaline from the adrenal medulla may play a more important role in regulation of bronchomotor tone (Barnes 1986). Similarly, pharmacological agents on the beta$_2$ adrenoceptors relax the smooth muscle resulting in bronchodilation.

These drugs are called beta$_2$ agonists and examples are salbutamol and terbutaline, often prescribed in obstructive disorders.

Nonadrenergic noncholinergic (NANC) nerves

A third branch of nerves supplying the airways have been identified called nonadrenergic noncholinergic (NANC) nerves and these can be either inhibitory or excitatory. Inhibitory NANC nerves appear to run in the vagus nerve and the neurotransmitters have been identified as vasoactive intestinal polypeptide (VIP) (Barnes et al 1991) and nitric oxide (NO) (Belvisi et al 1992), although NO appears to be the major neurotransmitter for bronchodilation.

Nitric oxide (NO) was identified as the endothelial relaxing factor (EDRF) (Ignarro et al 1987, Palmer et al 1987) and there has been a great deal of research over the last decade exploring its regulatory role in various organs of the body. NO is synthesized by a group of enzymes called nitric oxide synthases (NOSs) through the L–argenine–NO pathway. It is now known that NO is released by many different cells in the body but is oxidized very quickly, having a half-life of less than 5 seconds. It has a variety of physiological functions in almost all body systems and it appears that all airway epithelial cells are capable of producing NO (EpDRF) (Al-Ali & Howarth 1998).

Because NO has vasodilatory effects on pulmonary arterial and venous endothelial cells, and also bronchodilatory effects, it has been used therapeutically to improve $\dot{V}/\dot{Q}$ matching in the adult respiratory distress syndrome (ARDS). When inhaled NO has been shown to result in selective pulmonary vasodilation, improving oxygenation and haemodynamic variables (Rossaint et al 1993).

Studies involving groups of patients with obstructive lung disease have also produced some interesting findings regarding NO. There is evidence that chronic hypoxia results in a decrease in NO release and this may contribute to a rise in pulmonary vascular resistance. In COPD, therefore, it is suggested that chronic hypoxia impairs the release of NO, contributing to pulmonary hypertension and structural vascular changes (Al-Ali & Howarth 1998).

It must not be assumed, however, that NO has only beneficial effects. In fact NO is a free radical and can be quite toxic, resulting in epithelial damage and bronchial hyper-responsiveness (Sadeghi Hashjin et al 1996). Higher levels of NO are found in the exhaled air of asthmatics and this has been regarded as an important marker of airway inflammation (Kharitonov et al 1996).

In addition to autonomic and nonadrenergic noncholinergic nerve fibres there are a number of sensory nerves and receptors in the airways, including non-myelinated C-fibres. Receptors in the airways include stretch receptors, irritant receptors and C-fibre receptors. Irritant receptor activation results in coughing, bronchoconstriction and tracheal mucus secretion. Receptors in the airways may be triggered by inhaled irritants such as sulphur dioxide and cigarette smoke and also by a number of inflammatory mediators to be outlined in the next section. Reflex coughing and bronchoconstriction are mediated by different kinds of sensory nerves (Karlsson et al 1988). Whilst sensory C-fibre receptors are less sensitive to mechanical stimulation such as changes in lung volume, they are triggered by inflammatory mediators such as bradykinin, histamine and prostaglandins (Spina 1996). A number of neuropeptides, including substance P, are released by sensory nerves and these have been shown to increase airway responsiveness in asthma (Joos et al 1995).

Chemical mediators and airway function

At one time it was thought that the epithelial cells lining the respiratory tract simply acted as a protective barrier. However, many different cells in the lungs, including epithelial cells lining the airways, are an important site for the synthesis of metabolically active substances. These metabolites are formed from the breakdown of arachidonic acid in the membrane of cell walls. There are two metabolic pathways resulting in the formation of prostaglandins and leukotrienes, some of which are pro-inflammatory (Fig. 1.12). The prostaglandins, for example, exert different effects on the airways and pulmonary blood vessels.

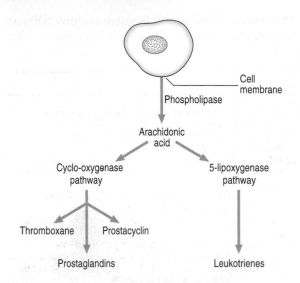

Figure 1.12 Synthesis of inflammatory mediators from arachidonic acid. Many of these mediators from the arachidonic cascade are pro-inflammatory and responsible for maintaining the inflammatory response in a number of disorders, particularly asthma.

Some prostaglandins such as PGI_2 and PGE_1 are vasodilators, whilst PGH_2 and $PGF_{2\alpha}$ are pulmonary vasoconstrictors and bronchoconstrictors (Barnes 1998).

A huge number of different cells in the airways are also able to synthesize mediators called cytokines which are important protein messengers enabling cells to 'talk' to each other. There are well over a hundred different cytokines with new ones being identified all the time. Cytokines are active as immune and inflammatory regulators in areas of inflammation. In earlier research it was assumed that only lymphocytes synthesized these chemical messengers and the term lymphokine was used. It is now known that many different cells produce these messengers, hence the term cytokine. It is the arachidonic metabolites outlined earlier and the cytokines which maintain the inflammatory response in bronchial asthma. A number of new pharmacological agents which target these inflammatory mediators are being studied. Currently, however, there is no real alternative to corticosteroids.

Two inflammatory cells are worthy of note. Mast cells are found throughout the respiratory tract in the airway walls, airway lumen and alveoli, and are also a source of the pro-inflammatory mediators identified earlier. In addition, the walls of mast cells have receptors for the immunoglobulin IgE. If an antigen enters the airways this complex of mast cell, IgE and antigen results in degranulation of the mast cell with the release of preformed mediators such as histamine. Histamine acts on receptors in smooth muscle fibres causing bronchoconstriction and increasing vascular permeability with resulting mucosal oedema. The result is narrowing of the lumen and increased airway resistance. The effects of histamine are seen in the early phase of bronchial asthma. Other pro-inflammatory mediators are also released from mast cells via the arachidonic pathway. Eosinophils are white cells found in the blood and also in the airway tissue spaces and these have also been identified as key inflammatory cells in asthma, their numbers increasing markedly during acute episodes.

Throughout life our lungs perform remarkably, ensuring that enough oxygen is obtained from the atmosphere and carbon dioxide is removed. The lungs and airways are open to the atmosphere, yet despite inhaling all manner of noxious substances almost with each breath, the lungs normally remain relatively sterile. A number of mechanisms involving nerves, cells, mediators and neurotransmitters act in concert in order that the integrity of the pulmonary system is maintained.

Normal defence mechanisms in the lungs are by and large adaptive, but at times these processes appear to go into overdrive. Although some precipitating factor is usually responsible for initiating the inflammatory response, e.g. smoking in COPD, virus and/or allergen in asthma, in many cases such a factor cannot be identified. Nor is it really known why these inflammatory processes, once initiated, are often maintained over time.

This chapter has provided an overview of physiology relevant to chronic respiratory illness. Knowledge of the complexity of pulmonary function has increased greatly over the last 20 years. Although some mysteries remain, with new insights into molecular and genetic mechanisms increasing all the time more effective pharmacological agents are a real possibility in the very near future.

REFERENCES

Al-Ali M K, Howarth P H 1998 Nitric oxide and the respiratory system in health and disease. Respiratory Medicine 92: 701–715

Barnes P J 1986 Neural control of human airways in health and disease. American Review of Respiratory Disease 134: 1289–1314

Barnes P J 1990 Neural control of airway function: new perspectives. Molecular Aspects of Medicine 11(5): 351–423

Barnes P J 1993 Non adrenergic non cholinergic nerves in airways. In: Andrews P, Widdicombe J (eds) Pathophysiology of the gut and airways. An introduction. Portland Press, London

Barnes P J 1998 Pharmacology of airway smooth muscle. American Journal of Respiratory and Critical Care Medicine 158(5/3): S123–S132

Barnes P J, Baraniuk J N, Belvisi M G 1991 Neuropeptides in the respiratory tract. Part 1. American Review of Respiratory Disease 144: 1187–1189

Bateman N T, Leach R M 1998 ABC of oxygen: acute oxygen therapy. British Medical Journal 317(7161): 798–801

Belvisi M G, Stretton C D, Barnes P J 1992 Nitric oxide is the endogenous neurotransmitter of bronchodilator nerves in human airways. European Journal of Pharmacology 210: 221–222

Chatte G, Sab J M, DuBois J M et al 1997 Prone position in mechanically ventilated patients with severe acute respiratory failure. American Journal of Respiratory and Critical Care Medicine 155: 473–478

Cherniack R M 1992 Pulmonary function testing, 2nd edn. W B Saunders, Philadelphia, p. 21

Dettenmeier P A 1992 Pulmonary nursing care. Mosby Year Book, London

Douglas N J, Flenley D C 1990 Breathing during sleep in patients with obstructive lung disease. American Review of Respiratory Disease 141: 1055–1070

Ferguson G T, Cherniack R M 1993 Management of chronic obstructive pulmonary disease. New England Journal of Medicine 328: 1017–1022

Ganong W F 1993 Review of medical physiology. The McGraw-Hill Companies, New York

Gibson A 1997 Surfactant and the neonatal lung. British Journal of Hospital Medicine 58(8): 381–384

Ignarro L J, Buga G M, Wood K S et al 1987 Endothelium derived relaxing factor produced and released from artery and vein is nitric oxide. Proceedings of the National Academy of Sciences of the United States of America 84(24): 9265–9269

Jenkins S C, Soutar S A, Moxham J 1988 The effects of posture on lung volumes in normal subjects and in patients pre- and post-coronary artery surgery. Physiotherapy 74: 492–496

Joos G F, Germonpre P R, Pauwels R A 1995 Neurogenic inflammation in human airways: is it important? Thorax 50: 217–219

Karlsson J A, Saint'Ambrogio G, Widdicombe J 1988 Afferent neural pathways in cough and reflex bronchoconstriction. Journal of Applied Physiology 65: 1007–1023

Kharitonow S A, Yates D H, Barnes P J 1996 Inhaled glucocorticoids decrease nitric oxide in exhaled air of asthmatic patients. American Journal of Respiratory and Critical Care Medicine 153: 454–457

Krayer S, Rehder K, Vettermann J et al 1989 Position and motion of the human diaphragm during anaesthesia paralysis. Anaesthesiology 70: 891–898

Levitzky M G, Cairo J M, Hall S M 1990 Introduction to respiratory care. W B Saunders Company, London

Nunn J F 1993 Nunn's applied respiratory physiology. Butterworth Heinemann, Oxford

Palmer R M J, Ferrige A G, Moncada S 1987 Nitric oxide release accounts for the obligatory activity of endothelium derived relaxing factor. Nature 327: 524–526

Rossaint R, Falk K J, Lopez F et al 1993 Inhaled nitric oxide for the adult respiratory distress syndrome. New England Journal of Medicine 328: 399–405

Sadeghi Hashjin G, Folkerts G, Henricks P A J et al 1996 Peroxynitrite induces airway hyperresponsiveness in guinea pigs in vitro and in vivo. American Journal of Respiratory and Critical Care Medicine 153: 1687–1701

Spina D 1996 Airway sensory nerves: a burning issue in asthma? Thorax 51(3): 335–337

Thompson N C, Dagg K D, Ramsay S G 1996 Humoral control of airway tone. Thorax 51(5): 461–464

Weibel E R 1963 Morphology of the human lungs. Springer-Verlag, Berlin

West J B 1992 Pulmonary physiology. Williams & Wilkins, Baltimore

Widdicombe J G 1998 Autonomic regulation i-NANC/e-NANC. American Journal of Respiratory and Critical Care Medicine 158: S171–S175

Widdicombe J, Davies A 1983 Respiratory physiology. Physiological principles in medicine. Edward Arnold, London

Widdicombe J G, Davies A 1991 Respiratory physiology. Edward Arnold, London

Respiratory assessment

Carol Lynn Cox

INTRODUCTION

The purpose of a respiratory assessment is to ascertain the health status of the respiratory system. The assessment is accomplished by taking a sound health history from the patient, family or significant other and undertaking a step-by-step process to achieve a full and comprehensive respiratory examination. This step-by-step process involves inspection, palpation, percussion and auscultation of respiratory structures. Through this process, whilst undertaking the assessment and preparing to prescribe care, the respiratory nurse can identify many of the problems that patients may have.

The body depends on the respiratory system to survive. Primary functions of the system include the exchange of oxygen and carbon dioxide in the lungs and tissues and the regulation of acid–base balance. Acid–base balance is the stable concentration of hydrogen ions in body fluids. Changes in the respiratory system affect every other system in the body, therefore a respiratory assessment constitutes a critical component of a patient's health evaluation.

Assessment of the respiratory system was once seen as the remit of the medical profession alone. However, due to changes in the delivery of health care, nurses are expanding their practice to incorporate history-taking and physical assessment in this area (Cox & McGrath 1999).

Assessment of patients is a major role in nursing and by expanding assessment techniques respiratory nurses can ensure patients receive the care most appropriate to their needs. Nurses working in respiratory care are well placed to obtain the health history and perform a detailed assessment that can focus nursing care. These nurses are becoming increasingly knowledgeable and proficient in the complex care of patients with respiratory problems. The ability to undertake and document a clear, concise and systematic respiratory assessment of a patient is an essential skill for respiratory nurses that enhances and expands their practice. Various approaches to respiratory assessment have been developed to aid this process. In this chapter the Cox Model (Cox 1997) is described, which respiratory nurses can use to readily identify and prioritize patient care.

As respiratory nurses enhance their roles through use of physical assessment models, it is imperative that they also expand their practice based on the use of evidence discovered through research. By undertaking a full and systematic assessment of the respiratory system, the respiratory nurse is in a unique position to act upon findings from the assessment by utilizing the latest recommendations from research publications to ensure that appropriate medical and nursing intervention occurs (McGrath & Cox 1998).

In order to undertake a full health history and physical assessment of the respiratory system it is essential that the respiratory nurse has a complete and full understanding of the underlying physiology associated with the system. It is beyond the scope of this chapter to describe in depth the anatomy, physiology and pathophysiology of this system and its many deviations from the normal which impact on health; however a brief review of the respiratory system structures is offered, along with a description of the mechanics of respiration. In addition, the respiratory nurse is referred to texts and articles that describe anatomy, physiology and pathophysiology in depth.

THE STRUCTURES OF THE RESPIRATORY SYSTEM

The respiratory system is comprised of the upper and lower airways and the thoracic cage. These structures work together in effecting the ex-change of oxygen and carbon dioxide in the lungs. The upper airways include the nose, mouth, nasopharynx, oropharynx, laryngopharynx and larynx. The lower airways include the trachea, bronchi, lungs, bronchioles and alveoli. The thoracic cage includes the ribs, sternum and vertebrae. These structures act as geographic landmarks that help identify underlying structures in the chest.

The base of each lung is positioned anteriorly at the level of the sixth rib at the midclavicular line and the eighth rib at the midaxillary line. The apices of the lungs extend 2–4 cm above the inner aspects of the clavicles. Posteriorly the lungs extend from the cervical area to the level of the tenth thoracic spinous process. On deep inspiration the lungs may descend as far as the twelfth thoracic spinous process. There are three lobes in the right lung and two lobes in the left. In the anterior thorax the right upper lobe ends level with the fourth rib in the midclavicular line and with the fifth rib in the midaxillary line. The right middle lobe extends triangularly from the fourth to the sixth rib in the midclavicular line and to the fifth rib in the midaxillary line. The left lobe does not have a middle lobe, therefore the upper lobe ends level with the sixth rib in the midclavicular line and at the fifth rib in the midaxillary line. In the posterior thorax, an imaginary line can be drawn from the level of the third thoracic spinous process to the inferior border of the scapulae and over to the fifth rib at the midaxillary line. The upper lobes are located at about the third thoracic spinous process and the lower lobes are located below this line of demarcation, extending to the level of the tenth thoracic spinous process.

THE MECHANICS OF RESPIRATION

The muscles of respiration help to expand and contract the chest cavity. Air pressure differences between the outside air and the lungs help to produce air movement. These processes together allow inspiration and expiration to occur. During normal quiet breathing the main muscle of inspiration is the diaphragm, which contracts causing its descent and a lengthening of the thoracic cavity. With increased effort the external intercostal muscles are also used in inspiration. Conversely, rising of the diaphragm and relaxation of the intercostal muscles causes expiration. During exercise, when the body requires increased oxygenation, and in some disease states like chronic obstructive pulmonary disease, in which forced inspiration and active expiration are required, the accessory muscles of respiration are also used. These include the intercostals on the inner surface of the ribs, the sternocleidomastoids on the sides of the neck, the scalenus in the neck and the abdominal rectus muscles. In forced inspiration, the sternocleidomastoid muscles raise the sternum and the scalenus muscles elevate and expand the upper chest. During active expiration, however, the internal intercostals contract to decrease the transverse diameter of the chest, and abdominal muscles pull the lower chest down whilst the lower ribs are depressed.

Air pressure differences allow the movement of air in and out of the lungs. All gases move from an area of greater pressure to one of lesser pressure. Breathing consists of inspiration, in which there is negative intrapulmonary pressure, expiration, in which there is positive intrapulmonary pressure, and a resting phase in which there is negative intrapleural pressure. The medulla in the brain controls breathing primarily through stimulating the contraction of the diaphragm and the external intercostals. As the diaphragm descends and expands the length of the chest cavity, the external intercostals contract to expand the anteroposterior diameter. These actions produce intrapulmonary pressure changes that result in inspiration.

During inspiration, air flows through the right and left mainstem bronchi into smaller bronchi and then into the bronchioles, alveolar ducts and alveolar sacs until it reaches the alveolar membrane. This airflow pattern may be altered by an obstruction, the volume and location of functional reserve capacity, the amount of intrapulmonary resistance or the presence of lung disease. Airflow follows the path of least resistance. In intrapulmonary obstruction or forced inspiration air is distributed unevenly (Landis 1993).

Musculoskeletal and intrapulmonary factors can affect respiration. For example, forced breathing such as in emphysema requires the use of the accessory muscles and that in turn requires additional oxygen so that these muscles can work. The result is less efficient breathing with an increased workload. An increased workload in respiratory disease may be due to several factors, including changes in compliance (lung tissue and thoracic cage distensibility), elastance (recoil of the lungs and chest wall to their resting state) and resistance. In emphysema, for example, although compliance is increased there is a decrease in elastance and an increase in airway resistance. In some pulmonary disorders where there is a restrictive pattern it is a decrease in compliance which increases the workload.

TAKING THE HEALTH HISTORY

A patient with respiratory problems or disease may have a wide range of symptoms. Some symptoms may be dissociated from the respiratory system directly, such as when in pregnancy the enlarged uterus and increased levels of circulating progesterone interact to create changes in respiratory function (Morton 1993, Ogilvie & Evans 1997, Seidel et al 1995). Conversely, there is a range of symptoms that are associated with respiratory problems and disease that should be explored fully if a tentative diagnosis and plan of care is to be made (Box 2.1) (Carpenito 1995, Cox 1997, Hope et al 1995, Ruch 1999, Seidel et al 1995).

Obtaining a good health history is the basis of discerning a diagnosis of respiratory problems or disease, particularly as a physical examination may show nothing abnormal even in quite advanced stages of some disease (Epstein et al 1997). Through the history, the respiratory nurse can gather an impression of the patient and identify issues of relevance to the plan of care. A good history can aid in focusing the respiratory nurse's mind during the respiratory examination. The process followed in the respiratory assessment is:

- inspection
- palpation
- percussion
- auscultation.

Box 2.1 Symptoms of respiratory problems or disease

- Cyanosis
- Stridor
- Wheezing
- Snoring
- Coughing
  - dry/moist/wet
  - brassy
  - hoarse
  - harsh
  - barking/whooping
  - bubbling
  - productive/non-productive
  - paroxysmal

- Gurgling
- Adventitious breath sounds
  - rhonchi (sonorous and sibilant)
  - crackles (rales)

- Friction rub
- Mediastinal crunch (Hamman sign)
- Barrel shaped chest
- Pigeon shaped chest (pectus carinatum)
- Funnel shaped chest (pectus excavatum)
- Tracheal shift
- Retraction and accessory muscle use
- Bulging intercostal muscles
- Pain
- Alteration in respiration
  - dyspnoea
  - tachypnoea
  - Cheyne–Stokes
  - Biot

The history serves as a primary vehicle through which the respiratory nurse establishes rapport with the patient. Before beginning to ask the patient, family or significant other questions about the patient's health history, the nurse should look at the patient and quickly assess whether he is experiencing any signs of respiratory distress, such as restlessness, anxiety, inability to focus on the conversation or noisy or laboured respirations. If the patient exhibits any of these signs, the nurse should ensure the patient's immediate problem is addressed and he is breathing comfortably before proceeding with the full health history. The health history is undertaken in two phases: firstly the interview, which elicits information, and secondly documentation of the data (Barkauskas et al 1994). The history is normally taken in a systematic manner. Through practice, the respiratory nurse will develop a personal scheme for taking a health history and will be ready to alter the sequence and nature of the data collected according to the condition of the patient.

The nurse should organize the environment so that it is quiet, ensures privacy and increases the physical and psychological comfort of the patient. The patient will have certain ideas about the purpose and content of the interview. Clarification of the patient's expectations and orientation of the patient to the goals of the interview will minimize the potential for misunderstanding and frustration. The interviewer must clarify any discrepancies and strive for a balance between allowing the patient, family or significant other to talk freely and tell their stories and using time efficiently in order for the history to be productive. According to Barkauskas et al (1994) the suggested order for the health history is:

1. Biographical information.
2. Patient's reason for seeking care (chief complaint).
3. Present health and present illness status.
4. Past health history/problems.
5. Current health information.
6. Family health history.
7. Review of systems:
   a) physical systems
   b) functional systems
   c) sociological system
   d) psychological system.
8. Developmental data.
9. Nutritional data.

Biographical information

This should include the patient's full name, address, telephone numbers, birth date, sex, race, religion, marital status, occupation (present or past), birthplace, source of referral, usual source of health care (e.g. Western orthodox or non-traditional), source and reliability of information and the date of the interview. If the patient is not the primary source providing the information, the person providing the information should be identified in the health history record. The patient's reason for seeking care should be written in the patient's, family's or significant other's own words.

Present health/illness status

This describes information associated with the reasons why the patient seeks care. This will include usual health, symptoms in chronological order including onset (date), manner (gradual or sudden), duration, precipitating factors, course since onset (frequency of incidence), patterns of remission and exacerbation, location, quality, quantity, associated phenomena (setting/environment), alleviating or aggravating factors, relevant family information and disability.

Past health history

This should include past general health, childhood illnesses, accidents and disabling injuries, hospitalizations, past surgery, acute and chronic illnesses, immunizations, medications and transfusions and allergies. Current health information addresses the current health-related activity of the patient. It will include asking questions about the use of drugs, alcohol, tobacco and caffeine as well as any medications taken regularly as prescribed by a doctor and those that are self-prescribed, exercise patterns, sleep patterns and any environmental factors that may be influencing the problem.

Current health information

This should include all major factors that influence the health of the respiratory system. These include allergies associated with the environment, animals, drugs or other substances; habits such as the consumption of alcohol, tobacco, drugs or caffeine; medications including their generic name, dosage, frequency of use, compliance of the patient in taking the medications and identification of the provider of the prescription (e.g. GP or self-prescription); exercise regime and sleep pattern. If allergies are reported, it is essential that the respiratory nurse ascertains the nature of the causative factor, the reaction of the patient to the factor, any therapies that have been used to alleviate the reaction and the sequelae of the reaction. Caution should be exercised when obtaining information about drug allergies.

A reaction to a drug may not always be an allergic response. The reaction may be due to the interaction of the drug with other drugs, misdosage or a side effect of the medication regimen. When recording information about habits such as the use of tobacco, it is important to note the number of cigarettes or cigars/amount of pipe tobacco used in a day. When obtaining information about the use of illegal substances, such as mood-altering drugs, the record should include the duration of usage, how much (in ounces or tablets) is taken in a day, when the activity occurs and whether it is regarded as recreational or other.

Patients often forget to admit that they also use non-prescription therapies such as aspirin or antacids, therefore the respiratory nurse should specifically ask about non-prescription items. Barkauskas et al (1994) and Morton (1993) indicate that this is a prime opportunity to educate patients about the appropriate use of non-prescription items.

Family health history

This is taken to obtain information about the patient's blood relatives (grandparents, parents, siblings and children) and to identify genetic, familial or environmental illnesses that have implications for the patient's present or future health problems. The respiratory nurse may choose to construct a genogram (Morton 1993) that provides a visual summary of the health of the patient, children and parents. To develop the genogram (Fig. 2.1) the respiratory nurse draws the relationship of family members to the patient, then writes in the ages of living family members and notes deceased members and the age at which they died. The respiratory nurse then records diseases that have a familial tendency such as asthma, or a genetic tendency such as cystic fibrosis, or an environmental cause such as lung cancer from exposure to carcinogens. Genetic illnesses are those that are inherited through the genes whilst familial illnesses are those that have not been demonstrated to be genetic but appear more often in some families. Environmental illnesses are due to exposure to toxic substances and may be occupationally related, i.e. shared by families

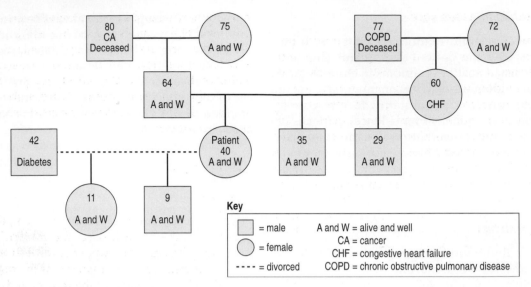

Figure 2.1   Genogram.

such as father and son working in coal mines or asbestos factories.

The health status of the family is important because the patient's health can be affected by the health conditions of other family members: for example a communicable disease such as tuberculosis may affect the entire family. Heredity and constitutional factors are associated with many respiratory illnesses, therefore a strong family history of an illness will offer important information in assessing and diagnosing the patient's problem. The respiratory nurse should always ask whether or not the patient's family members have a diagnosed health problem. A patient with a chronic respiratory disease such as chronic obstructive pulmonary disease may eventually need considerable family assistance in relation to the activities of daily living.

Review of systems

This includes collecting information about the present and past health of each system. This portion of the health history is organized from head to foot in body direction and from physical to psychosocial factors. Physical systems should be addressed first, beginning with the neurological and ending with the musculoskeletal. A check list

may be used to facilitate questioning and to ensure that all systems are addressed. The respiratory nurse should ask questions about the patient's symptoms and allow the patient, family or significant other enough time to think so that they can answer thoroughly. It is important to ask questions in language that is easy to understand, therefore medical terminology should be avoided. For example, the respiratory nurse would ask the patient, 'Do you have any cramp-like feelings in your legs when you walk?' rather than asking, 'Do you have intermittent claudication?'.

The developmental history

The developmental history should include a summary of the patient's development to date and a statement of the current developmental functioning of the patient. Recent life changes and life experiences may reveal important information about the patient's present or past health problems. There are a number of assessment tools that can facilitate assessment of the developmental history of the patient. Two useful tools are the Life Changes Questionnaire (Rahe 1975) and the Life Experiences Survey (Sarason et al 1978).

The nutritional assessment

The nutritional assessment includes a description of an average day's food intake. This section of the health history involves identifying the adequacy, inadequacy or excess of consumption of the four basic food groups and the presence or past experience of any nutritional problems. The goals of a nutritional assessment are to identify whether there are any associated problems due to malnutrition or over-consumption leading to obesity, hypertension and cardiovascular disease and to identify nutritional parameters for optimal health and fitness. For example, a side effect of alcoholism is malnutrition (Bridges et al 1999). Thiamine deficiency is common in patients who are alcoholics as are a number of other health problems such as iron deficiency anaemia. Thiamine deficiency and anaemia affect the respiratory system. Anaemia results when the consumption of alcohol is excessive and the variety of foods in the diet is limited. Anaemia is associated with a reduction in the number of red blood cells (RBCs) and/or haemoglobin in the blood. A decrease in the ability of the blood to carry oxygen occurs because of reduced RBCs and haemoglobin. The patient with this problem will exhibit signs of fatigue, breathlessness and orthopnoea.

PREPARATION FOR RESPIRATORY ASSESSMENT

Assessment of the respiratory system is best undertaken in a quiet, well-lit environment. This is not always easy to accomplish in the clinical setting. As a minimum, privacy should be provided so that a discreet interview can be conducted and the chest can be exposed for examination. Selective listening must be employed during auscultation; this can be readily undertaken even in the busiest clinical environment. For a basic assessment, positioning of the patient is essential. If possible, the patient should be placed in a sitting position that allows access to the anterior and posterior thorax. The nurse should ensure the patient is not exposed to cold because shivering may alter breathing patterns, and that tubing such as ventilator tubing is not resting on the chest where sounds can be transferred and be confused with what is transpiring within the thorax. If the patient cannot sit up, the supine semi-Fowler's position can be used to assess the anterior thorax and the side-lying position to assess the posterior thorax. Nurses should be aware that these positions may create some distortion in findings.

Inspection

Cyanosis

Before assessing the respiratory system, the respiratory nurse must inspect the patient's skin, including the chest and upper and lower extremities. This permits an assessment of the degree of peripheral oxygenation of the tissues. A dusky or bluish colour to the skin (cyanosis) is reflective of a decrease in oxygen content of the arterial blood. A differentiation must be made between central and peripheral cyanosis. Central cyanosis results from prolonged hypoxia (Morton 1993) that affects all body organs in patients with right to left shunting, a common cause of hypoxaemia in patients with pulmonary disorders. The oral mucosa, tongue and lips, as well as the nail beds, should be inspected for cyanosis. Peripheral cyanosis results from vasoconstriction, vascular occlusion and/or reduced cardiac output. The patient's extremities will feel cool to touch, the nail beds, lips and sometimes the skin will appear bluish or mottled. Peripheral cyanosis is often seen in patients who have been exposed to the cold. In peripheral cyanosis, however, the oral mucosa is not affected. It is important for the respiratory nurse to know that dark skinned patients may be more difficult to assess. In these patients the best places to assess for cyanosis are the oral mucosa and lips. In central cyanosis these areas will appear ashen grey rather than bluish in colour.

Clubbing

After the assessment for central and peripheral cyanosis has been completed, assess the patient's fingertips and toes for abnormal enlargement, nail thinning and an abnormal alteration in the angle of the finger and toe bases. This is termed clubbing. Clubbing results from chronic tissue hypoxia (Wilkins et al 1988). To assess for finger clubbing, ask the patient to place the first phalange of the index finger on each hand together, finger nail facing finger nail. Normally when the fingers are placed in this position there is a diamond shaped space between them. However with clubbing, the angle at the nail base is greater than 180° and so when the phalanges of the fingers are placed together no space is left between them.

Quality of breathing

The nurse should continue with the assessment by determining the rate, rhythm and quality of breathing as well as discerning the configuration of the thorax. The respiratory nurse may find that assessment is managed more expeditiously by assessing the anterior chest first, including inspection, palpation, percussion and auscultation, and then assessing the posterior chest. During inspection, chest symmetry, skin condition and accessory muscle use should be assessed. Nurses should determine whether nasal flaring is present, which could be a response from exposure to smoke or chemicals. Respiratory rates vary with age, and the respiratory nurse should be aware of normal rates in the patient's age group. The respiratory rate is increased in many conditions, such as acute and chronic pulmonary disease, cardiac failure and anxiety. Conversely, the respiratory rate is decreased with depression of the respiratory centre occurring from narcotic overloading and cerebral lesions. The respiratory nurse should note whether the patient is eupnoeic, which means the respiratory rate is within the normal range for that particular patient's age group. She/he should consider the quality of respiration by assessing type and depth of breathing. Awake female adult patients normally exhibit thoracic breathing which involves an upward and outward motion of the thorax, whereas in the male respiration is primarily abdominal (Bates 1995, Morton 1993). Respiration in females is primarily

costal whereas in males it is diaphragmatic. Sleeping patients normally exhibit abdominal breathing using the abdominal muscles.

Chest movement

Next, the nurse should inspect the anterior thorax for symmetry of movement by standing in front of the patient or at the foot of the bed and carefully observing the patient's breathing. Nurses should look for equal expansion of the chest wall and be alert for the abnormal collapse of part of the chest wall during inspiration along with an abnormal expansion of the same area during expiration, which is called paradoxical movement. Paradoxical movement is indicative of a loss of normal chest wall function, such as in flail chest. Flail chest occurs when two or more ribs are broken in two or more places and frequently results from an injury sustained during closed chest cardiac massage or from a blow to the chest. A unilateral absence of chest movement may indicate previous surgical removal of a lung, bronchial obstruction, or a collapsed lung as in the case of pneumothorax, haemothorax or haemopneumothorax. Delayed chest movement may indicate congestion or consolidation of the underlying lung tissue. The nurse should check for the use of accessory muscles by observing the movement of the sternocleidomastoid, scalenus and trapezius muscles in the shoulders and neck. Hypertrophy of the accessory muscles may indicate frequent use, such as in chronic obstructive pulmonary disease in which the accessory muscles replace the work of the diaphragm and external intercostal muscles (Ruch 1999).

Breathing patterns

Note the position the patient assumes to breathe. A 'tripod position' that involves patients resting their arms on their knees, the arms of a chair or an over-bed table may be an early sign of impending respiratory embarrassment. Nurses should determine whether the patient is experiencing orthopnoea, which is evidenced by the patient becoming breathless when lying flat, or platypnoea, which is evidenced by the patient becoming short of breath when sitting upright. Orthopnoea is frequently caused by increased blood return to the lungs. Platypnoea, along with signs like tachypnoea (rate greater than 20 respirations per minute) and hypopnoea (abnormally shallow respirations) may occur from protective splinting associated with pain from surgery or pleurisy. Liver enlargement and abdominal ascites may prevent the diaphragm from descending and produce a similar pattern. Conversely, bradypnoea (rate less than 12 respirations per minute) may indicate neurologic or electrolyte disturbance in a critically ill patient.

External thorax

The nurse should observe the patient's skin on the anterior and posterior thorax and look for signs of unusual colour, lumps, scars and lesions. If these are present, their location should be noted. The skin should normally match the rest of the patient's complexion. Scars may be indicative of previous thoracic surgery. The location of underlying ribs, sternum and xiphoid process should be inspected. An abnormality may reflect a problem within the thorax. For example, deformities resulting from defects in the sternum, such as pectus excavatum (funnel chest) or pectus carinatum (convex chest), can hinder breathing by preventing full expansion of the thorax (Seidel et al 1995). Deformities of the posterior thorax that may affect ventilation include curvatures of the spine such as lordosis, scoliosis, kyphosis and kyphoscoliosis. In each instance, these deformities can compress one lung whilst allowing over-expansion of the opposite lung.

Palpation

Palpation is a sophisticated skill used in respiratory assessment that involves use of the hands and fingers to gather information through the sense of touch. Touch is considered therapeutic, and is the actuality of 'laying on of hands' (Ashcroft 1994, Cox & Hayes 1997, 1998, Seidel et al 1995). Palpation is the moment in which the respiratory nurse begins to invade the patient's body. This is a particularly sensitive time and therefore the approach should be gentle. The respiratory nurse's hands should be warm as this is not only practical

in terms of the approach to the patient but also symbolic of the respect in which the patient is held and the privilege the patient gives in allowing the respiratory nurse to examine his body.

Technique

Various parts of the hands and fingers are used for specific types of palpation (Box 2.2) due to their variance in sensitivity associated with position, vibration and temperature.

Generally both hands are used simultaneously in palpation in order to compare the right and left sides of the patient's thorax. The palmar surface of the hand and fingers is more sensitive than the fingertips and is used to discern size and shape, whereas the ulnar surface of the hand and fingers is used to assess the vibration caused by the transfer of sound waves from inside the chest to the chest wall. The backs of the hands are used to discern hot and cold.

Palpating the trachea

The trachea should be palpated to ensure that it is midline. The nurse should stand in front of the patient, or to the right side. He/she should ask the patient to bend their head forward slightly, placing two fingers on either side of the trachea just above the suprasternal notch. The fingers should slide gently out and to the sides of the trachea toward the patient's clavicles until the sternocleidomastoid muscles are reached. Each finger should have covered an equal distance, indicating a midline trachea. The nurse should explain carefully to the patient what is happening and care should be taken to ensure that fingers are not

---

Box 2.2 Areas of the hand used in palpation

- Palmar surface of the hand and finger pads – to assess size, consistency, texture, fluid, surgical emphysema and the texture and form of a mass or structure.
- Ulnar surface of the hand and fingers – to assess vibration.
- Dorsal surface of the hands – to assess temperature.

(Source: Cox 1997)

wrapped around the patient's neck whilst performing this manoeuvre as the patient may perceive this as an attempt to occlude her airway.

Palpating the thorax

The entire thoracic area should be palpated for pulsations, tenderness, depressions, bulges and paradoxical movement. Bilateral symmetry should be felt, with some elasticity of the rib cage, whilst the sternum and xiphoid process remain inflexible and the spine rigid. Surgical emphysema may be felt (as well as heard on auscultation) under the skin. Surgical emphysema is indicative of the introduction of air from a rupture somewhere in the respiratory system or from infection produced by gas-producing organisms. Surgical emphysema, upon discovery, always requires immediate attention (Hudak & Gallo 1994). A coarse popping or grating which occurs on inspiration may be palpated and auscultated. This suggests a pleural friction rub. Pleural friction rubs are caused by inflammation of the pleural surfaces. They are a frequent occurrence in lobar pneumonia and, due to associated pain, are disconcerting for the patient.

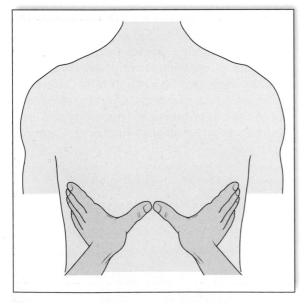

Figure 2.2 Assessing respiratory excursion.

Respiratory excursion

Respiratory excursion (thoracic expansion) can be assessed by standing behind the patient and placing the thumbs next to each other along the spinal processes at the level of the tenth rib (Fig. 2.2). The palms of the hands should be kept lightly in contact with the posterolateral surfaces of the patient's back. The nurse should watch the separation that occurs between the thumbs during quiet and deep breathing. A loss of symmetry in the distance between the thumbs indicates a problem on one or both sides of the thorax.

Respiratory excursion cannot be assessed whilst the patient is in a supine position, therefore it may not be assessed in the intensive care unit. However, this assessment can be done in situations in which the patient may sit or stand. Any absence or delay in chest movement or asymmetry in separation of the thumbs from the spinal processes may be indicative of a previous surgical removal of a lung, complete or partial obstruction of the airway or underlying lung, or diaphragmatic dysfunction on the affected side.

Tactile fremitus

Tactile (vocal) fremitus may be assessed in patients who are not intubated or receiving mechanical ventilation. Tactile fremitus can be discerned by placing the ulnar aspects of the hands parasternally at the second intercostal space at the level of bifurcation of the bronchi (Cox 1997) (Fig. 2.3). Fremitus is the palpable vibration of the chest wall that occurs during speech.

A decrease in fremitus occurs in pleural effusion and pneumothorax. This is reflective of an inability of the chest wall to transmit the vibrations of sound (Wilkins et al 1988). An increase in vibration is indicative of consolidation and can be palpated in conditions like lobar pneumonia.

Shifts to the mediastinum

Finally, by determining the position of the apex beat of the heart (point of maximal impulse) and the trachea, any shifts to the mediastinum can be discerned. As previously described, the position of

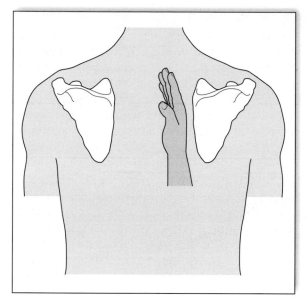

Figure 2.3 Assessing tactile fremitus.

the trachea should be palpated at the area of the suprasternal notch. The trachea should be moved gently from side to side, and the nurse should feel along the upper edges of each clavicle to the borders of the sternocleidomastoid muscles. Although a slight, barely noticeable deviation to the right is not unusual, any deviation should be noted. A shift of the mediastinum towards the side of a lesion indicates shrinkage of the lung due to collapse or fibrosis. Displacement away from the lesion occurs with fluid or air in the pleural space. Displacement of the trachea alone is more likely following contraction of an upper lobe, whereas a shift of the apex beat alone may be due to a lesion of a lower lobe. There may be problems within the chest such as atelectasis, pleural effusion, tension pneumothorax, tumour or thyroid enlargement which can cause the trachea to deviate (Hudak & Gallo 1994).

Percussion

Percussion involves striking one object against another to produce percussion sounds (sound waves). These sounds are termed forms of resonance and arise from vibrations 4–6 cm deep in the body's tissues (Bates 1995, Seidel et al 1995). In percussion the finger of one hand functions as a hammer (plexor) and strikes the dorsal surface of the opposite hand's finger on the interphalangeal joint (Fig. 2.4)

To perform this form of indirect percussion, as opposed to direct percussion, which is when the hand strikes the patient's chest directly, the non-dominant hand is placed on the surface of the patient's chest with the fingers slightly spread. The distal phalanx of the middle finger is placed firmly on the chest surface of the patient whilst the other fingers are held slightly off the surface of the patient's chest. The wrist of the other hand is snapped downward and the tip of the middle finger, which is being used as the hammer, sharply taps the interphalangeal joint of the finger that is pressing on the patient's chest. Table 2.1 classifies percussion sounds and where these may be heard.

The loudness of the sound gives an indication of the density of the medium. A quiet, or dull, percussion sound reflects a dense medium. Therefore, percussion sounds over air are loud and over fluid are less loud. Over solid areas percussion sounds will be soft.

There are several points to consider when percussing the chest. The tap of the striking finger (plexor) should be done quickly, lifting the finger

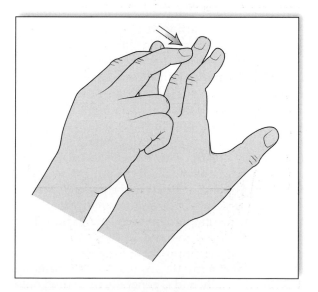

Figure 2.4 Percussion technique.

Table 2.1   Percussion sounds

Sound	Intensity	Pitch	Duration	Quality	Location
Dullness	Soft	Moderate	Moderate	Thud-like	Liver area
Flatness	Soft	High	Short	Quiet/Dull	Muscle area
Tympani	Loud	High	Moderate	Drum-like	Epigastric bubble
Resonance	Loud	Low	Long	Hollow	Air-filled healthy lungs
Hyper-resonance	Very Loud	Low	Long	Boom-like	Emphysematous lungs

(Source: Cox 1997)

to prevent dampening of the sound. Only one location should be percussed at a time, and this should be repeated several times in each area in order to facilitate interpretation of the sound. Is the sound flat and dull as would be heard in a solid mass tumour, or is it hyper-resonant, i.e. very loud and boom-like, as is found in the lungs of a patient who has emphysema? When the patient is ventilated and the sounds associated with percussion change to hyper-resonance, the respiratory nurse should consider the possibility that the patient has sustained a pneumothorax (Morton 1993). Hyper-resonance also results from overinflation of the lungs such as occurs with chronic obstructive pulmonary disease.

Diaphragmatic excursion should be assessed through percussion. To perform this procedure, nurses should ask patients to inhale deeply and hold their breath. Percuss down the midscapular line on one side starting at T7 or at the end of the scapula in the midscapular line until the lower edge of the lung is identified by the sound changing from resonance to dullness. Mark this point with a felt tip pen. This is the location of the diaphragm at full inhalation. Patients should be asked to breathe normally for a few moments and then take a deep breath, exhale fully and hold their breath. The nurse should percuss upwards from the mark on the patient's back at the midscapular line towards the patient's scapula. Where dullness ends and resonance begins is the level of the diaphragm at full expiration. This point should be marked and the procedure repeated on the opposite side of the patient's chest. Diaphragmatic excursion is normally 3–5 cm bilaterally and is generally measured only on the posterior thorax. Due to the location of the liver on the right, it is not abnormal for diaphragmatic excursion to be slightly less on the right than on the left. As in respiratory excursion, minimal excursion of the diaphragm is indicative of underlying pathology such as may be found in tumour or cystic fibrosis.

Auscultation

Technique

Auscultation provides critical information about the condition of the lungs and pleura. Sounds heard upon auscultation can be characterized in the same fashion as in percussion (location, intensity, pitch, quality and duration). The patient should be in a sitting position, if at all possible, so that the anterior, lateral and posterior thorax can be assessed. It is usually preferable for the diaphragm of the stethoscope to be used to hear normal as well as abnormal (adventitious) breath sounds (Cox & McGrath 1999). The diaphragm of the stethoscope transmits high-pitched sounds better and provides a broader area of sound, whereas the bell transmits softer sounds. When the bell is used, pressure on the bell will, by stretching the patient's skin underneath the bell, create a diaphragm effect. The diaphragm of the stethoscope should be pressed firmly on the patient's skin so that there is no movement of the skin on the diaphragm. Normally the patient should be approached from the right side for auscultation, and the tubing of the stethoscope should be taut so that there are no bends that may distort the conduction of sound. In addition, care should be taken to ensure the tubing does not brush against clothing, bed clothing or cot sides because these extraneous sounds may distort sounds being conducted from the chest. If the

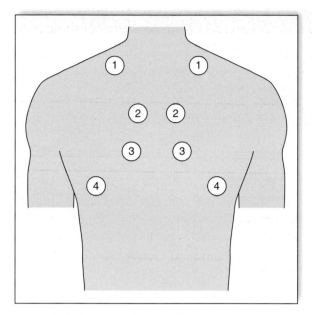

Figure 2.5 Sequence for auscultation.

patient has a considerable amount of hair in the areas to be auscultated, wetting the hair with water will flatten it out and subsequently reduce the effect of the hair scratching on the diaphragm. The patient should be asked to take deep breaths (if not intubated and ventilated) through the mouth, exaggerating the normal respiration. Demonstration of the deep breathing technique by the respiratory nurse will help the patient understand how to deep breathe correctly, so that hyperventilation does not occur. Exaggerated breathing is tiring. Elderly and critically ill patients generally experience problems which are pathologic in the lung bases, so with these patients it is best to begin auscultation at the bases before fatigue sets in (Cox & McGrath 1999, Oh 1991, Seidel et al 1995).

A systematic approach should be used during auscultation (Fig. 2.5). Each position should be listened to throughout inspiration and expiration. A side-to-side comparison approach should be used as the diaphragm of the stethoscope is moved downward on the thorax, at intervals of several centimetres, from where the apices of the lungs are located to the bases. Comparison should be from right to left or left to right. Sounds from the right middle lobe and the lingula on the left are heard best in the patient's respective axillae (Bates 1995,

Epstein et al 1997, Seidel et al 1995). When auscultating the posterior thorax, the nurse should ask the patient to bend her head forward and downward slightly to enlarge the listening area. The nurse should not auscultate over bones such as the scapulae and sternum because bone blocks the transmission of sound.

Normal breath sounds

Breath sounds are made as air flows through the respiratory tree and are attenuated by distal lung structures which they pass. Sounds are characterized by their intensity, pitch, duration on inspiration and expiration and quality. Normal breath sounds are classified as bronchial (tubular), bronchovesicular and vesicular. The characteristics and location of normal breath sounds are outlined in Table 2.2.

Bronchial or tubular breath sounds are heard over the tracheal area and have a harsh quality. They are high in pitch and intensity, and the expiratory phase is longer than the inspiratory phase with a short gap between the two phases. Although these sounds are normal when heard over the tracheal area, when heard over peripheral lung tissue (e.g. the basilar area) they would be indicative of a pathological process that is enhancing the transmission of the sound to the chest wall. Examples of conditions in which this type of sound may be heard are consolidation related to lobar pneumonia, provided a patent bronchus is present, or fibrosis. To discern consolidation, voice sound assessment techniques can be used. These include testing for whispered pectoriloquy or egophony by asking the patient to whisper 'ninety-nine' or say 'e-e-e' repeatedly. Normally the whispered sound is non-distinct. However, in whispered pectoriloquy the sound is clearly audible. In egophony the spoken letter 'e' sounds like 'a'. A bronchus that is obstructed will block transmission of bronchial sounds and lead to absent or markedly diminished breath sounds.

Bronchovesicular breath sounds are heard over the major bronchi and are medium in pitch and intensity. Bronchovesicular sounds would be considered abnormal if they were heard over peripheral lung tissue areas and may be indicative of

Table 2.2   Normal breath sounds

Sound	Intensity of expiration	Pitch of expiration	Duration of inspiration and expiration	Location
Bronchial	Usually high	High	Expiration longer than inspiration	Trachea
Bronchovesicular	Medium	Medium	Inspiration and expiration equal	Near the bronchi below the clavicles and between the scapulae, especially on the right side
Vesicular	Soft	Low	Inspiration longer than expiration	Healthy lung

(Source: Cox 1997)

atelectasis. Vesicular breath sounds are low in pitch and intensity and are heard over healthy lung tissue.

Breath sounds will be more difficult to hear or may even be absent when fluid, such as blood or pus, has accumulated in the pleural space. Breath sounds will also be more difficult to hear or may be absent when secretions or a foreign object, such as a suction catheter or a peanut, obstruct the bronchi, when the lungs are hyperinflated through manual hyperinflation with a re-breathing bag or through ventilation, or when breathing is shallow due to splinting. When listening for breath sounds, it is necessary to eliminate superimposed sounds. One frequently superimposed sound in the critical care unit is the sound of water bubbling in ventilator tubing. This can be transmitted to the patient's chest and could lead to a misdiagnosis during auscultation. Therefore, before undertaking auscultation, the respiratory nurse should listen to the environmental sounds created by equipment supporting the patient so that random sources of sounds are not confused with what is transpiring in the patient's chest during auscultation (Lane 1990, Thurnock 1994).

Abnormal breath sounds

Adventitious sounds (Table 2.3) are abnormal breath sounds that occur when air passes through narrowed airways, due to constriction or partial obstruction, when fluid accumulates in the lungs,

or when the lining of the chest cavity becomes inflamed. Adventitious breath sounds include crackles or rales as they were previously termed (Barkauskas et al 1994, Seidel et al 1995), wheezes, rhonchi, which may be identified as sibilant (high-pitched) or sonorous (low-pitched snoring sounds), pleural friction rubs and mediastinal crunch.

Crackles are heard more often on inspiration than on expiration in the critically ill patient. Crackles are discrete discontinuous sounds lasting only a few milliseconds, which occur on inspiration when atelectasis is present. Upon inspiration a fine crackling sound, similar to the crinkling of cling film or strands of hair being rubbed together between the fingertips, can be heard as the alveoli pop open. Crackles heard on inspiration and expiration are related to fluid being present in the alveoli. This form of crackles can be classified as fine, medium or coarse dependent upon the amount of fluid present. Fine crackles are high-pitched and relatively short in duration whereas coarse crackles are low-pitched and relatively long in duration. In pneumonia and fibrosing alveolitis crackles have a high-pitched sound and start later in the inspiratory phase.

Wheezes are high-pitched sounds which may occur anywhere in the chest during inspiration or expiration. Wheezes which clear with coughing generally come from the trachea or larger upper airways and are frequently associated with exposure to a cigarette's nicotine, tar and smoke.

Table 2.3 Adventitious sounds

Sound	Intensity	Pitch	Quality	Duration	Location
Crackles	Soft	High	Fine	Short/discontinuous/ dry/end of inspiration	Lung bases
Crackles	Medium	Medium	Medium	Medium/moist/bubbly by during inspiration & expiration	Lung tissue
Crackles	Loud	Low	Coarse	Long/harsh throughout inspiration & expiration	Lung tissue
Sonorous rhonchi	Loud	Low	Snoring	Continuous throughout inspiration & expiration	Large bronchi/ bronchioles
Sibilant rhonchi	Soft	High	Squeak	Continuous throughout inspiration & expiration	Small bronchi/ bronchioles
Wheeze	Medium/loud	Medium/high	Musical	Continuous throughout inspiration & expiration	Large/medium/ small bronchi/ bronchioles
Friction rub	Medium/loud	Low/medium	Grating	Continuous throughout inspiration & expiration	Pleural surfaces
Crunch	Medium/loud	Low/medium	Clicking/gurgling	Synchronous with the heartbeat	Mediastinum

(Reproduced with permission from Cox & McGrath 1999)

However, some wheezes are actually classified as rhonchi. This form of wheeze does not clear with coughing and may be related to bronchospasm or constriction of the airways associated with an allergic reaction, such as from an insect sting. In status asthmaticus, wheezes (sibilant rhonchi) are prolonged on expiration and may be heard as soon as the nurse approaches the patient's bedside.

Rhonchi are classified as sonorous or sibilant. Sonorous rhonchi are low-pitched, rumbling sounds which are more pronounced during expiration. They originate in larger bronchi. The sounds are caused by the passage of air through an airway obstructed by mucus, muscular spasm, tumour or external pressure. Tracheobronchitis causes sonorous rhonchi to occur. Sibilant rhonchi originate in smaller bronchi and, as noted above, produce a high-pitched sound which is related to bronchospasm.

Friction rubs occur outside the respiratory tree and have a dry, grating, low-pitched sound. Frequently the description given for a friction rub is the sound of two pieces of leather rubbing together. Pleural friction rubs are heard on inspiration and expiration and may be confused by the respiratory nurse with pericardial friction rubs. If in doubt as to whether the patient has a pleural or pericardial friction rub, the nurse should ask the patient to hold his breath. If the rub is pleural it will cease, whereas the pericardial rub will continue as the patient's heart beats (Barkauskas et al 1994, Cox 1997, Cox & McGrath 1999, Seidel et al 1995). Friction rubs are caused by inflamed, roughened surfaces rubbing together. Over the lungs the sound is associated with pleurisy. Over the pericardium the sound suggests pericarditis.

Mediastinal crunch, or Hamman sign, is associated with mediastinal emphysema (Seidel et al 1995). Loud crackles, clicking and gurgling sounds can be heard over the mediastinum. The sounds are synchronous with the patient's heartbeat and are not related to respirations. However, it may be noted that the sounds can be more pronounced at the end of expiration and are due to air and fluid in the pleural cavity or large cavities in the lungs. If there is doubt regarding the sound, the nurse should help the patient to lean to the left or to lie on the left side as it will then be easier to discern.

DOCUMENTATION OF THE RESPIRATORY ASSESSMENT

Documentation should describe what has been discerned from the health history and from the physical assessment including inspection, palpation, percussion and auscultation. The health history forms the foundation for the patient's plan of care. Deviations from the normal should be recorded. Adventitious sounds should be recorded in terms of their location (e.g. anterior right base), intensity (e.g. soft or loud), pitch (e.g. high or low), characteristic sound (e.g. crackles), duration on inspiration and expiration and quality (e.g. fine or medium). All nursing interventions employed to treat what has been found should be documented. For example, in the case of fine crackles being heard on inspiration, the respiratory nurse would document that the patient was instructed on deep breathing techniques and given medication for discomfort when splinting, hypopnoea and tachypnoea were present. Following treatment, an evaluation of the outcome of the treatment administered by the respiratory nurse is documented along with any further plans for care.

CONCLUSION

This chapter has described the pertinent aspects of taking a sound health history related to the respiratory system and explained the step-by-step process involved in undertaking a full and comprehensive respiratory physical assessment. It has described respiratory structures, the mechanics of respiration and the four processes of respiratory physical assessment which are inspection, palpation, percussion and auscultation. A systematic approach has been stressed and areas have been highlighted in which respiratory nurses may enhance their knowledge and practice. Many of the problems that patients may have and the signs and symptoms that the respiratory nurse may note whilst undertaking the assessment and preparing to prescribe care have been explored. By undertaking a full and comprehensive assessment, which includes taking a health history of respiratory problems and disease and undertaking a physical assessment, respiratory nurses can detect problems in the early stages of development and take appropriate action. It has been postulated in this chapter that it is essential for respiratory nurses to expand their assessment skills to provide a comprehensive and holistic assessment of patients under their care. This enhances the care patients receive.

REFERENCES

Ashcroft R 1994 Complementary therapy in the critical care unit. In: Millar B, Burnard P (eds) Critical care nursing. Baillière Tindall, London

Barkauskas V, Stoltenberg-Allen K, Baumann L, Darling-Fisher C 1994 Health and physical assessment. Mosby, London

Bates B 1995 Physical examination and history taking, 6th edn. J B Lippincott, Philadelphia

Bridges K, Trujillo E, Jacobs D 1999 Nutrition: alcohol-related thiamine deficiency and malnutrition. Critical Care Nurse 19(6): 80–85

Carpenito L 1995 Nursing care plans and documentation: nursing diagnoses and collaborative problems, 2nd edn. J B Lippincott, Philadelphia

Cox C L 1997 Advanced practice: physical assessment. City University, London

Cox C, Hayes J 1997 Reducing anxiety: the employment of therapeutic touch as a nursing intervention. Complementary Therapies in Nursing and Midwifery 3(6): 163–167

Cox C, Hayes J 1998 Experiences of administering and receiving therapeutic touch in intensive care. Complementary Therapies in Nursing and Midwifery 4(5): 128–133

Cox C, McGrath A 1999 Respiratory assessment in critical care units. Intensive and Critical Care Nursing 15(4): 226–234

Epstein O, Perkin G, de Bono D, Cookson J 1997 Clinical examination. Mosby-Wolfe, London

Hope R, Longmore J, Hodgetts T, Ramrakha P 1995 Oxford handbook of clinical medicine, 3rd edn. Oxford University Press, Oxford

Hudak C, Gallo B 1994 Critical care nursing: a holistic approach, 6th edn. J B Lippincott, Philadelphia

Landis K 1993 Respiratory system. In: Morton P (ed) Health assessment in nursing, 2nd edn. F A Davies, Philadelphia

Lane G 1990 Pulmonary clinical assessment. In: Thelan L, Davie J, Urden L (eds) Textbook of critical care nursing: diagnosis and management. C V Mosby, St Louis

McGrath A, Cox C 1998 Cardiac and circulatory assessment in intensive care units. Journal of Intensive and Critical Care Nursing 14(6): 283–287

Morton P 1993 Health assessment in nursing, 2nd edn. F A Davies, Philadelphia

Ogilvie C, Evans C 1997 Symptoms and signs in clinical medicine: an introduction to medical diagnosis. Butterworth-Heinemann, Oxford

Oh T 1991 Intensive care manual, 3rd edn. Butterworths, London

Rahe R 1975 Epidemiological studies of life change and illness. International Journal of Psychiatry in Medicine 6(1–2): 133–146

Ruch V 1999 Pulmonary disorders. In: Gawlinski A, Hamwi D (eds) Acute care nurse practitioner, clinical curriculum and certification review. W B Saunders Company, London

Sarason I, Johnson J, Siegal J 1978 Assessing the impact of life changes: development of life experiences survey. Journal of Consultant Clinical Psychology 46(5): 932–946

Seidel H, Ball J, Dains J, Benedict G 1995 Mosby's guide to physical examination, 3rd edn. Mosby, London

Thurnock C 1994 Technology in critical care nursing. In: Millar B, Burnard P (eds) Critical care nursing. Baillière Tindall, London

Wilkins R, Hodgkin J, Lopez B 1988 Lung sounds. C V Mosby, St Louis

3 Smoking and smoking cessation

Jennifer Percival

Smoking represents the single most preventable cause of premature death, chronic disease and general ill health in the United Kingdom (UK). Despite this fact there are over 10 million regular cigarette smokers in England (over 12 million in the UK) and 1 in 4 adults smoke regularly. Smoking causes 1 in 5 of all deaths, equivalent to 220 men and 110 women dying every day because of their smoking. Helping smokers to give up is therefore vital because smoking is the largest single cause of death and disability in this country. There are several issues that need to be explored in relation to smoking and smoking cessation:

- the current prevalence and distribution of smoking
- the health consequences of smoking
- the social and psychological factors associated with smoking

- helping smokers to stop – a review of effective interventions
- the role of the health professional – guidelines for practice
- using nicotine replacement therapy
- enabling smokers to move through the cycle of change.

THE CURRENT PREVALENCE AND DISTRIBUTION OF SMOKING

The extent of the problem

Tobacco is currently the leading cause of ill health and disability in the UK, causing 1 in 5 of all deaths. Cigarette smoking killed 121 700 people in the UK in 1995. The death rate in the age group 35–64 was an estimated 40% higher because of smoking and about half of all regular cigarette smokers will eventually be killed by their smoking (Doll et al 1994).

The prevalence of smoking

The prevalence of adults who smoke varies across England, ranging from 24% in the South West, East Anglia and the West Midlands to 29% in Greater London. Currently 27% of the population of Great Britain are smokers (28% men, 26% women). Cigarette smoking levels also vary according to age, the highest levels being amongst men and women in their early twenties and falling thereafter as some of them quit smoking (Fig. 3.1). In the age group 16–19, 30% of men and 31% of women are cigarette smokers rising to 42% and 39% when aged 20–24 and falling after that. Only about 10% of people aged 75 years or more are smokers. Cigarette smoking varies more with age amongst men than amongst women. In the 16–19 age group women are more likely than men to be cigarette smokers and men are more likely to be smokers in the years between 20 and 44.

When do people start smoking?

The great majority of smokers take up the habit when they are young and it is relatively unusual

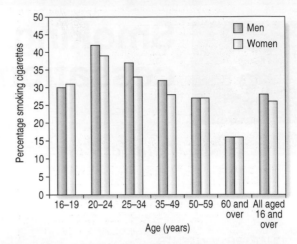

Figure 3.1 Prevalence of cigarette smoking by age and sex amongst adults in 1998. Reproduced with permission from Living in Britain 1988, National Statistics, © Crown Copyright 2000.

for someone to start smoking in their twenties. Working to discourage people from ever starting to smoke is very worthwhile and there are many prevention programmes operating in schools. Teenage smoking has been rising in recent years (Fig. 3.2) and this poses a new threat to the otherwise downward trends in consumption that had been seen in the UK.

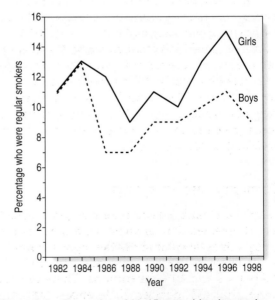

Figure 3.2 Proportion of 11–15 year-olds who smoke 1982–1998. Reproduced with permission from Living in Britain 1988, National Statistics, © Crown Copyright 2000.

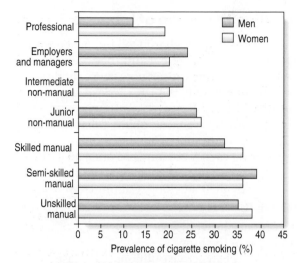

Figure 3.3 Prevalence of cigarette smoking by sex and socio-economic group (1996). Reproduced with permission from Smoking – related behaviour and attitudes 1997, National Statistics, © Crown Copyright 2000.

Social class and smoking

The decline in smoking prevalence has been steeper in non-manual occupations and social class has now become a clear differentiating factor in smoking behaviour (Fig. 3.3). Currently 21% of professional men smoke compared to 35% of men in unskilled manual occupations; 12% of professional women smoke compared to 34% of women in unskilled manual occupations. A survey of low income families found that smoking was related closely to the social features of deprivation such as manual work, marital status, lone parenthood, low educational attainment, housing tenure and receiving means tested benefit (Marsh & Mackay 1994).

Ethnicity and smoking

In 2000 a Health Development Agency (HDA) report revealed that amongst the different Asian groups Bangladeshis show the highest smoking prevalence of 18%. This falls to 15% for Pakistanis and 10% for Indians. There are also some marked gender differences: amongst South Asian women smoking rates are generally very low, for example only 2% of Pakistani women smoke. The smoking prevalence rate for both Afro-Caribbean and Pakistani men is 34%. Indian men show the lowest smoking prevalence (18%) but amongst Bangladeshis a significantly higher rate of smoking is recorded (49%) (Health Development Agency 2000).

Summary

- The smoking of tobacco is currently the greatest cause of ill health and disability in the UK.
- Smoking is responsible for 20% of the annual deaths in the UK.
- Smoking prevalence varies across various socio-economic groups.
- Unskilled manual workers are more likely to smoke than people in the professional groups.
- Cigarette smoking is widening the social class divide in mortality.
- 28% of women smoke during pregnancy.
- 1 in 2 men who continue to smoke will die prematurely as a result.

THE HEALTH CONSEQUENCES OF SMOKING

The constituents of tobacco smoke

Tar, carbon monoxide and nicotine are all found in tobacco smoke, along with 4000 chemicals. Tar is a complex mixture of chemicals which is slowly absorbed when deposited in the lungs during smoking. The sulphurous substances produced in smoke irritate the lung and are closely associated with inflammation of the airways and emphysema. Nicotine stimulates the central nervous system, increasing the heart rate and blood pressure. Nicotine is a powerful and fast acting drug and it is the substance in tobacco which causes addiction. Nicotine alone does not cause cancer. There has been much publicity of low nicotine products but smokers tend to inhale more deeply when using them and have as much nicotine in the body as smokers of standard nicotine cigarettes, and they also inhale similar levels of chemicals and tar.

Nicotine acts on the body in a number of ways. It causes the smoker's heart rate to go up by 10–20 beats per minute and temporarily narrows the smoker's blood vessels, which can cause the body's temperature to drop in the extremities. This same narrowing also causes blood pressure to rise. Carbon monoxide, a known poisonous gas, cuts down the efficiency of the lungs to find oxygen and smokers often become breathless sooner than non-smokers. Tar, formed when the tobacco smoke condenses, collects in the lungs. This damages the cilia which normally help protect the lungs from infection. Tar is also responsible for the yellow/brown colour that heavy smokers may have on their fingers or that can be seen around the ceilings of their homes. In the short term smoking affects the facial skin, which can lose its pink complexion and have increased wrinkling. Finally, there is the smoker's cough which many smokers just take for granted.

Box 3.1   Diseases linked to smoking

Respiratory

- Chronic bronchitis
- Emphysema
- Lung cancer
- Recurrent infections in the airways
- Damage and loss of efficiency in the lungs

Heart and circulation

- Coronary heart disease
- Atherosclerosis – this is the build-up of fatty deposits and loss of elasticity in the artery walls which can lead to a range of diseases including strokes, peripheral vascular disease and gangrene, and aortic and other aneurysms
- Buerger's disease, which can also lead to gangrene

Cancers

- Lungs
- Mouth, nose and throat
- Larynx
- Oesophagus
- Pancreas
- Bladder
- Stomach
- Blood, e.g. leukaemia
- Kidney

Other disorders

- Peptic ulcers – both in incidence and the time they take to heal
- Tobacco amblyopia (defective vision)
- Adverse effects on fertility

The health burden of tobacco

In 1950 Professor Richard Doll published the first study to show the clear link between cigarette smoking and lung cancer; now every single packet of cigarettes sold in the UK carries a government health warning. Research continues to prove the association between smoking tobacco and the disease and mortality related to it.

Smoking causes obvious and often fatal diseases and about half of all regular cigarette smokers will be killed by their smoking (Callum 1998). The most common of these are:

- coronary heart disease
- cancer of the lung
- chronic obstructive pulmonary disease (chronic bronchitis and emphysema).

Although these are the most common diseases, there are many other diseases linked to smoking (Box 3.1). Smoking can also increase the incidence and severity of everyday complaints that people often do not realize are related to their smoking, such as coughing, sneezing and shortness of breath on exertion.

Passive smoking

Breathing in other people's cigarette smoke is called passive smoking. The smoke inhaled by the passive smoker is a combination of the sidestream smoke from the burning end of the cigarette and the smoke inhaled and exhaled by the smoker (mainstream smoke). The US Environmental Protection Agency has declared passive smoking or exposure to environmental tobacco smoke (ETS) to be a Class A carcinogen, which means it is capable of causing cancer in humans.

Passive smoking may cause the following in adults:

- irritation to the eyes, nose and throat
- aggravation of asthma and allergies
- increased risk of coronary heart disease
- increased risk of lung cancer for non-smokers who are exposed to passive smoking over long periods.

A Health Education Authority survey showed that half of the children in England live in a household with at least one smoker. Children do not have any choice about whether they are exposed to tobacco smoke and the US Surgeon General has concluded that children whose parents smoke develop respiratory symptoms more frequently and show small but measurable differences in lung function tests when compared with children of non-smoking parents (US Department of Health and Human Services 1986). In addition, children of smokers have also been shown to be particularly affected by chronic middle ear effusions (glue ear) and to have an increased prevalence of asthma.

Women and smoking

Women took up smoking later in the 20th century than men (Fig. 3.4). Due to the time lag between starting to smoke and the onset of smoking related disease, the effects of smoking on women's health are still emerging. Lung cancer is now rising in women and falling in men and in Scotland it has already overtaken breast cancer as the lead cause of cancer deaths in women. Smoking reduces bone density and women who smoke 20 cigarettes a day throughout adulthood will probably have reduced their bone density by 5–10% by the time they reach menopause, compared to non-smokers, and consequently run a greater risk of fracture (Law & Hackshaw 1997).

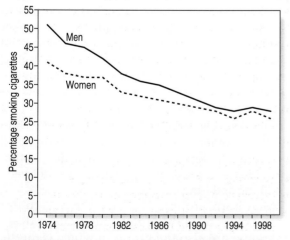

Figure 3.4   Comparison of men and women smokers 1974–1998. Reproduced with permission from Living in Britain 1998, National Statistics, © Crown Copyright 2000.

Summary

- Smoking is not an immediate cause of death but is the cause of the disease from which the smoker eventually dies.
- Smokers are at greater risk of illness and early death than non-smokers.
- Smoking 25 cigarettes a day makes you 25 times more likely to die from lung cancer and almost twice as likely to die from coronary heart disease.
- Stopping smoking has immediate benefits for men and women of all ages irrespective of them having a smoking related disease.
- Ex-smokers live longer than continuing smokers.

THE SOCIAL AND PSYCHOLOGICAL FACTORS ASSOCIATED WITH SMOKING

Smoking is associated with being an adult. When young people see adults smoking and are surrounded by positive images of the habit and tobacco advertising and promotion, some will want to experiment with cigarettes and unknowingly will be running the risk of becoming addicted to smoking.

The Health Education Authority (1992) showed that 93% of adults think that smokers are more likely than non-smokers to get lung cancer and 80% of people think smokers are more likely to get heart disease. This shows that there is a conflict between the health warning on the cigarette packet, the common knowledge of the population that smoking is a factor in lung cancer and heart disease, and the desire of young people to take up the habit. It is interesting to look into the factors that lead somebody to start smoking. The UK tobacco industry spends about £100 000 a year on advertising and generates about £6.5 billion in tobacco product tax and £1.5 billion in

Activity 3.1

- List the reasons why you think people start smoking.
- List the reasons why you think people continue to smoke after they have started.
- List the reasons why people stop smoking.
- List the reasons why people relapse.

VAT for the Treasury (ASH 1993). Rising taxation has reduced tobacco consumption and increased revenue; however studies of smokers on low income have shown that these smokers cut back on other spending to absorb price increases (Marsh & Mackay 1994).

Young people and smoking

The tobacco industry needs to recruit new smokers for the loss of around 330 smokers a day through death. Most smokers take up the habit when they are teenagers. About one-third of adult smokers start smoking regularly from the age of 14–15. One of the problems with this is that the younger people are when they first start to smoke, the more likely they are to suffer from a smoking related illness and the harder they will find it to stop. A smoker starting at the age of 15 is 3 times more likely to die from lung cancer than someone who starts in their twenties.

There is a strong relationship between image and smoking and many factors affect a young person's self-image. Sociability, maturity, independence, conformity and attractiveness are the intangible reasons young people give for smoking. Non-smokers are sometimes viewed as lacking in these qualities. Although legally not for sale to those under 16, cigarettes are widely available to young smokers through newsagents, confectioners or vending machines. The majority of under 16-year-olds do not find it difficult to buy cigarettes.

This, then, is a product which is heavily advertised, easily available and seen by peers as socially acceptable, and which very quickly leads to an addiction to a very powerful substance, nicotine, and to a delivery method that is known to cause cancers and heart disease. The biggest problem with smoking is that it is a habit that is acquired early by young people who have far more pressing concerns in their day-to-day existence than the thought of their future mortality and the risk of death through smoking. The cavalier attitude of 'you have to die of something' or 'you could get run over by a bus' seems to prevail against the heavy scientific evidence demonstrating the real consequences of starting to smoke.

Summary

- Young people are susceptible to becoming addicted very quickly to nicotine and they are more likely to smoke if their parents, older brothers and sisters or friends smoke.
- The tobacco industry spends £100 000 a year advertising the product.
- The majority of smokers take up the habit whilst in their teens and have rarely made the free choice associated with being an adult.
- Smokers give financial savings and improvements to health as the two main advantages to giving up smoking.
- Among those who have tried to quit, health reasons are the main motivation.

THE HEALTH BURDEN OF SMOKING OVER THE GENERATIONS

In the 1930s cigarette consumption by women doubled from 5% to 10% and ready made cigarettes accounted for 75% of tobacco production. At that time doctors began to suspect a link between smoking and lung cancer but it wasn't until 1950 that Sir Richard Doll published a study linking cigarette smoking to lung cancer, so people who started smoking before the 1950s were unaware of the fatal consequences of taking up the habit. It was in the 1960s that low tar and low nicotine cigarette brands were introduced after major reports on smoking and health by the Royal College of Physicians. However, it was not until 1971 that the first health warning was put on the side of a cigarette packet. This was a voluntary agreement between the government and the tobacco industry that is still in place today. The peak of popularity for smoking was around the mid 1970s when 50% of men and 40% of women in the UK were regular smokers. By 1984 smoking levels had dropped to 36% for men and 32% for women. It is the comparison of trends in cigarette smoking and lung cancer deaths that provides evidence of the direct link between smoking and lung cancer.

Men born around 1900 are the age cohort who experienced the highest lung cancer death rates and are also the group in which cigarette smoking reached its peak. The picture is even clearer for women, amongst whom the smoking epidemic occurred more recently, with the highest death rates being seen in women born in the mid 1920s, in the group in which cigarette smoking reached its peak. By 1995 lung cancer mortality for men had passed its peak and was falling for all age groups. Lung cancer deaths for women aged 65–69 had also peaked. In women the rates were falling for younger age groups but still increasing for older age groups as those born in the 1920s reached the highest ages of mortality.

In 1992 the government published the first health strategy for England, *Health of the nation* (DOH 1992). Targets were introduced to reduce the prevalence of smoking. In 1994 adult smoking levels had reached 28% for men and 26% for women. Levels were highest amongst 20–24-year-old men and women, at 48% and 38% respectively. In 1997 the newly elected Labour Government pledged to introduce a series of tobacco control measures, including a ban on advertising and sponsorship.

REDUCING SMOKING IN THE FUTURE – TOBACCO CONTROL

To ensure a healthier future smokers must be encouraged, motivated and enabled to give up, new generations must be prevented from starting to smoke, and all non-smokers must be protected from passive smoking. Given the complex nature of smoking behaviour and the way in which cigarettes are a feature of our society, a comprehensive tobacco control policy is needed to help reduce public acceptability of smoking. A comprehensive tobacco control policy is made up of five areas:

- ending all tobacco promotion
- providing health education and support for those who want to quit
- using the well-established methods of fiscal policy and keeping prices up to encourage people to quit and to deter young people from starting
- extending smoke-free provision in public places
- limiting young people's access to tobacco.

HELPING SMOKERS TO STOP
The role of the healthcare professionals

The burden on the National Health Service (NHS) of disease and ill-health created by smoking is enormous and costs approximately £1.76 million every year in England (Buck et al 1997). On the basis of research evidence, national guidelines for practice have been developed to ensure that NHS staff can contribute to a smoking cessation strategy which fits in with the overall tobacco control requirements (West et al 2000). Giving smoking cessation advice is much better value than providing a medical intervention such as long term oxygen therapy for COPD. The recommendations listed below have been made on the basis of proven, effective cessation interventions and the systematic review of advice given in primary care settings.

The role of the healthcare professional is fundamental if smoking cessation targets are to be achieved and therefore it is recommended that healthcare professionals should:

- assess the smoking status of patients at every opportunity
- advise all smokers to stop
- assist those interested in stopping smoking
- offer follow up
- refer to specialist cessation services if necessary
- recommend smokers who want to stop to use nicotine replacement therapy (NRT)
- provide accurate information and advice on nicotine replacement therapy (NRT).

The essential features of individual smoking cessation advice are, where appropriate, to:

- **Ask** about smoking at every opportunity
- **Advise** all smokers to stop
- **Assist** the smoker to stop
- **Arrange** follow up.

Ask

All patients should have their smoking (or other tobacco use) status established and checked at every visit. A system should be devised to record smoking status in the notes. The guidelines suggest noting a patient as a:

- smoker
- non-smoker
- recent ex-smoker or
- interested in stopping.

This can be assessed with an open-ended question such as 'Have you ever tried to stop?' followed by 'Are you interested at all in stopping now?'. This will allow monitoring of motivation to quit over a period of time.

Advise

Even if they do not currently wish to quit, all smokers should be advised of the value of stopping and the risks to health of continuing. The advice should be clear, firm and tailored to their personal situation.

Assist

If the smoker would like to stop, help should be offered. The key points, which can be covered in 5–10 minutes, are:

- Set a date to stop and stop completely on that day.
- Review past experience: what helped, what hindered?
- Plan ahead: identify likely problems and make a plan to deal with them.
- Tell family and friends and enlist their support.
- Plan what you are going to do about alcohol.
- Try NRT, using whichever product suits best.

Further support that could be offered to someone wanting to quit can be obtained from the NHS smoking helpline on 0800 169 0169 where practical advice is available on:

- making an action plan
- reasons for stopping
- avoiding relapse
- coping with stress.

Further smoking cessation resources can usually be obtained from local health promotion units.

Arrange

Depending on facilities it is useful to arrange a follow-up visit in about a week, and further visits after that if possible. Most smokers make several attempts to stop before finally succeeding (the average is around 3–4 attempts), thus relapse is a normal part of the process. If a smoker has made repeated attempts to stop and has failed, and/or experienced severe withdrawal, and/or requested more intensive help, consider referral to a specialist cessation service.

Guidelines recommend that health commissioners invest in providing a service to smokers which will result in cost-effective health gain for the population (DOH 1998). In primary care the potential for helping smokers is enormous. However, many GPs do not intervene with smokers (Health Education Authority 1995).

Summary

- Smoking cessation interventions should be delivered by as many health professionals in different services as possible, provided they have the necessary skills, experience and commitment.
- Pregnant smokers should be given firm and clear advice to stop smoking opportunistically throughout pregnancy and should be given as much support as possible.
- Training increases the likelihood of health professionals to intervene with smokers and may increase smoking cessation rates.
- Hospital patients who smoke should, where appropriate, be offered help in stopping smoking, including the offer of nicotine replacement therapy.
- The smoking status of all hospital patients should be established on admission and recorded in their notes.
- Ideally people should be warned of a hospital's smoke-free status before admission.

SMOKING CESSATION

The effect of nicotine on the body

When tobacco smoke is inhaled nicotine is absorbed into the bloodstream and its effects on the brain are felt within 7–8 seconds. The immediate physiological effects are:

- increased heart rate and blood pressure
- constriction of small blood vessels under the skin
- changes in hormonal levels and metabolism
- affected mood and behaviour.

Throughout the day the level of nicotine in the bloodstream of the average smoker rises.

Addiction

Addiction involves not only a physical dependence upon the drug nicotine, but also a psychological and emotional dependence upon smoking as a means of coping with stress, boredom, anxiety or anger. Smoking becomes an automatic habit and the association of smoking with everyday activities contributes to the difficulties smokers experience when giving up. The effects of addiction on the mood and behaviour of smokers are complex and depend on their general constitution, how long they have been smoking, the kind of smoking habit they have, the number of puffs they take, how deeply they inhale, and the situation they are in at the time. The complexity of the addiction to nicotine makes the one-to-one, person-centred approach the most effective when offering brief advice and support, as it is impossible to predict the responses any individual smoker may have upon receiving unsolicited advice to completely change their behaviour.

Nicotine causes the addiction to smoking and the withdrawal of nicotine causes the withdrawal symptoms when someone stops smoking. These begin within a few hours, peak within a few days and typically last 4–6 weeks. The symptoms are:

Activity 3.2

Smokers often quote stress relief as a reason for continuing. Write down your thoughts on this particular justification.

Activity 3.3

How much weight would you expect somebody giving up smoking to put on and what advice would you give somebody who was concerned about this to the extent of choosing not to give up smoking?

- agitation or depression
- insomnia
- irritability
- frustration or anger
- anxiety
- difficulty in concentrating
- restlessness
- increased appetite or weight gain
- decreased heart rate.

Weight gain

Many smokers are anxious about gaining weight when they give up smoking. Women are more concerned than men about putting on weight if they try to give up (Health Education Authority 1996). Twice as many women as men are motivated to give up for aesthetic or cosmetic reasons such as the lingering smell of tobacco smoke and the effect of smoke on skin and teeth.

NICOTINE REPLACEMENT THERAPY

In June 1998 an expert panel called for a more effective UK public policy on smoking cessation and the use of nicotine replacement therapy (NRT) (DOH 1998). The panel's report stated that tobacco addiction should be taken as seriously as drug or alcohol addiction and that combating it represented a major opportunity to improve the health of the nation. It also called for NRT to be made available on prescription, in particular for those in lower income groups. The report noted that since the 1970s about half a million people have stopped smoking every year. However, while the percentage of affluent men and women who have stopped smoking has more than doubled from around 25% to nearly 60%, amongst the poorer groups the prevalence remains as high as 70% and these groups have the lowest rates of cessation. Consequently, the people in the most disadvantaged social groups suffer most from smoking related morbidity and mortality, are least likely to be aware of the benefits of NRT, or may perceive themselves as being unable to afford NRT when attempting to stop. It is these groups that would gain the most from NRT being available on prescription.

Nicotine replacement therapy (NRT) can help smokers to give up smoking. Clinical trials have shown that NRT doubles the chance of success of smokers wishing to give up. However, NRT is not a magic cure and does not provide a complete replacement for cigarettes. It reduces but does not eliminate withdrawal symptoms such as irritability and depression, it reduces but does not remove the urge to smoke, and those using it to help them give up smoking will need a great deal of determination to get through the first few weeks. Dependence on NRT products has not been found to be a serious problem. Some smokers continue to use the gum and nasal spray for a year or more but this appears to be mostly out of concern about the possibility of returning to smoking.

Nicotine replacement products help smokers give up by offering them a chance to break their addiction to nicotine with a gradual dose reduction. Nicotine replacement therapy (NRT) is available in:

- skin patches
- gum
- nasal sprays
- inhalers.

For maximum effect, NRT must be used in sufficient quantity and for a long enough period and smokers must follow the instructions in the package.

Nicotine skin patches

Transdermal patches release nicotine which is slowly absorbed through the skin over a period of hours and provides a steady level of nicotine. This method is the easiest to use as smokers just apply one patch each morning. Some patches are designed to be worn for 24 hours and others are worn for 16 hours. Both come in different dosages. Unless they smoke fewer than 10 cigarettes per day, smokers should normally use the highest dose patch available. This method is most useful for smokers who smoke more than 15 cigarettes a day.

Nicotine gum

In the gum formulations nicotine is released through chewing and is absorbed in the lining of the mouth. There are 2 mg and 4 mg dosages which come in traditional, mint or other flavours. People use between 10 and 15 pieces a day for up to 3 months and after this time there should be a gradual reduction in usage. When used properly the gum is at least as effective as the patch. Smokers often complain of the taste at first but if they persevere for a week or so most get used to it. It is important to chew the gum slowly to get the most out of this therapy. Nicotine that is swallowed is wasted as the nicotine has to be absorbed through the lining of the mouth. Smokers should try the 2 mg gum first and if they find the taste acceptable but are still experiencing severe cravings and withdrawal symptoms they should switch to the 4 mg gum.

Nicorette nasal spray

Nicorette nasal spray (NNS) consists of a small bottle of nicotine solution whose top delivers a dose of nicotine in a spray when pressed down. The nasal spray works more rapidly than gum or a patch and replicates the way that a smoker experiences nicotine being absorbed from a cigarette. However, this method can be difficult to get used to because the spray irritates the nose. The nasal spray is only available on private prescription.

Nicorette inhalator

The Nicorette inhalator consists of a plastic mouthpiece and a supply of nicotine cartridges that attach to the end. Smokers puff on it like a cigarette. Despite its name, nicotine from it does not get into the lungs – it stops in the mouth and throat. Its nicotine delivery is very similar to that of nicotine gum.

The cost of each of these nicotine replacement products is roughly similar, and approximately the same as the cost of smoking.

Summary

- Although making NRT available on prescription would have financial implications for the NHS, the benefit in the substantial reduction in the cost of treating smoking related disease would be great.
- Nicotine replacement therapy has been found to double the success rate of a single smoking cessation attempt.
- The majority of smokers are in the most disadvantaged social groups and are the least likely to purchase NRT.
- NRT works by reducing the severity of many of the physiological withdrawal symptoms experienced during smoking cessation attempts.
- NRT can be administered by a gum, patches, vapour inhalator or nasal spray and the active ingredient is pure nicotine.
- NRT products are licensed as pharmaceutical medicines for use in smoking cessation and therefore may only be purchased from a pharmacy by people over 18 years of age. The nicotine spray is only available on private prescription.
- The advantage of NRT is that its only active ingredient is nicotine and it is therefore devoid of the 4000 noxious elements found in cigarette smoke.
- The weekly cost of NRT is less than the weekly cost of 20 cigarettes per day and it is intended to be used for a limited period up to a maximum of 3 months.
- There is no evidence that nicotine is carcinogenic.
- During a period of complete abstinence from cigarettes NRT effectively reduces and controls the addiction formed from smoking.

Bupropion

Bupropion (Zyban) is a non-nicotine-based treatment which has been shown in trials to be highly effective in helping smokers to quit (Hurt et al 1997, Jorenby et al 1999). It is indicated as an aid to smoking cessation in combination with motivational support for nicotine-dependent patients. Bupropion is an antidepressant that reduces the smoker's withdrawal symptoms and the desire to smoke, and it works by desensitizing the brain's nicotine receptors. For a lot of smokers, it

will provide a different way to help them overcome their addiction to cigarettes. The standard dose of bupropion is 300 mg per day and the course lasts 2 months, with the stopping smoking date set at around day 8 of the course. It is important that only smokers motivated to quit should be prescribed the drug.

Some of the press coverage positioned bupropion as a 'wonder drug' and there have been claims that it is (almost) twice as effective as NRT. In fact, it is too soon to make comparisons between NRT and bupropion. Both products have an important role to play and will meet smokers' needs in different ways. A Cochrane review (Silagy et al 2000) says of bupropion and nicotine replacement:

Nicotine replacement therapy (NRT) has proven efficacy in over 80 studies and has a very benign side-effect profile. The early results for several antidepressants, especially bupropion, are sufficient to endorse their use in medical practice. There is insufficient published evidence to recommend bupropion in preference to NRT or vice versa. Bupropion may also be helpful in those who fail nicotine replacement.

The most serious side-effect risk with bupropion is seizures – but this is estimated at less than 1 in 1000 risk. There are other possible more common side-effects (> 1 in 100 risk) including, among others, dry mouth, gastrointestinal problems, insomnia, tremor, headaches and increased skin sensitivity. It is contraindicated for people with hypersensitivity to bupropion, seizure history, bulimia or anorexia, hepatic cirrhosis and bipolar disorder, and for users of monoamine oxidase inhibitors. Bupropion should not be used in pregnancy or while breast feeding, and caution is advised while driving.

Bupropion is available on normal NHS reimbursable prescriptions – so it will be up to health authorities and Primary Care Groups/Trusts to decide whether to spend part of their drugs budget on bupropion as part of their smoking cessation strategy. Users of bupropion have access to a free support service, funded by the drug's makers, Glaxo Wellcome, that includes regular 'motivational mailings' sent to their home address and personalized letters reminding them why they decided to quit and encouraging them to stick at it. This support package, called 'Right Time', includes access to a telephone helpline run by QUIT.

Patients who self-refer and express a wish to try bupropion need to be assessed as being motivated to quit and to ensure that the drug is clinically appropriate for them. Smokers should be encouraged to return to the service for further help. On the negative side, if they ask for bupropion and are refused a prescription, they may decide that 'if the NHS doesn't give me the new treatment, then they obviously don't think I need to stop that much'. Helping people prepare to stop is an essential part of the process of quitting. Premature attempts lead to quick relapses.

The trials of bupropion in America are impressive and there is no doubt that the product is an effective smoking cessation aid and a very welcome addition to the tools available to help people stop smoking. It is not, however, the magic bullet that smokers dream of finding to stop their addiction to nicotine.

ENABLING SMOKERS TO MOVE THROUGH THE CYCLE OF CHANGE

The approach suggested takes note of a model of behaviour change developed by Prochaska and DiClemente. The 'stages of change' model (Prochaska & DiClemente 1984, Prochaska et al 1992) assumes that individuals' behaviour change attempts can be categorized into several stages. It proposes that assessing a person's stage of change helps professionals to use an appropriate strategy that matches the individual's stage of change (Fig. 3.5).

The stages of change

Precontemplation

The person is not interested in change. Some people may never have considered change or may not be aware of the risks their behaviour may carry. Others may understand the risks and may have considered change, but are not interested in changing their behaviour at this time.

Contemplation

This involves thinking about change. People at this stage are considering the possibility of change but have not yet made a decision to change.

Preparation

People at this stage are preparing to change. They have made a commitment to change but have not yet made plans to do so.

Making change

People at this stage are making changes to aspects of their behaviour.

Maintenance

This involves maintaining change. People at this stage are continuing to make changes. For some this remains a struggle for some time and others relapse into their old behaviour patterns.

Using the cycle of change with smokers

Some smokers think that stopping smoking is simply a matter of will power and that when the time is right they will be able to throw away their

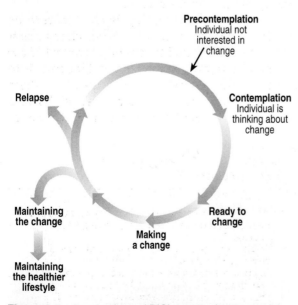

Figure 3.5 Prochaska and DiClemente change model. Adapted from Prochaska & DiClemente 1984.

cigarettes and never want to smoke again. This is optimistic because smoking is a complex habit and the smoker has to deal with the addiction to nicotine as well as the psychological and social aspects of the habit.

Smoking cessation is a process not an event and, because smoking is a personal habit, no two smokers will move through the process in exactly the same way. Providing factual information on the dangers to health may increase clients' knowledge about the choices they are making, but there is no evidence that this will help them change. The model shows that change is a process which happens over considerable time, with people's attitudes changing before their behaviour and frequent relapse being a common feature.

No amount of force can make a person change and this is not the role of the helping professional. The approach most useful to the smoker is where the discussion closely matches the stage the smoker is in. The key skills needed for this are the ability to listen and willingness to work with the information the smoker is giving you, not your own agenda. Pushing the issue too far with a reluctant client can lead either to an aggressive response or to collusion. Collusion is when the smoker will make a statement as a way of ending the discussion, for example 'Yes, I will try to cut down the number I smoke', but in reality has no intention of following through on this statement.

Although at any one time two-thirds of smokers have said that they would like to give up their smoking, the proportion who are actually trying to stop is only about 1 in 6. Consequently, offering all smokers information about the practicalities of cessation will fail to help 5 out of 6 of them. The Health Education Authority showed that of those smokers who had seen a GP in the last year, 29% said that they had discussed smoking either at the surgery or elsewhere, and over two-thirds (68%) said they had not discussed it at all. Of the people who had discussed smoking, only one-third (35%) had found it helpful (Health Education Authority 1996).

Most smokers entering health service premises will expect to be asked if they smoke. There is evidence that when the issue is not raised, an endorsement of the habit may be assumed by

Activity 3.4

What opportunities are there in your current working environment to raise the issue of smoking status?

the smoker: 'It must be OK – they would have told me if it wasn't.' It is therefore important that systems are set up in hospitals to ensure that smoking status is assessed and the result recorded at every visit.

When it has been established that a person is a smoker, it is necessary to use open-ended questions to help gain more insight into their current stage of change. Questions that may be useful are:

- How important is your smoking to you?
- Have you ever considered stopping?
- Are you interested at all in stopping now?
- What is the longest time you have managed to go without a cigarette?
- What do you enjoy most about smoking?
- Has anyone ever suggested to you that you stop smoking?

It is important that a record of the person's smoking status and, where possible, readiness to change is made in their notes.

This way of working has been shown to be effective in supporting behaviour change as it allows the individual to remain in control of the decision-making process. The 'helper role' is to support the individual by guiding them through the processes, using key skills and strategies to facilitate discussion. Evidence

Activity 3.5

- What replies have you heard from smokers who are asked, 'Have you ever considered giving up smoking?'
- List some of the things that smokers may say to justify their smoking.
- When asked if they would like help to give up, some smokers become defensive. Why do you think this is?
- If you found yourself in this situation how would you handle it?

suggests that the qualities of the helper and his interpersonal skills when working with clients, regardless of training or intervention type, determine his effectiveness as a helper. Using this approach is likely to take longer than simply giving advice, but can be achieved in short sessions of 5–30 minutes.

Summary

- Using communication skills appropriate to each stage will reduce the client resistance that many health professionals associate with offering opportunistic advice to smokers.
- The use of open-ended questions and the person-centred approach is essential.
- Using the appropriate approach makes a significant difference to the way smokers relate to healthcare professionals.

Assessing a smoker's stage of change

When smokers are unsure about whether or not they are ready to think about stopping smoking it is useful for them to have a chance to weigh up their thoughts about smoking in a constructive manner by writing down all the conflicting aspects. Helping them make a list of everything they like about smoking and then everything they dislike helps create a picture of the choice they are currently making (Fig. 3.6). The simple act of considering their smoking in this depth may bring about a shift in attitude.

If they say they are not interested in stopping (precontemplation):

- Reinforce their knowledge about the health risks and about the benefits of stopping.
- Correct any misconceptions such as the belief that 'the damage is already done'.
- Provide appropriate support material.
- Invite them to discuss smoking again with you or a colleague at any time, and tell them that support is available should they decide to try to stop.
- Record your findings in the notes.

If they are thinking about stopping smoking (contemplation):

- Discuss in detail any ambivalence and go through the results of the scales exercise.
- Try to help them establish why they are undecided. Is one of the reasons they wish to continue smoking more heavily weighted than they are acknowledging to themselves? Using open-ended questions and a facilitative approach will help them clarify the situation.
- Check their knowledge about the health risks and personalize the benefits of stopping.

Are they aware of any changes in their health that are attributable to their smoking?

- Encourage your clients to believe that they can succeed in stopping if they really want to. Let them know what further help is available including telephone helplines.
- Discuss the advantages of using nicotine replacement therapy and check any misconceptions they may have about the products.
- Record smoking status and offer an open ended invitation to discuss the subject again.

Preparing to change (preparation)

To help smokers move towards the next change, health workers can suggest a change in current behaviour around the smoking habit, such as switching brands, smoking only in one place in the home, or buying one pack at a time. Removing cigarettes from the automatic place they now occupy in the smoker's life will start the change by separating smoking from other routine activities. Action plans will be successful if they

Activity 3.6

Ask current smokers to fill out the scales in Figure 3.6 and when they have finished ask them to indicate at the bottom where they are now as they review what they have written.

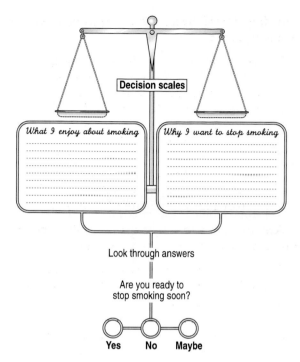

Figure 3.6   Decision scales.

have a timetable and a stop date, are designed by the smoker, are realistic and include a form of external support.

Ready to stop (making changes)

Keeping a diary page (Fig. 3.7) can make it clear to smokers where their danger points are and will help to identify where they need to develop other diversions or distractions to fill the gaps. The diary needs to cover all the work, home and leisure situations experienced in a typical week.

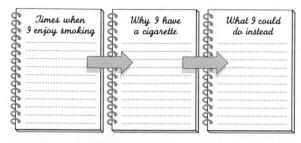

Figure 3.7   Diary sheet.

Going through the completed diary sheet and offering to work through the results in order to inform a cessation attempt is a useful tool. It can highlight which cigarettes could easily have been done without and which cigarettes were most needed. This discussion will help form the basis for the action plan as anticipating a future situation in which there may be a strong smoking cue will allow smokers time to develop an alternative plan. For example, if a cigarette at the end of a meal has been highlighted as important, what will they plan to do at the end of a meal on the first cessation day, since giving up eating is not a long term strategy?

Helping smokers make an action plan

Using information about the smoking habit gleaned from the diary keeping exercise, the next stage is actively to work towards the stop date. By now smokers should have more reasons for giving up smoking than for continuing. They should also be clear about the benefits to themselves from giving up smoking. The key is for them to anticipate likely problems, plan ahead for difficult situations and identify who or what will support them. Some smokers may like to join a 'stop smoking' group and get their support through this means. The health professional can help by informing them of the specialist services for smokers available in the area. The key to success is wanting to stop. Although smokers are being helped, it is important that *they* remain in charge of how and when they are going to change their habits.

An action plan needs the following components:

- A stop date – when is the best time, a holiday, weekend or work day?
- Support – who or where will this come from?
- Rewards – in addition to the longer term benefits, having a distinct reward at the end of the first week or month has been shown to help, e.g. buying a treat.
- Knowledge of the triggers and cues and a plan for alternative coping behaviours.
- Strategies to handle unexpected problem situations.

- Management of the addictive component and handling the withdrawal symptoms.
- Awareness of current diet and how the cessation attempt may impact on it.

Actually stopping

The main reasons people give for wanting to quit are to improve their health, to save money and to protect their family and children from passive smoking. The main barriers to quitting given by smokers are:

- withdrawal symptoms
- lack of will power
- inability to cope in social situations without cigarettes
- boredom.

By now the smokers you are working with should know exactly why they want to stop, when they are going to do it, what help is available to them, including NRT products, and how they are going to manage the first few days without cigarettes. Once these decisions have been made they are ready to take action. Listing changes that could be made to assist with stopping smoking can be helpful and can increase insight into the complex nature of giving up smoking.

These are some of the changes that could be made:

- cope with the urges to smoke, e.g. do deep breathing exercises
- deal with the temptations to smoke, e.g. get rid of all smoking apparatus

Activity 3.7

- Make a list of the possible rewards that smokers could give themselves at the end of the first day, week and month.
- What questions could you ask that would help them develop their plans for coping on a daily basis or if unexpected problems arise?

- change your routine, e.g. go for a walk after a meal
- change the way you feel about smoking, e.g. 'I am choosing not to smoke'.

Self-image

Many smokers say they will miss being a smoker because they believe that most of the 'fun' people are smokers and that non-smokers can be boring. This attitude can contribute towards an unsuccessful attempt to quit, and addressing the issue of self-image before the stop date is helpful.

Ask smokers to list three or more qualities about themselves that they think will improve when they stop smoking. Encourage them to focus on how good it will feel to have managed the change and to be free of the old restrictions imposed by smoking. Ask them to close their eyes and see themselves smoke-free, healthier and more in control of their lives. Encourage them to be patient with themselves and proud of their progress.

Coping with relapse

Even with the best laid plans some smokers may be unprepared for a high risk situation and may have a cigarette, thinking that just one won't hurt and that it will help them cope right now. Lapses are part of life and yet for some smokers they are used as an opportunity to convince themselves that they have no will power, or that maybe smoking isn't so bad for them after all, or they may just feel very guilty and give themselves a hard time.

Some tips for handling a lapse are:

- stop smoking again immediately
- remind yourself of all the reasons for not wanting to be a smoker
- talk to somebody who can get you back on track.

Asking what led up to the lapse and how the cigarette helped is useful. Check if smoking made the problem manageable or not as sometimes the sense of guilt that a motivated quitter may feel will leave them with a sense of failure. Help by encouraging them not to feel guilty and not to let one mistake distract them from their main plan, which is to become a non-smoker. Help them decide how they will handle the problem differently next time.

Helping prepare for the next attempt to stop

As relapse is part of the cycle of change it is worth drawing a smoker's attention to this possibility and working through the situations most likely to cause a relapse, such as drinking after work with a social group. Alcohol, tea and coffee are all associated with cigarettes and can all weaken a person's resolve to stay stopped. Help smokers to plan for what they will do if a relapse occurs and to look at where smoking fits into the wider context of their lives.

Some smokers express strong feelings of grief and loss around the time of giving up smoking and many people will confess to feeling as if they have lost their best friend. Since many comfortable routines involve smoking, the many changes needed to cope without cigarettes can feel strange and can produce a definite sense of loss. Smokers may feel they have lost part of how they think they are supposed to look or act. These feelings are normal and a grief reaction can occur whenever something important is taken away from our lives. Grief reactions tend to follow a certain pattern and denial, anger, bargaining and depression may all occur when someone stops smoking, although not necessarily in any specific order.

Maintaining change (staying stopped)

Having managed to withdraw from nicotine dependence and the social and psychological habit associated with smoking, a smoker will begin to feel victory over the habit. Many ex-smokers say that they still think about smoking and occasionally feel tempted to have a cigarette, although they know they never would.

If you are working with smokers who have stopped within the last 6 months they may still be liable to relapse. You can support them by offer-

Activity 3.8

Think of something you have lost, either a possession or the end of a relationship. Go back to that time and try and remember what you felt like and the sort of things that you told yourself at the time.

- Did your health change in any way at the time?
- Were you aware of any symptoms of stress?
- What might smokers say to you that would show they were experiencing loss/grief?
- What responses might you make in this situation?

ing follow-up sessions reinforcing their determination to stay stopped and helping them remain positive about being ex-smokers. This is a crucial stage and encouragement and reassurance will help smokers to stay stopped.

Try asking them to tell you their reasons for stopping and check whether their expectations of the actual results were realistic. The active support of a helping relationship can really help maintain a smoker's morale and determination. Some smokers are vulnerable to relapse for years and it is always worth checking how long smokers have been stopped for, asking how confident they feel about staying stopped and applauding their efforts. Your continued offer of help and support may be invaluable.

Lifestyle changes

To help motivate your patients to change their risk-carrying lifestyles you should:

- Find out what the patient already knows and believes about lifestyle and health.

Activity 3.9

Talk to some smokers you know who have given up and ask them if they are ever tempted to have just one cigarette. Think through their answers and decide if they are vulnerable to relapse or just remembering an old friend with fondness.

- Develop a partnership with your patient in which you act as an expert who can help, and the patient remains in control of the choices concerning health.
- Recognize that not all patients are ready for change and many may need help to understand the impact their chosen lifestyle has before overcoming their barriers to change.
- Let the patient decide what, when and how to change, and elicit from the patient a commitment to change. Tackling one aspect of behaviour at a time is usually more successful than trying to remove several risk factors simultaneously.
- When patients want to and are ready to change, facilitate them to develop an action plan with specific, achievable goals. This should be written by the patients themselves. If they get stuck finding alternative behaviours, encourage them to re-examine why they want to change.
- The role of the health professional is to build up patients' belief in their ability to carry out change and to succeed in achieving the goals they have set for themselves, and to provide support during the process.

Summary

People are likely to succeed in stopping smoking:

- when they have thought about stopping for a period of time before attempting it.
- when they are ready, not when someone else tries to coerce them.
- when they know enough about their smoking habit and why they want to stop.
- when they are prepared for how they will feel and have developed alternatives to put in the place of smoking.
- when they learn how to cope in different ways with situations in which they would normally have turned to cigarettes.
- when they have built up a positive image of themselves as a non-smoker and can control their lives without needing a cigarette.
- when they make quitting the most important thing they are doing and make staying stopped a priority.

CONCLUSION

Over and above the risk of premature death, smoking has a very great impact on the day-to-day health of the individual. The disability that breathlessness brings and its effect on the quality of life of those suffering from smoking related disease are often underestimated. The only way to counteract this is to prevent the young from starting to smoke and to ensure that smokers have every opportunity to stop smoking.

REFERENCES

ASH 1993 Tobacco advertising – the case for a ban, 4th edn. ASH, London

Buck D, Godfrey C, Parrott S, Raw M 1997 Cost effectiveness of smoking cessation interventions. Health Education Authority, London

Callum C 1998 The UK smoking epidemic: death in 1995. Health Education Authority, London

Department of Health (DOH) 1992 Health of the nation. HMSO, London

Department of Health (DOH) 1998 Smoking kills: a White Paper on tobacco. The Stationery Office, London

Doll R, Peto R, Wheatley K et al 1994 Mortality in relation to smoking: 40 years observation on male British doctors. British Medical Journal 309: 901–911

Health Development Agency 2000 Tobacco and England's ethnic minorities. Health Development Agency, London

Health Education Authority 1992 Health and lifestyle survey. Health Education Authority, London

Health Education Authority 1995 Health in England. Health Education Authority, London

Health Education Authority 1996 National adult smoking campaign tracking survey. Health Education Authority, London

Hurt R D, Sachs D P, Glover E D et al 1997 A comparison of sustained release bupropion and placebo for smoking cessation. New England Journal of Medicine 337: 1195–1202

Jorenby D E, Leischow S J, Nides M A et al 1999 A controlled trial of sustained release bupropion, a nicotine patch, or both for smoking cessation. New England Journal of Medicine 340: 685–691

Law M R, Hackshaw A K 1997 A meta-analysis of cigarette smoking, bone mineral density and risk of hip fracture: recognition of a major effect. British Medical Journal 315: 841–846

Marsh A, Mackay S 1994 Poor smokers. Policy Studies Institute, London

Office of National Statistics 1997 Prevalence of cigarette smoking, by sex and socio-economic group. In: Smoking-related behaviour and attitudes. National Statistics, London, table 3, p. 11

Office of National Statistics 1998a Prevalence of cigarette smoking by sex and age: 1974 to 1998. In: Living in Britain. National Statistics, London, table 8.1, p. 123

Office of National Statistics 1998b Proportion of pupils who were regular smokers by sex and age. In: Smoking, drinking and drug use among young teenagers. National Statistics, London, vol 1, table 3.4, p. 23

Prochaska J O, DiClemente C 1984 The transtheoretical approach: crossing traditional foundations of change. Dow Jones-Irwin, Homewood, IL

Prochaska J O, DiClemente C, Norcross J C 1992 In search of how people change. American Psychologist 47: 1102–1114

Silagy C, Mant D, Fowler G et al 2000 Nicotine replacement therapy for smoking cessation. Cochrane Database Systematic Review 2: CD000146

United States Department of Health and Human Services 1986 The health consequences of involuntary smoking: a report of the Surgeon General. GPO, Washington DC

West R, McNeill A, Raw M 2000 Smoking cessation guidelines for health professionals. Thorax 55(12): 987–999

4 Diagnostic investigations

Liz Dunn   Cecilia Connolly

When a patient presents with cough, breathlessness, wheeze, stridor or chest tightness it is important to recognize and differentiate the pathology or disordered physiology most likely to be the clinical reason for the symptoms. Clinical knowledge provided by patients and by those closely involved in their care assists in identifying the most appropriate investigation to confirm diagnosis and to determine appropriate treatments for different patients presenting with respiratory symptoms.

Respiratory diagnostic investigations include:

- lung function testing
- arterial blood gas analysis and pulse oximetry
- imaging
- bronchoscopy
- thoracoscopy
- needle biopsy.

LUNG FUNCTION TESTING

Lung function testing has several important uses and includes:

- diagnosis of respiratory disease
- screening for presence of respiratory impairment
- assessing objectively effectiveness of treatment
- monitoring progression and control of disease.

Lung function testing is performed on patients with obstructive or restrictive respiratory disease (Box 4.1). The normal airway is thin walled and stays open on both inspiration and expiration.

Obstructive respiratory diseases

- Chronic obstructive pulmonary disease (COPD)
  - chronic bronchitis
  - emphysema
- Asthma
- Bronchiectasis
- Cystic fibrosis

Restrictive respiratory disorders

- Chest wall disease
  - kyphoscoliosis
  - scoliosis
- Neuromuscular diseases
  - muscular dystrophies
  - motor neurone disease (MND)

Obstructive pulmonary disease reduces the area of the cross section of the airway, reducing the flow of air through to that particular area of the lung, and is usually a result of intrinsic lung disease. Restrictive disorders prevent the lungs expanding to their full extent and are usually as a result of chest wall or neuromuscular diseases.

Spirometry

Spirometry allows screening of lung function to assist in both the diagnosis and the ongoing mon-itoring of pulmonary disease. The indications for spirometry referral may include:

- smoking history > 10 years
- exposure to occupational hazards (e.g. asbestos, dust, chemicals)
- suspected obstructive or restrictive disorders
- wheeze or breathlessness
- assessment of the progress of a disorder
- preoperative assessment
- to establish appropriateness of long term oxygen therapy.

Spirometry is the measurement of breathing volumes and capacities and normal values are dependent on age, height, sex and ethnic origin. In people with normal lungs, resting breathing volume or functional residual capacity (FRC) is about 50% of the total lung capacity (TLC) (Fig. 4.1)

To measure residual volume (RV), TLC and FRC requires complex equipment and Kendrick & Smith (1992a) suggest that simple spirometry is often sufficient as it measures the volumes of air between TLC and RV, providing the following values:

- vital capacity (VC)
- forced vital capacity (FVC)
- forced expiratory volume in 1 second (FEV_1)
- forced expiratory flow (FEF).

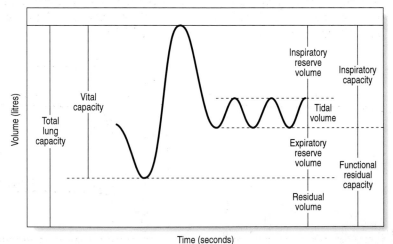

Figure 4.1 Normal lung volumes and capacities. Tidal volume = volume of air in or out per breath. Vital capacity = sum of the tidal volume, inspiratory and expiratory reserve volumes. Functional residual capacity = volume remaining in the lungs at the end of a normal tidal expiration (about 3 L in a healthy adult). Reproduced with permission from Cherniack 1992.

Vital capacity and forced vital capacity

Vital capacity (VC) is the maximum amount of air that can be exhaled from the lungs after maximal inspiration. VC is a measure of the size of the lungs. This can be measured in two ways:

• In slow vital capacity (SVC) or relaxed vital capacity (RVC), air is slowly exhaled from maximal inspiration to full expiration. When air is exhaled slowly there are no effects from narrow tubes or damaged lungs. Some authorities prefer to use this measurement using total inspiration, as the result will be the same. The definitions for VC and SVC are both technically correct and in practice either can be used, as they are interchangeable.

• In forced vital capacity (FVC) air is exhaled rapidly from maximal inspiration to maximal expiration. When the air is being forced out of the lungs under pressure, this pressure within the chest may cause premature closure of the smaller airways, trapping air in the alveoli. If this is the case, the FVC may be less than the SVC because less air is exhaled.

Forced expiratory volume in 1 second

A spirometer measures lung volumes through the forced expiration of air from the lungs. Flow can also be calculated by measuring the amount of air expired in one second (FEV_1), proportional to the total volume of expiration (FVC) (see Fig. 4.2). The ratio of FEV_1/FVC is expressed in per-

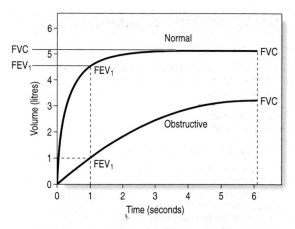

Figure 4.3   Obstructive volume/timed curve.

centage terms. This gives the proportion of the total volume that can be expired in 1 second. The majority of people with normal lungs can expel 80% or more of their FVC in 1 second. The FEV_1 ratio is calculated thus:

$$\frac{FEV_1}{FVC \text{ or } VC} \times 100 = FEV_1/VC \text{ ratio}$$

The physiological diagnosis of obstructive abnormalities is airflow limitation, as demonstrated when the FEV_1/VC ratio is below the lower level of normal (see Fig. 4.3). Early in obstructive disease the FVC may be normal, but is demonstrably reduced as the disease progresses and the RV increases because of trapped air. The progress of obstructive disease in the lungs is quantified by the fall of FEV_1.

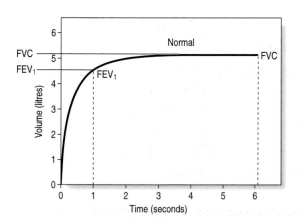

Figure 4.2   Normal volume/timed curve.

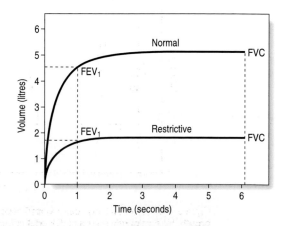

Figure 4.4   Restrictive volume/timed curve.

In restrictive lung disease (see Fig. 4.4), there is a reduction in TLC. This can be inferred in spirometry where there is a fall in FVC and FEV_1, but the FEV_1/VC ratio is normal or even high. When FVC and FEV_1 both fall, diagnosis of restrictive disease can only be made by a further assessment of TLC.

Reversibility testing

Reversibility testing relates to the extent to which airflow obstruction can be reversed with bronchodilators. A greater than 15% increase in FEV_1 or peak expiratory flow rate (PEFR) from baseline indicates a positive response (Fig. 4.5). When present, reversibility with bronchodilators is a means of diagnosing asthma as distinct from chronic obstructive pulmonary disease (COPD). However, although the majority of patients with COPD have fixed airflow obstruction, some reversibility can be produced by bronchodilators or corticosteroids (British Thoracic Society 1997).

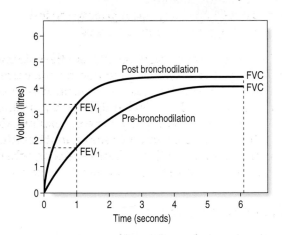

Figure 4.5   Volume/timed curve demonstrating reversibility testing.

Flow volume loops

The flow volume loop or curve (Fig. 4.6) produces a visual representation of the rate of airflow in and out of the lungs, plotted on the y-axis, against the volume of air from maximal inhalation to maximal exhalation, plotted along the x-axis. Nose clips should be worn by the patient undergoing this test (Simonds 1999).

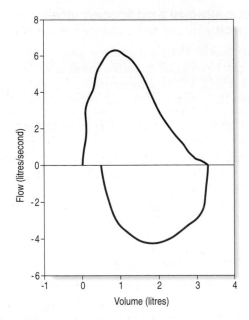

Figure 4.6   Normal flow volume loop.

Many extra readings can be plotted from these loops, for example FEF 50 (maximal expiratory flow (MEF) 50) and FEF 75. These represent flow when half and when three-quarters of the air has

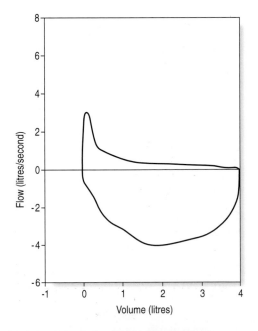

Figure 4.7   Obstructive flow volume loop.

been exhaled and these measurements were at one time thought to be markers of smaller airways disease.

Obstructive respiratory disease changes the appearance of the flow volume curve (Fig. 4.7). There is a rapid peak expiratory flow but the curve descends more quickly than normal and takes on a concave shape. This reflects the airway collapse which occurs as the conducting airways are compressed during forced expiratory effort.

In restrictive respiratory disease the changes in the flow volume loop are relatively unaffected (Fig. 4.8), but the overall size of the curve will appear smaller than normal.

Performing spirometry

The patient's age, height, weight, sex and ethnic origin must be recorded before the initial spirometry so that their predicted normal values can be calculated (Figs 4.9 and 4.10). As it is advisable to omit bronchodilators for 6 hours prior to performing spirometry, the time and dose of the patient's last bronchodilator should be recorded.

The American Thoracic Society (1987) issued guidelines to pre-test conditions. These include

the following recommendations that prior to the test the patient should avoid:

- vigorous exercise for at least 30 minutes
- alcohol for at least 4 hours
- wearing tight clothing or anything restricting the chest
- taking bronchodilators for 6 hours
- smoking for 24 hours.

Spirometry relies upon patient understanding, cooperation and commitment. It is of the utmost importance that the patient is informed of the reasons for the test and understands the significance of the technique required. It is essential that the patient is encouraged to participate actively whilst performing spirometry. To obtain accurate results from spirometry the nurse must ensure that the patient:

- sits upright in a chair
- maintains good posture
- has an empty bladder
- has not eaten a large meal prior to the test
- is in an appropriate environment.

To obtain a satisfactory result from the spirometer, the patient must be prepared for measurements to be taken. The patient must breathe in as far as possible, place his/her lips tightly around the mouthpiece and rapidly force the expired air into the spirometer until he/she cannot breathe out any more or until the flow ceases or, when expiration is really slow, for at least 10 seconds.

Types of equipment

Flow measuring spirometers

This group of spirometers measure airflow from the patient. The measurement of airflow (litres per second) is integrated to give a volume measurement and is performed by computer. The basic theory is that when a flow signal is measured against time, the area under the curve is theoretically the volume. The graph displays the area of the curve divided into sections. The more sections there are, the greater the accuracy. The volume from 0 seconds to 1 second is the FEV_1 and the total area under the curve is the FVC. The

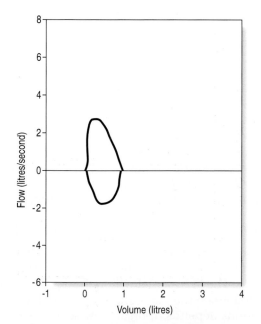

Figure 4.8   Restrictive flow volume loop.

	Height(cm)	150	155	160	165	170	175	180	185	190	195
18 - 25	FVC	3.65	3.94	4.23	4.51	4.80	5.09	5.38	5.67	5.95	6.24
	FEV1	3.24	3.45	3.67	3.88	4.10	4.31	4.53	4.74	4.96	5.17
	FEV1%	83%	83%	83%	83%	83%	83%	83%	83%	83%	83%
	PEF	497	516	534	552	571	589	608	626	644	663
26 - 29	FVC	3.55	3.83	4.12	4.41	4.70	4.99	5.27	5.56	5.85	6.14
	FEV1	3.12	3.33	3.55	3.76	3.98	4.19	4.41	4.62	4.84	5.05
	FEV1%	82%	82%	82%	82%	82%	82%	82%	82%	82%	82%
	PEF	487	505	524	542	560	579	597	616	634	653
30 - 33	FVC	3.44	3.73	4.02	4.31	4.59	4.88	5.17	5.46	5.75	6.03
	FEV1	3.00	3.22	3.43	3.65	3.86	4.08	4.29	4.51	4.72	4.94
	FEV1%	81%	81%	81%	81%	81%	81%	81%	81%	81%	81%
	PEF	476	495	513	532	550	569	587	605	624	642
34 - 37	FVC	3.34	3.63	3.91	4.20	4.49	4.78	5.07	5.35	5.64	5.93
	FEV1	2.89	3.10	3.32	3.53	3.75	3.96	4.18	4.39	4.61	4.82
	FEV1%	81%	81%	81%	81%	81%	81%	81%	81%	81%	81%
	PEF	466	485	503	521	540	558	577	595	614	632
38 - 41	FVC	3.23	3.52	3.81	4.10	4.39	4.67	4.96	5.25	5.54	5.83
	FEV1	2.77	2.99	3.20	3.42	3.63	3.85	4.06	4.28	4.49	4.71
	FEV1%	80%	80%	80%	80%	80%	80%	80%	80%	80%	80%
	PEF	456	474	493	511	530	548	566	585	603	622
42 - 45	FVC	3.13	3.42	3.71	3.99	4.28	4.57	4.86	5.15	5.43	5.72
	FEV1	2.66	2.87	3.09	3.30	3.52	3.73	3.95	4.16	4.38	4.59
	FEV1%	79%	79%	79%	79%	79%	79%	79%	79%	79%	79%
	PEF	446	464	482	501	519	538	556	574	593	611
46 - 49	FVC	3.03	3.31	3.60	3.89	4.18	4.47	4.75	5.04	5.33	5.62
	FEV1	2.54	2.75	2.97	3.18	3.40	3.61	3.83	4.04	4.26	4.47
	FEV1%	78%	78%	78%	78%	78%	78%	78%	78%	78%	78%
	PEF	435	454	472	490	509	527	546	564	583	601
50 - 53	FVC	2.92	3.21	3.50	3.79	4.07	4.36	4.65	4.94	5.23	5.51
	FEV1	2.42	2.64	2.85	3.07	3.28	3.50	3.71	3.93	4.14	4.36
	FEV1%	78%	78%	78%	78%	78%	78%	78%	78%	78%	78%
	PEF	425	443	462	480	499	517	535	554	572	591
54 - 57	FVC	2.82	3.11	3.39	3.68	3.97	4.26	4.55	4.83	5.12	5.41
	FEV1	2.31	2.52	2.74	2.95	3.17	3.38	3.60	3.81	4.03	4.24
	FEV1%	77%	77%	77%	77%	77%	77%	77%	77%	77%	77%
	PEF	415	433	451	470	488	507	525	543	562	580
58 - 61	FVC	2.71	3.00	3.29	3.58	3.87	4.15	4.44	4.73	5.02	5.31
	FEV1	2.19	2.41	2.62	2.84	3.05	3.27	3.48	3.70	3.91	4.13
	FEV1%	76%	76%	76%	76%	76%	76%	76%	76%	76%	76%
	PEF	404	423	441	459	478	496	515	533	552	570
62 - 65	FVC	2.61	2.90	3.19	3.47	3.76	4.05	4.34	4.63	4.91	5.20
	FEV1	2.08	2.29	2.51	2.72	2.94	3.15	3.37	3.58	3.80	4.01
	FEV1%	76%	76%	76%	76%	76%	76%	76%	76%	76%	76%
	PEF	394	412	431	449	468	486	504	523	541	560
66 - 69	FVC	2.51	2.79	3.08	3.37	3.66	3.95	4.23	4.52	4.81	5.10
	FEV1	1.96	2.17	2.39	2.60	2.82	3.03	3.25	3.46	3.68	3.89
	FEV1%	75%	75%	75%	75%	75%	75%	75%	75%	75%	75%
	PEF	384	402	420	439	457	476	494	513	531	549

(Age — left vertical label)

Figure 4.9 Normal predicted spirometry for males. Reproduced with permission of Vitalograph Ltd.

loop includes information on respiratory flow and different types of airflow limitation can be identified from the expiratory portion of the graph.

Flech pneumotachograph

This device monitors airflow and is measured using the following relationships:

$$\text{Flow} = \frac{\text{Pressure difference}}{\text{Resistance}}$$

These measurements are usually taken in the laboratory, where the machinery can measure airflow at various levels of sophistication.

Turbines

These are airflow sensing devices. When the patient exhales into the turbine a low inertia vane rotates. The light signal within the device is interrupted when the vane rotates. The frequency of rotations depends upon airflow so a flow signal is generated.

Age	Height(cm)	150	155	160	165	170	175	180	185	190	195
18 - 25	FVC	3.11	3.33	3.55	3.77	3.99	4.21	4.43	4.66	4.88	5.10
	FEV1	2.70	2.90	3.10	3.29	3.49	3.69	3.89	4.08	4.28	4.48
	FEV1%	84%	84%	84%	84%	84%	84%	84%	84%	84%	84%
	PEF	383	400	416	433	449	466	482	499	515	532
26 - 29	FVC	3.00	3.22	3.44	3.67	3.89	4.11	4.33	4.55	4.77	4.99
	FEV1	2.60	2.80	3.00	3.19	3.39	3.59	3.79	3.98	4.18	4.38
	FEV1%	84%	84%	84%	84%	84%	84%	84%	84%	84%	84%
	PEF	376	393	409	426	442	459	475	492	508	525
30 - 33	FVC	2.90	3.12	3.34	3.56	3.78	4.00	4.23	4.45	4.67	4.89
	FEV1	2.50	2.70	2.90	3.09	3.29	3.49	3.69	3.88	4.08	4.28
	FEV1%	83%	83%	83%	83%	83%	83%	83%	83%	83%	83%
	PEF	369	386	402	419	435	452	468	485	501	518
34 - 37	FVC	2.79	3.01	3.24	3.46	3.68	3.90	4.12	4.34	4.57	4.79
	FEV1	2.40	2.60	2.80	2.99	3.19	3.39	3.59	3.78	3.98	4.18
	FEV1%	82%	82%	82%	82%	82%	82%	82%	82%	82%	82%
	PEF	362	378	395	411	428	444	461	477	494	510
38 - 41	FVC	2.69	2.91	3.13	3.35	3.58	3.80	4.02	4.24	4.46	4.68
	FEV1	2.30	2.50	2.70	2.89	3.09	3.29	3.49	3.68	3.88	4.08
	FEV1%	81%	81%	81%	81%	81%	81%	81%	81%	81%	81%
	PEF	355	371	388	404	421	437	454	470	487	503
42 - 45	FVC	2.59	2.81	3.03	3.25	3.47	3.69	3.91	4.14	4.36	4.58
	FEV1	2.20	2.40	2.60	2.79	2.99	3.19	3.39	3.58	3.78	3.98
	FEV1%	81%	81%	81%	81%	81%	81%	81%	81%	81%	81%
	PEF	347	364	380	397	413	430	446	463	479	496
46 - 49	FVC	2.48	2.70	2.92	3.15	3.37	3.59	3.81	4.03	4.25	4.47
	FEV1	2.10	2.30	2.50	2.69	2.89	3.09	3.29	3.48	3.68	3.88
	FEV1%	80%	80%	80%	80%	80%	80%	80%	80%	80%	80%
	PEF	340	357	373	390	406	423	439	456	472	489
50 - 53	FVC	2.38	2.60	2.82	3.04	3.26	3.48	3.71	3.93	4.15	4.37
	FEV1	2.00	2.20	2.40	2.59	2.79	2.99	3.19	3.38	3.58	3.78
	FEV1%	79%	79%	79%	79%	79%	79%	79%	79%	79%	79%
	PEF	333	350	366	383	399	416	432	449	465	482
54 - 57	FVC	2.27	2.49	2.72	2.94	3.16	3.38	3.60	3.82	4.05	4.27
	FEV1	1.90	2.10	2.30	2.49	2.69	2.89	3.09	3.28	3.48	3.68
	FEV1%	78%	78%	78%	78%	78%	78%	78%	78%	78%	78%
	PEF	326	342	359	375	392	408	425	441	458	474
58 - 61	FVC	2.17	2.39	2.61	2.83	3.06	3.28	3.50	3.72	3.94	4.16
	FEV1	1.80	2.00	2.20	2.39	2.59	2.79	2.99	3.18	3.38	3.58
	FEV1%	78%	78%	78%	78%	78%	78%	78%	78%	78%	78%
	PEF	319	335	352	368	385	401	418	434	451	467
62 - 65	FVC	2.07	2.29	2.51	2.73	2.95	3.17	3.39	3.62	3.84	4.06
	FEV1	1.70	1.90	2.10	2.29	2.49	2.69	2.89	3.08	3.28	3.48
	FEV1%	77%	77%	77%	77%	77%	77%	77%	77%	77%	77%
	PEF	311	328	344	361	377	394	410	427	443	460
66 - 69	FVC	1.96	2.18	2.40	2.63	2.85	3.07	3.29	3.51	3.73	3.95
	FEV1	1.60	1.80	2.00	2.19	2.39	2.59	2.79	2.98	3.18	3.38
	FEV1%	76%	76%	76%	76%	76%	76%	76%	76%	76%	76%
	PEF	304	321	337	354	370	387	403	420	436	453

Figure 4.10   Normal predicted spirometry for females. Reproduced with permission of Vitalograph Ltd.

Lung volumes

Simple spirometry can only measure subdivisions of lung volume that lie within the VC range. To measure other lung volumes (RV, TLC and FRC) more complex equipment and procedures are required, such as:

- helium dilution
- nitrogen washouts
- body plethysmography.

Helium dilution

This measurement is taken with the patient attached to a closed circuit spirometer containing a known volume and concentration of helium, usually 10%. The patient is connected to the machine via a mouthpiece with a nose clip in position.

The measurement is taken during normal respiration. Within a few minutes the gas in the patient's lungs equilibrates with the helium concentrated gas in the spirometer. The helium concentration is monitored continuously and falls to a lower, steady state level through the patient's respiration. Carbon dioxide is removed from the system by soda lime absorption and a low flow of oxygen is added to allow for the ongoing consumption, thereby maintaining the volume chamber or spirometer volume constant. FRC is calculated by measuring the ratio of the initial concentration to the final concentration of helium present in the system.

This can be a very frightening experience for a breathless patient who may wish to be accompanied for the procedure. The patient may feel anxious and perhaps claustrophobic due to the mouthpiece and the nose clip. It is essential that the nurse gives the patient exact details of the procedure prior to the test. The patient must be informed that:

- the test will be performed whilst he is sitting upright in a chair
- a tight fitting mouthpiece will be used
- a nose clip will be applied
- normal breathing is required.

Nitrogen washout

This test is based upon the principle of conservation of an inert gas, in this case nitrogen. The patient is attached to a mouthpiece, which is connected to an inspiratory source of 100% oxygen at the end of normal expiration. The patient exhales via one-way valves into a collection bag previously filled with oxygen so that there is no nitrogen present. The patient breathes out the nitrogen present in the lungs, and as it is washed out the content of nitrogen is continuously measured. When the nitrogen concentration falls to less than 2%, the test is complete and the volume of nitrogen in the bag is measured. The FRC can be calculated on the basis that this nitrogen volume represents 80% of the lung gas contained at the beginning of the test.

New machines fitted with microprocessors use a calculation based upon instantaneous, breath-by-breath measurement of exhaled volume times nitrogen concentration. The test can take up to 4 minutes for patients with normal

---

Box 4.2	Reasons for peak flow monitoring

- Diagnosis
- Reversibility testing
- Determine treatment plan
- Monitor response to treament
- Integral part of asthma self-management plan

---

lungs but may take up to 15 minutes for patients with severe obstructive disease.

The nurse must explain the details of all tests requested before the patient goes to the laboratory. The technician in the laboratory is trained to alleviate the patient's anxieties and will know when the patient needs a break between tests.

Peak expiratory flow rate

Peak expiratory flow rate (PEFR) detects airflow obstruction in the larger airways, is one of the simplest lung function measurements and is most useful for diagnosing and monitoring asthma. Kendrick & Smith (1992b) suggest that a single one-off measurement is of limited use and recommend that serial measurements are required to gain information about disease severity, provoking factors and response to treatment.

To interpret the PEFR the result needs to be compared with the reference values (Fig. 4.11) as these vary according to age, height and sex.

 Case study 4.1

Gregory is a 35-year-old financial advisor who was diagnosed asthmatic in childhood. He attends the asthma clinic run by a practice nurse. His treatment consists of 800 mcg beclomethasone twice per day inhaled using a turbohaler and he takes salbutamol as required, usually 3–4 times per week. He monitors his peak flow as part of his self-management plan. He develops a cold and begins to notice a change in his peak flows (Fig. 4.12). He doubles his inhaled steroid dose and increases his salbutamol; however there is a further dip in his peak flow so he initiates a 5-day course of oral prednisolone once a day. He begins to notice an improvement in his peak flows over the next few days (Fig. 4.13). Gregory makes a note of treatment initiated so that he can discuss this with the practice nurse at his next appointment.

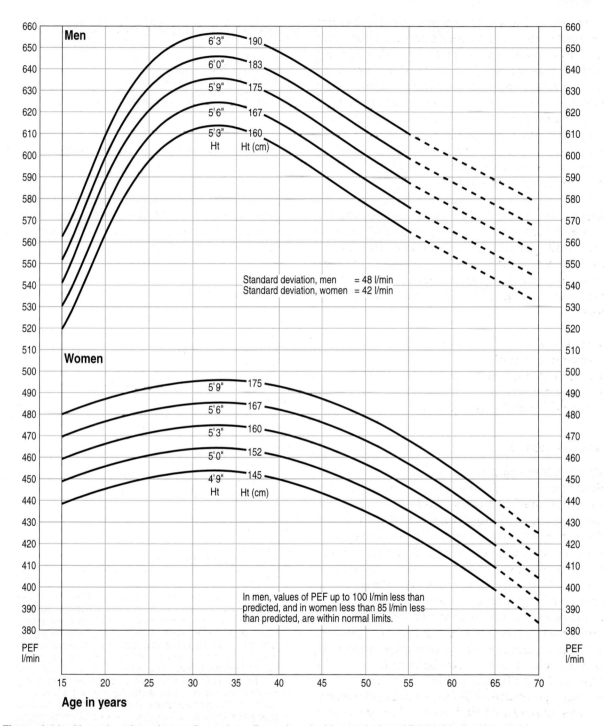

Figure 4.11 Normal peak expiratory flow values. Reproduced with permission of British Medical Journal.

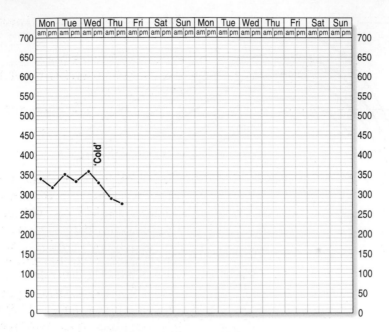

Figure 4.12 Peak flow chart begins to change.

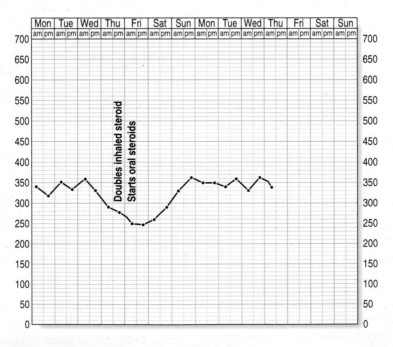

Figure 4.13 Peak flow chart begins to improve.

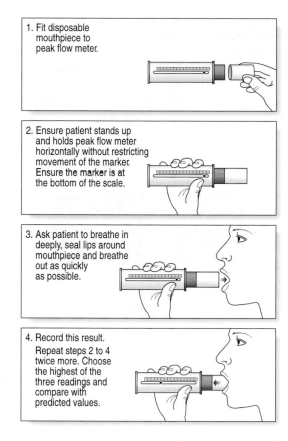

1. Fit disposable mouthpiece to peak flow meter.

2. Ensure patient stands up and holds peak flow meter horizontally without restricting movement of the marker. Ensure the marker is at the bottom of the scale.

3. Ask patient to breathe in deeply, seal lips around mouthpiece and breathe out as quickly as possible.

4. Record this result. Repeat steps 2 to 4 twice more. Choose the highest of the three readings and compare with predicted values.

Figure 4.14 Measuring peak expiratory flow using a peak flow meter.

Peak flow meters

The Wright peak flow meter and mini Wright peak flow meter measure peak flow of air on forced expiration. The mobile vane within the meter is balanced against a constant tension spring.

The patient exhales forcibly into the mouthpiece of the handheld device (Fig. 4.14). The vane rotates, a ratchet holds the vane at the maximal point reached and a reading is taken. Air is allowed to escape through an aperture along the length of the meter. The greater the volume of air exhaled into the meter, the further the vane will rotate, exposing more of the aperture. This ensures that resistance to the blow is constant and a peak flow can be measured accurately.

These readings may be taken before and after the administration of bronchodilators to measure the efficacy of treatment. The nurse must ensure that the patient:

- sits upright in a chair
- seals his lips tightly around the mouthpiece
- exhales forcibly
- repeats the test 3 times, with the highest result recorded.

PULSE OXIMETRY

Pulse oximetry is an extremely useful and simple way to monitor the peripheral oxygen saturation (SpO_2) of arterial blood and contributes greatly to the patient's initial respiratory assessment and subsequent observations. Continuous evaluations of responses to clinical interventions are possible, particularly since arterial oxygen saturation changes are often rapid.

Pulse oximeters (Fig. 4.15) are compact and light in weight and provide a continuous digital display of:

- oxygen saturation
- heart rate
- plethysmographic waveform.

The quality of this waveform and subsequent accuracy of the readings is dependent upon the strength of the pulse and the peripheral perfusion at the point at which the oxyhaemoglobin saturation is being measured. The strength of the pulse is proportional to the amplitude of the waveform and it is largely from this waveform

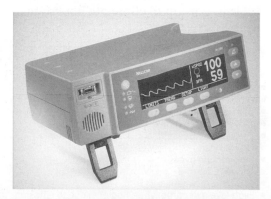

Figure 4.15 Pulse oximeter. Reproduced with permission of Mallinckrodt, Nellcor Oximetry, Pleasanton, California.

that the percentage measurement of oxyhaemo-globin saturation is generated.

The oximeter probe is usually attached to a person's finger or earlobe. The site should be chosen for the quality of the peripheral circulation reflected in the plethysmographic waveform and for the comfort of the patient. It is worth noting that although oximetry is a non-invasive technique, clip-on probes used for continuous monitoring can cause pressure and discomfort. The position of these should be changed regularly and in some cases this begs the question as to whether continuous monitoring is essential. Hourly readings may suffice and reduce the disturbance to the patient, particularly if the sound of the alarm has added to this. Visitors are then more likely to focus their attention on the patient than be distracted by or concerned with the monitor's visual displays! However, the patient's condition and the value of continuous assessment in detecting hypoxaemia should not be underestimated here.

The probe consists of a small light-emitting diode on one side and a light detector on the other. The technique works because of the light-absorbing characteristics of haemoglobin. If hypoxaemia is experienced by patients the blueness of their blood will be measured by the oximeter. Based on the amount of light absorbed by the vascular bed, the oximeter calculates the amount of blueness and displays it in terms of percentage oxyhaemoglobin saturation.

The sensitivity of the probe is dependent on the translucence of the skin at the point of contact and it is important to eliminate impediments to

measurements such as nail varnish or bright fluorescent light. Poor peripheral perfusion and anaemia will affect the accuracy of measurements as will any movement of the patient, such as shivering, fitting or movements associated with confusion. If there are any suspicions of inaccuracy the probe itself should be checked for damage and the power supply established to be intact.

Pulse oximetry should be used with caution for patients with high levels of carboxyhaemoglobin owing to smoking, since oxygen saturations may be recorded as falsely high. Exposure to carbon monoxide (CO), for instance in a person suffering from smoke inhalation, results in the formation of a high proportion of carboxyhaemoglobin molecules in a short space of time. Reliance on pulse oximetry in this instance could prove fatal for the patient. Similarly, this type of monitoring is contraindicated for patients suffering from hypothermia and vasoconstriction leading to poor peripheral perfusion or damaged skin.

Although peripheral oxygen saturation correlates well with arterial blood gas analysis of oxyhaemoglobin saturation (SaO_2), laboratories are

Case study 4.2

Stephanie is 24 years of age and suffers from cystic fibrosis. She is a receptionist and lives with her boyfriend.

She was admitted to the adult cystic fibrosis unit with an acute infective exacerbation. Her SpO_2 on admission was 91% so she was administered 28% oxygen, which increased her SpO_2 to 96%. She was also initiated on intravenous antibiotics and bronchodilators in addition to her regular treatments. She was reviewed by the dietitian and had chest physiotherapy. The next morning she complained of a severe headache, so after being given paracetamol, she had arterial blood gases (earlobe method) taken on 28% oxygen. The results were PaO_2 9.4 kPa, $PaCO_2$ 6.7 kPa, pH 7.37, which indicated that although her oxygen was corrected there had been an increase in her $PaCO_2$. Her oxygen was decreased to 24% and earlobe gases were taken after 1 hour. These were: PaO_2 8.6 kPa, $PaCO_2$ 5.8 kPa, pH 7.39. Her SpO_2, taken on the pulse oximeter, was 95%.

She continued to be monitored using pulse oximetry as the carbon dioxide level was known. She was discharged after a week to finish her 2 week course of intravenous antibiotics at home.

Box 4.3 Possible reasons for false readings

- Peripheral vasoconstriction
- Anaemia
- High bilirubin blood levels
- Skin pigment
- Movement (e.g. shivering or fitting)
- Dysrhythmias resulting in inadequate perfusion
- Nail varnish
- Intravenous dyes
- Damaged probe
- Severe hypoxaemia
- High levels of carboxyhaemoglobin due to smoking
- Exposure to carbon monoxide

Box 4.4 Limitations of pulse oximetry

- Unable to detect carbon dioxide levels
- Inaccurate readings due to patient's condition

---

advised to validate their oximetry readings with arterial oxygen saturation and to establish a predicted linear regression. Some pulse oximeters have been shown to over- or underestimate SaO_2 by + or − 4%, especially when saturations are below 82% (Carter 1998, Severinghaus et al 1989).

The value of continuous accurate monitoring of SpO_2 is that responses to interventions such as tracheal suctioning, turning, mobilizing and oxygen therapy can be observed and acted upon swiftly. The normal SpO_2 for an adult breathing room air is 95–100% and concerns would generally be raised if it fell below 90%. The brain is the most sensitive organ to oxygen depletion and signs of hypoxaemia such as confusion and visual and cognitive impairment usually occur when SaO_2 is between 80 and 85% and cyanosis occurs at around 75%.

As with any patient monitoring device, the pulse oximetry should contribute to the overall clinical picture and complement other observations and clinical signs. Lung performance, the effectiveness of treatment and the level of respiratory distress cannot be detected without other diagnostic tests. Additionally, the adequacy of carbon dioxide elimination will need to be assessed by full arterial blood gas analysis or the use of a carbon dioxide monitor. It is possible to have a normal SaO_2 but to have a raised $PaCO_2$ (Davidson & Hoise 1993) which, if not treated, will result in a respiratory acidosis (low pH).

Table 4.1 Normal arterial blood gas values

PaO_2	12–14 kPa
$PaCO_2$	4.6–6.0 kPa
pH	7.35–7.45
HCO_3	22–26 mmol/L
SaO_2	95% +
Base excess	−2 to +2

ARTERIAL BLOOD GAS ANALYSIS

Arterial blood gas analysis can reveal vital information regarding a patient's respiratory state (Table 4.1). Acid–base imbalance can be an indicator for life saving interventions and treatments such as oxygen therapy, hydration, non-invasive ventilation (NIV), intermittent positive pressure ventilation (IPPV) and renal dialysis.

Effective communication and explanation of blood gas analysis and resulting implications are an essential component of care for the patient in respiratory distress. Equally, family and friends will require an understanding of the patient's condition in order to support the patient and each other. In the critical care setting the emphasis is necessarily on the patient's physiological state, particularly in order to reach as stable a condition as possible. Psychological and spiritual care may take an inevitable second place but are none the less essential considerations in the holistic care of both the individual patient and relatives and carers (encompassing all healthcare workers, friends and family involved).

Withdrawal of arterial blood can be obtained using different sampling methods:

- arterial line
- arterial 'stab'
- earlobe.

An arterial line is common in the intensive care unit (ICU) or high dependency unit (HDU) environment, particularly when regular blood gas analysis is required. Arterial 'stabs' for less frequent testing are usually taken from the radial or brachial arteries. Femoral stabs and lines into the femoral artery are contraindicated due to a higher infection risk, though they may be necessary due to difficulties in accessing an alternative artery. Capillary blood can be taken from the earlobe, which has been demonstrated to be within 2% accuracy of an arterial 'stab', and has proven less painful than radial sampling and less invasive (Pitkin et al 1994). The risk of bleeding, bruising and ongoing discomfort is reduced and this method is arguably an easier and safer procedure to learn and perform effectively.

The value of knowing a patient's baseline blood gas analysis cannot be underestimated. Disturbances such as low oxygen or increased carbon dioxide are more meaningful when compared to the individual's 'norm'. Also, the additional information gained from full blood gas analysis compared to pulse oximetry is essential in many cases.

Case study 4.3

Jack is a 72-year-old man with known chronic obstructive pulmonary disease. His FEV_1 is 1.1 L, FVC is 1.6 L and his oxygen saturation was 92% when breathing room air. He had recently suffered a virus which had caused him to be anorexic. Over the next couple of weeks his sputum became yellow/green in colour and was more tenacious and difficult to expectorate. He had smoked for over 30 years but had reduced the number he smoked a day from 25 to 5 during his recent illness. He could normally walk 100 yards before becoming breathless but had been housebound for a month and was breathless at rest. He had swollen ankles and the veins in his neck were more prominent.

One evening he became increasingly breathless, cyanosed and delirious, causing his wife to call an ambulance. He was taken on a stretcher to his local hospital and given 35% oxygen through a Venturi oxygen mask during transit. On arrival at the accident and emergency department Jack's SpO_2 was 95% on 35% oxygen, but he was slipping in and out of consciousness. Blood gas analysis taken on 35% oxygen revealed a PaO_2 of 8.9 kPa and a $PaCO_2$ of 8.3 kPa, identifying that although his SpO_2 performed using an oximeter was within the normal range, the oxygen therapy administered was causing hypercapnia. His oxygen was reduced to 28% via a Venturi oxygen mask and repeat arterial blood gases after 30 minutes were PaO_2 7.8 kPa and $PaCO_2$ 7.1 kPa. He became more alert and less confused as his $PaCO_2$ reduced.

He was treated with 28% oxygen, diuretics, intravenous antibiotics and nebulized salbutamol. A few hours later he was no longer drowsy or confused and his hospital notes were available to make comparisons with his previous baseline blood gases, spirometry and chest X-rays. Oxygen therapy was used with caution in view of his hypercapnia but as his condition improved it was possible to monitor his progress with oximetry.

A few days later, Jack had recovered sufficiently to walk around the ward without oxygen, the oedema of his ankles had significantly reduced and he was able to take his antibiotics orally. His blood gas and spirometry measurements were more comparable with his baseline.

DIAGNOSTIC RADIOLOGY
Chest X-ray

Chest X-ray is a valuable aid to diagnosis of respiratory disease. The information provided is not restricted to the heart and lungs as liver and lymph node abnormalities may also be detected. The radiation dose required for a chest X-ray is small, but must be considered carefully, particularly for pregnant women and young children.

A normal chest X-ray (Fig. 4.16) will show the:

- shape and size of the heart
- lung fields and pleura
- rib cage
- diaphragm
- bony structures
- soft tissue of the breasts.

The heart size is calculated using the cardiothoracic ratio. The widest diameter of the heart is divided by the widest horizontal diameter of the lungs. This is normally less than 50%. Chest X-ray is the primary examination performed when patients present with persistent cough, chest pain, unexplained breathlessness, the presence of blood in sputum, weight loss and pyrexia of unknown origin.

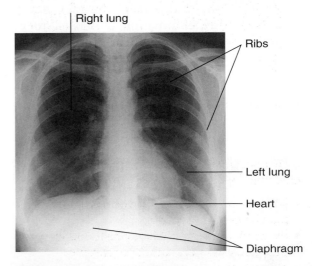

Figure 4.16   Normal chest X-ray.

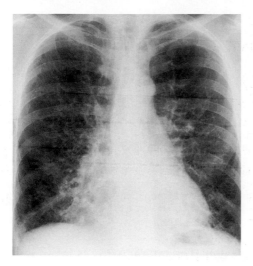

Figure 4.17 Chest X-ray showing bronchiectasis.

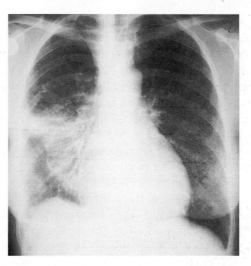

Figure 4.18 Chest X-ray showing a shadow indicative of lung cancer.

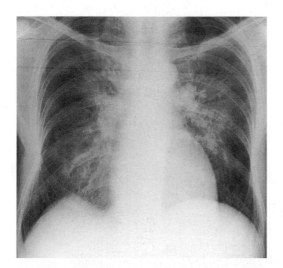

Figure 4.19 Chest X-ray showing a pneumonia.

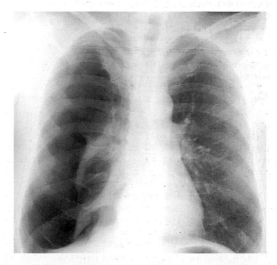

Figure 4.20 Chest X-ray showing a pneumothorax.

Abnormalities found using chest X-rays include the following:

- patients with hypertension or heart failure may have an enlarged heart
- over inflated lung field may be found in people with severe asthma or chronic obstructive pulmonary disease
- pneumothorax
- consolidation or shadowing indicating infection or the presence of a tumour
- specific shadowing that may indicate a primary or secondary tumour
- cavities that may indicate active tuberculosis (TB)

- calcification may indicate that the patient has previously suffered TB which is not presently active
- pleural effusion (fluid in the pleural cavity).

(see Figs 4.17, 4.18, 4.19, 4.20.)

Performing chest X-ray

Chest X-ray is best performed with the patient standing. The anterior chest is positioned against the film cassette and the patient holds on to each side of the machine. This rotates the scapulae away from the posterior chest. The patient is asked to take a deep breath in and hold that breath at maximum lung capacity.

When a patient is too ill to stand for a posteroanterior view, films will have to be taken in an anteroposterior view (from front to back). This reduces the efficacy of the X-ray technique, because a consequence of this view is that the heart is magnified, as it lies farther away from the film. Further restrictions are experienced when a portable X-ray machine is used. This is due to the shorter X-ray tube-to-film distance, which causes further magnification of the heart, and this must be taken into consideration when assessing the heart size on an anteroposterior chest radiograph.

It is impossible to reproduce a perfect exposure of the whole of the chest because of the wide range of densities (bone, soft tissues of the mediastinum, through to aerated lung tissue) within the thorax. The radiographer will alter the kilovoltage to highlight the specific area of the chest to be examined. For example, a high kilovoltage technique (120–150 kVp) allows greater penetration of the mediastinum, which improves visualization of the trachea and main bronchi, but restricts visualization of calcified structures, so that rib fractures or calcified pulmonary nodules are less conspicuous.

A lateral chest X-ray provides the third dimension and may help to determine the site of a lesion identified on the posteroanterior projection. It is interesting that often an opacity clearly visible on a posteroanterior film is not visible on a lateral X-ray. The lateral X-ray may allow accurate localization of lesions and may also reveal hidden abnormalities lying behind the heart or

Case study 4.4

Rina is referred to the chest clinic as she has had a cough for 4 weeks, weight loss and night sweats. She has a chest X-Ray (Fig. 4.21) which shows cavities that indicate active tuberculosis.

A sputum specimen is collected and she is commenced on 6 months of tuberculosis chemotherapy to treat her tuberculosis. A notification is sent to the Public Health Department. The tuberculosis nurse specialist contact traces and monitors Rina's treatment over the next 6 months. She makes a full recovery.

diaphragm. The lateral X-ray is taken with the patient standing at right angles to the film cassette. It is usually not relevant which side projects nearer to the cassette.

Within recent years the development of computer assisted tomography has been used to provide information about areas not easily seen on posteroanterior and lateral X-rays. There are still times when X-rays can provide further anatomical information by using the lateral decubitus view to demonstrate small pleural effusions. The patient lies on his side with the affected side downwards. The beam is passed horizontally onto the film behind the patient.

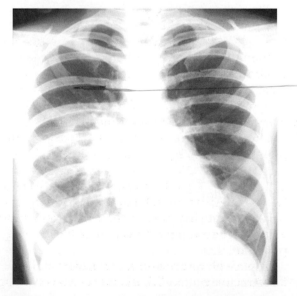

Figure 4.21   Chest X-ray showing a tuberculosis cavity.

Ultrasonography

This technique is limited in the chest because high frequency sound waves do not traverse air and are completely reflected at interfaces between soft tissue and air. This makes the technique of little use in normally aerated lungs. However, fluid can easily be detected through this method. It is therefore very useful in detecting localization of small or loculated effusions. Whereas a normal chest X-ray may be unable to distinguish between pleural thickening and pleural fluid, ultrasonography can differentiate these two conditions.

Computerized tomography

The image display of computerized tomography (CT) is fundamentally different to the image projected by a chest X-ray. CT is much more sensitive to differences in attenuation of X-rays by various tissues.

A CT machine consists of an X-ray source and a range of detectors which surround the patient. The X-ray source rotates around the patient and the detectors measure the consequential attenuated beam. The signals from the detectors are used to construct an image by a mathematical technique. The reconstructed images are transverse cross sections of the patient and are viewed so that the left side of the image is to the right side of the viewer. Each section of the image is a matrix of voxels (three dimensional elements) containing a measurement of X-ray attenuation, arbitrarily called Houndsfield units (HU): water measures 0 HU, air measures 1000 HU (so that lung parenchyma is approximately −600 HU), fat measures −80 HU, soft tissue measures 40–80 HU and bone measures 800 HU. If a voxel is completely occupied by a tissue of uniform density then the attenuation will be truly representative of that tissue. Yet if the section contains tissues of two different densities, for example half lung and half dome of diaphragm, then the attenuation value will be a weighted average of the two components.

Because of the cross-sectional nature of the CT, it can accurately localize lesions seen on only one

view on chest X-ray. CT produces exquisite images of various components of mediastinal anatomy (i.e. lymph nodes and vessels) and of density differentials, such as calcifications within a pulmonary nodule. The disadvantages of CT are high cost and the increased exposure to radiation. For these reasons CT of the thorax should only be used to solve questions unanswered by less sophisticated investigations.

Magnetic resonance imaging (MRI)

The most common use of MRI in respiratory disease is to take an image of suspected complications of existing disease. These may include cerebral metastases, spinal metastases and cord compression, retroperitoneal fibrosis and occasionally hypertrophic pulmonary osteoarthropathy.

The patient is placed in a very strong magnetic field (typically 0.2–1.5 T) and irradiated with radiofrequency waves, which excite atoms that then relax into a lower energy state once the source of radiation is turned off (Hall-Craggs & Goddard 1999). The atoms in lower energy state actually release small amounts of energy, which can be detected by a receiver to construct an image.

The advantages of MRI are:

- there are no known hazards to the patient compared to the attendant risk of ionizing radiation in CT scanning
- the ability to obtain sections in any plane
- the improvement of contrast resolution allows differentiation of soft tissues
- the use of special sequences which give functional information (e.g. velocity of blood flow).

The disadvantages of MRI are:

- long scan time
- reduced spatial resolution compared to CT
- inability to image calcium
- reduced acceptance to patients due to the magnetic cylinder (bore of the magnetic field) causing possible claustrophobia.

MRI scans can be very frightening with some patients finding the procedure intolerably noisy and claustrophobic. It is imperative that the nurse tells patients that they will be lying down and that their whole body will be inside a tubular machine which is magnetic and is taking the images. It should be explained that there is less danger associated with this procedure than CT scanning and images will only be taken of the particular area requested. About 15 minutes should be allocated for this explanation and patients given time to think about their fears and anxieties and invited to ask any questions they may have about the procedure. The nurse must ask if the patient experiences any particular problems when lying down, such as breathlessness or pain. If the patient does experience more pain when lying, then appropriate analgesics can be given prior to the procedure.

INVASIVE PROCEDURES

Bronchoscopy

Bronchoscopy is among the most commonly used diagnostic and therapeutic procedures in respiratory medicine. Diagnostic bronchoscopy and tissue biopsy are an integral part of investigations used to assess respiratory disease.

There are three types of bronchoscopy techniques:

- flexible fibre optic bronchoscopy
- rigid bronchoscopy
- laser bronchoscopy.

The development of fibre optic bronchoscopy and associated techniques of transbronchial lung biopsy and bronchoalveolar lavage have revolutionized the practice of respiratory medicine. Diagnosis at bronchoscopy is not confined to visible lesions as the simultaneous use of flexible instruments and fluoroscopy allow biopsy of distal bronchi or lung parenchyma (Muers 1996). In contrast, use of the rigid bronchoscope has become less common, although it may be essential in some circumstances, such as in the presence of a rigid mass which prevents insertion of the flexible bronchoscope. Neither of these investigations should be performed without simpler diagnostic tests indicating the need for further investigation.

Box 4.5 Common indications for bronchoscopy

- Mass, nodule, suspicious lesion or cancer
- Haemoptysis or bleeding
- Pneumonia or other infection
- Diffuse or interstitial disease in a non-immunocompromised patient
- Therapeutic bronchoscopy for lobar or segmental atelectasis
- Cough or wheeze
- Immunocompromised patient
- HIV or AIDS with respiratory symptoms
- Tracheal pathology or stridor
- Patient in intensive care or on a ventilator

The following situations may be considered as absolute contraindications, but the medical team will take the ultimate decision as to whether to perform bronchoscopic procedures. When a patient presents with any of the following (for either flexible or rigid bronchoscopy), comprehensive assessment is required:

- severe hypoxaemia which may worsen during the procedure
- an unstable cardiac status
- life threatening arrhythmias.

The following are added contraindications when using a rigid bronchoscope:

- an unstable neck
- a severely ankylosed cervical spine
- severely restricted motion of the temporomandibular joints.

Complications of bronchoscopy

Complications of rigid and flexible fibre optic bronchoscopy are similar. The flexible fibre optic bronchoscopy is usually carried out under local anaesthetic. Sedatives such as midazolam may cause respiratory depression, hypoventilation and hypotension and sometimes syncope. Local anaesthetics applied to the throat may lead to laryngospasm, bronchospasm, seizures and, rarely, cardiorespiratory arrest. The added complications when using a rigid bronchoscope include soft tissue damage, which can lead to airway perforation, or sub-glottal oedema and complications of general anaesthesia.

Bronchoscopy and related procedures, including brushing and lavage, may also be associated with:

- bronchospasm
- hypoxaemia
- cardiac arrhythmias
- fever
- pneumonia
- pneumothorax
- haemorrhage.

Almost one-third of patients develop fever and influenzae-like symptoms after a bronchoscopy and bronchoalveolar lavage. It has been shown that the fever is induced by proinflammatory cytokines derived from alveolar macrophages activated by instillation of fluid into the airways (Prakash 1999).

It is not generally necessary to admit patients to hospital after a bronchoscopic lung biopsy. The post-bronchoscopy patient should be carefully monitored for 6–8 hours after the procedure. Patients with significant post-bronchoscopic bleeding, pneumothorax and respiratory distress will be admitted for further monitoring and possible treatment.

Bronchoscopy and related procedures are among the safest diagnostic pulmonary procedures. Nurses must be mindful of the potential for complications for all patients following bronchoscopic investigations. There have been reported deaths from pneumothorax that developed many hours after bronchoscopic lung biopsy. On discharge, patients must be advised to contact their GP or the hospital immediately if they develop pain or breathlessness after they get home. A post-bronchoscopy leaflet should be given to patients on discharge, explaining how they should feel for the first 12 hours and detailing what to do if prevailing symptoms worsen or new symptoms develop. The proven safety of bronchoscopy must not lead to complacency when caring for these patients.

Laser bronchoscopy

Laser bronchoscopy is used to reduce the size of tracheobronchial tumours and can be used to treat both benign and malignant forms. Laser therapy through the bronchoscope causes cell death through intense heat, coagulation and evaporation of tissue. This procedure is usually palliative and indicated for relief of symptoms caused by airway obstruction. It is possible to insert a stent during the procedure to maintain patency of the airway.

Thoracoscopy

Thoracoscopy is the diagnostic treatment of choice when needle biopsy and aspiration fail to determine the cause of persistent empyema (exudative pleural effusion). The procedure involves the examination and sampling of the visceral and parietal pleura. This may be carried out under general anaesthetic or by a combination of sedation and local anaesthesia. A rigid thoracoscope is inserted into the pleural space through a small stab incision. For adults, a 9 mm rigid thoracoscope is generally used. The lung is collapsed by introducing about 200 ml of air, which allows the pleura to separate. This technique requires an experienced operator who can view the pleura

Case study 4.5

Brian, aged 56, is a smoker who has a history of weight loss, persistent cough and haemoptysis. At his outpatient appointment he was advised that he required a bronchoscopy. He was given the opportunity to discuss the reasons for this procedure and the potential risks and complications. He was given a date to have the daycase bronchoscopy and advised not to eat or drink for 4 hours prior to the investigation and that he would require somebody to escort him home.

The procedure was under local anaesthetic, consisting of intravenous midazolam and Xylocaine throat spray. The procedure was uncomplicated and post-bronchoscopy he remained nil by mouth until the local anaesthetic had worn off. His vital signs were observed during and post-procedure and compared with his baseline observations. He was able to go home, escorted by his partner, and given a post-bronchoscopy advice leaflet. He was specifically advised to report any signs of increased breathlessness or chest pain immediately as these could be associated with a pneumothorax. That evening he took 2 paracetamol, as advised, for a low grade temperature.

Brain returned to the outpatients department the following week where he was given a diagnosis of lung cancer and treatment options were discussed with him. At the time of diagnosis he was also seen by the lung cancer nurse specialist.

and take multiple biopsies. Mesothelioma remains difficult to diagnose but this technique has a sensitivity of over 90% for pleural malignancy and tuberculosis (Muers 1996).

Complications after this technique are rare and deaths following the procedure are extremely rare. An underwater seal drain is needed after thoracoscopy until the lung is fully inflated.

Videothoracoscopy

Videothoracoscopy is the insertion of a surgical telescope into the thorax via a stab incision. This allows inspection of the pleural cavity and visually directed biopsies to be taken from intrapleural abnormalities. Forceps for the biopsy may be introduced either through a channel in the instrument or through a separate incision. This technique offers a good surgical approach to clarify diagnosis in patients who have a negative transthoracic biopsy, particularly when mesothelioma is suspected.

This procedure is usually carried out under general anaesthetic, but in Europe and North America satisfactory results are reported under local anaesthetic and sedation (LoddenKemper 1998). Videothoracoscopy provides a far superior view of the thoracic cavity than a video monitor. The technique has further revolutionized thoracic surgical practice as well as diagnostic procedures.

Needle biopsy

Biopsy of the lung tissue and aspiration of pleural effusion or lung fluid is possible by the use of a range of fine needles. The procedure is less invasive than techniques such as bronchoscopy and thoracoscopy, though it is limited to areas that can be reached. A number of other investigations such as chest X-rays and scans will contribute to the information required to guide the use of this procedure.

The procedure may be diagnostic and palliative since a large volume of fluid (up to a litre) may be aspirated from the pleural space, negating the need for an intercostal chest drain to be inserted, and reducing breathlessness. The most significant findings from fluid specimens are infection, including tuberculosis and malignancy. Needle biopsy is particularly useful in confirming a diagnosis of mesothelioma, but is 50% less sensitive to other malignancies than pleural fluid cytology (Spiro 1999).

Complications such as pneumothorax are unlikely since the needles used are relatively blunt. If a rupture of the intercostal artery or vein occurs during the procedure a haematoma can quickly develop on the chest wall, though this seldom warrants any action at the time of procedure. A patient should be advised to observe the site following this and should be alerted to report signs of fever. In the case of malignant cells being present in the pleural fluid it is not uncommon for 'seeding' of these cells to occur along the needle track. A single fraction of radiotherapy controls developing nodules in most instances (Spiro 1999).

For this procedure patients are required to sit upright with their arms folded in front of them and resting on a pillow. Refinements to their position should be made to ensure maximum comfort, particularly with respect to breathing.

CONCLUSION

Diagnostic investigations to determine the nature of respiratory disease are becoming more sophisticated with advanced technology. Both non-invasive and invasive tests, in conjunction with presenting symptoms, history and respiratory assessment, assist in the diagnosis and management of respiratory disease. It is therefore essential that diagnostic investigations are not used in isolation.

REFERENCES

American Thoracic Society 1987 Standardisation of spirometry. American Review of Respiratory Disease 136: 1285–1295

British Thoracic Society 1997 Guidelines for the management of chronic obstructive pulmonary disease. Thorax 52 (suppl 5): S1–S28

Carter B G 1998 Accuracy of two pulse oximeters at low arterial haemoglobin oxygen saturation. Critical Care Medicine 26(6): 1128–1133

Cherniack R M 1992 Pulmonary function testing, 2nd edn. W B Saunders, Philadelphia, p. 21

Davidson J A H, Hoise H E 1993 Limitations of pulse oximetry: respiratory insufficiency – a failure of detection. British Medical Journal 307(6900): 372–373

Hall-Craggs M, Goddard P 1999 Magnetic resonance imaging. In: Albert R K, Spiro S G, Jett J R (eds) Comprehensive respiratory medicine. Mosby, London, ch 2

Kendrick A H, Smith E C 1992a Simple measurements of lung. Professional Nurse 7(6): 395–404

Kendrick A H, Smith E C 1992b Respiratory measurements 2: interpreting simple measurements of lung function. Professional Nurse 7(11): 748–754

LoddenKemper R 1998 Thoracoscopy – state of the art. European Respiratory Journal 11: 213–221

Muers M F 1996 Diagnostic bronchoscopy and tissue biopsy. In: Weatherall D J, Ledingham J G G, Warrell D A (eds) Oxford textbook of medicine, 3rd edn. Oxford University Press, Oxford, vol 12, sections 11–17

Pitkin A D, Roberts C M, Wedzicha J A 1994 Arterialised earlobe blood gas analysis: an underused technique. Thorax 49: 364–366

Prakash U B S 1999 Bronchoscopy. In: Albert R K, Spiro S G, Jett J R (eds) Comprehensive respiratory medicine. Mosby, London

Severinghaus J W, Naifeh K H, Koh S O 1989 Errors in 14 pulse oximeters during profound hypoxia. Journal of Clinical Monitoring 5: 72–81

Simonds A K 1999 Scoliosis and kyphoscoliosis. In: Albert R K, Spiro S G, Jett J R (eds) Comprehensive respiratory medicine. Mosby, London

Spiro S 1999 Closed pleural biopsy in comprehensive respiratory medicine. In: Albert R K, Spiro S G, Jett J R (eds) Comprehensive respiratory medicine. Mosby, London

5

Respiratory medication

Sadhna Murphy

Guidelines which recommend strategies for the treatment of respiratory diseases, such as those produced by the British Thoracic Society (BTS), include the medication used for the treatment of respiratory disease. When implementing such guidelines for respiratory care it is necessary to understand:

- the actions of drugs used in the treatment of respiratory disease
- the side effects of drugs used in the treatment of respiratory disease
- when and what medication to use in relation to the disease process
- how to select an appropriate inhaler device
- how and when to use nebulizers
- self-management and adherence to medication.

CATEGORIES AND EFFECTS OF RESPIRATORY MEDICATION

Bronchodilators

There are three groups of bronchodilators:

- sympathomimetic bronchodilators
- anticholinergics
- methylxanthines.

Sympathomimetic bronchodilators

Sympathomimetic bronchodilators are also referred to as beta$_2$ agonists. These agents mimic the actions of adrenaline on the smooth muscles of the airways. Short acting selective beta$_2$ agonists are used in the treatment of asthma (BTS 1997a) and chronic obstructive pulmonary disease (BTS 1997b). They affect mainly the airways and vascular smooth muscle and include:

- salbutamol
- terbutaline
- fenoterol.

At a molecular level, beta$_2$ agonists exert their effects by activating the beta receptors. This leads to activation of adenylate cyclase which converts adenosine triphosphate to cyclic 3′,5′-adenosine monophosphate (cyclic AMP). Cyclic AMP acts as a secondary messenger to produce protein kinase which causes smooth muscle relaxation by reducing intracellular calcium concentration.

Long acting beta$_2$ agonists include:

- salmeterol
- formoterol.

They exert their effect in a similar fashion to short acting beta$_2$ agonists. However, their long duration of action is due to the fact that, being more lipophilic, they are bound to the phospholipid layer of smooth muscles. Over a period of hours they then leach out and bind to the beta$_2$ receptors and continue to relax the smooth muscle of the airways. Long acting beta$_2$ agonists have been shown to improve asthma control and lung function when used regularly (Devoy et al 1995, Pauwels et al 1997).

Clinical pharmacokinetics and toxicity of sympathomimetic bronchodilators

Salbutamol and terbutaline are the most commonly used short acting agents in this group. They are usually given by inhalation of aerosol, dry powder or nebulized solutions, to cause bronchodilation within a few minutes. The rapid onset of action makes these the drugs of choice for quick relief of symptoms. A peak bronchodilator effect is reached within 15 minutes with a duration of action of 4 to 8 hours depending on the dose given, hence administration is every 6 hours. When given by the oral route, beta$_2$ agonists undergo extensive first pass metabolism in the liver and have a reduced duration of 3–4 hours. Modified release beta$_2$ agonists can be used orally at step 4 of the British guidelines for asthma (BTS 1997a).

The most common adverse effects seen with this group of drugs are tremor of the hands, tachycardia at high doses and hypokalaemia, particularly with concomitant administration of methylxanthines, diuretics and corticosteroids. Plasma potassium levels should be carefully monitored when using these combinations.

Anticholinergics

There are currently two anticholinergic drugs available:

- ipratropium bromide
- oxitropium bromide.

They are also referred to as anti-muscarinic agents since their main action is on the muscarinic receptors. In the parasympathetic system, the nerve endings of the postganglionic parasympathetic fibres normally release acetylcholine. The main muscarinic effects of acetylcholine on the lung tissues are to cause bronchoconstriction and to increase bronchial secretion. Anticholinergic agents block the cholinergic reflex of the vagus nerve that causes bronchospasm in some asthmatic patients by opposing the effects of acetylcholine. Hence, the net result is bronchodilation. Anticholinergic agents do not appear to affect sputum viscosity, sputum clearance and production of saliva. Muscarinic receptors are present in larger numbers in the proximal airways rather than in the small airways. They are also more densely located in the airways of young children and the older patient. Hence, in these patients, anticholinergics may be the bronchodilator of choice. In asthma patients, anticholinergics may be used if toxicity is observed with beta$_2$ agonists.

Clinical pharmacokinetics and toxicity of anticholinergics

Both agents can be given by inhalation of aerosol droplets from metered dose inhalers. Ipratropium bromide solution can also be nebulized when large doses are required. When inhaled, the peak bronchodilator effect is achieved up to 1 hour later. The slow onset of action makes this group of drugs not ideal when a quick relief is required. The duration of action of ipratropium bromide is similar to beta$_2$ agonists, i.e. 4–6 hours. Oxitropium bromide has a longer duration of action of 8 hours and can be administered two to three times daily.

At therapeutic doses ipratropium bromide and oxitropium bromide have few adverse effects. The most common complaint from patients is dry mouth and bitter taste. The dose administered can be reduced as long as therapeutic benefits are still apparent; alternatively other measures, such as frequent mouthwashes or artificial saliva, can be used to offset these adverse effects.

Methylxanthines

Theophylline is the only bronchodilator in this class of drug in clinical use for treating:

- acute and chronic asthma (BTS 1997a)
- exercise induced bronchospasm
- nocturnal asthma (Martin & Kraft 1996)
- chronic obstructive pulmonary disease (COPD) where reversible airways disease is present (BTS 1997b).

Aminophylline contains theophylline and ethylenediamine, a component which makes theophylline more water soluble and hence available in an injectable form. The mechanism of action of theophylline is not entirely clear. It is thought that theophylline increases the concentration of cyclic adenosine monophosphate (cAMP) by inhibiting phosphodiesterase, an enzyme involved in breaking down cAMP. An increased concentration of cAMP then leads to bronchodilation. Another mode of action is thought to be the antagonism of adenosine receptors. The pharmacological action of endogenous adenosine on respiratory smooth muscle is to cause constriction. Theophylline may also cause bronchodilation by releasing endogenous catecholamines from the adrenal medulla. Apart from its effect on smooth bronchial muscle, theophylline has actions on other organ systems. It stimulates the central nervous system, increasing alertness and sometimes causing sleep disturbances. It also has transient diuretic effects, increases gastric acid secretion, causes a transient increase in plasma glucose, stimulates the cardiovascular system, and may increase the efficiency of diaphragmatic contraction.

Clinical pharmacokinetics and toxicity methylxanthines

Both theophylline and aminophylline can be given orally as slow release (SR) preparations. Only aminophylline can be administered by the intravenous route. The intramuscular route is not recommended since the injection solution is too irritant. When given orally, theophylline is well absorbed from the gastrointestinal tract. The bioavailability is assumed to be 100% although this may vary for the various slow release preparations (Hendeles et al 1984). Slow release preparations have long half-lives necessitating once or twice daily administration to provide an adequate plasma concentration. The presence of food in the gastrointestinal tract may alter the absorption of some of the slow release preparations.

For optimal bronchodilation to occur, a plasma theophylline level of 10–20 mg/L is required. Individual response to prescribed dosages is variable, therefore theophylline plasma levels need to be monitored on an individual basis. After initiation of the treatment, the time to steady state varies from 4 to 7 days depending on the half-life of the drug. Levels at 8 hours post-dose within 1 week of treatment give a better representation of individual drug handling and allow dosage adjustments to be made. Several factors and drugs are known to affect the plasma level of theophylline (Box 5.1).

The toxicity of theophylline is dependent on the plasma concentration achieved. It is worthwhile noting that some patients have saturable kinetics where theophylline is concerned. This means that small dosage increases can cause a large increase in the plasma levels. Gastrointestinal symptoms of nausea, vomiting and diarrhoea and tremor are visible at therapeutic levels. Above 20 mg/L, a

Box 5.1 Factors affecting theophylline levels

Factors decreasing theophylline levels

- Smoking (effects can last up to 6 months after stopping)
- Young age (increased metabolism capacity)
- Alcohol consumption
- Cystic fibrosis
- Drugs: phenytoin, rifampicin, carbamazepine, phenobarbitone

Factors increasing theophylline levels

- Old age
- Liver disease and cirrhosis
- Congestive cardiac disease
- Viral infection and pneumonia
- Severe pulmonary obstruction
- Drugs: cimetidine, erythromycin, ciprofloxacin, allopurinol, oral contraceptives

large proportion of patients will experience convulsions and arrhythmias, particularly the life threatening ventricular tachycardia.

Corticosteroids

These are the most potent anti-inflammatory agents used in the treatment of asthma and in any lung disease where reversibility is present. They are not bronchodilators but are effective at reducing bronchial hyper-reactivity. The pharmacology of corticosteroids is complex. At a cellular level, corticosteroids interact with intracellular receptors to produce mediator proteins via a series of mechanisms. The mediator proteins are thought to be at the basis of the pharmacological effects of corticosteroids (for a detailed mode of action, the reader is referred to pharmacology textbooks). The overall effects are:

- stabilization of leukocyte lysosomal membranes
- prevention of accumulation of macrophages at the site of inflammation
- reduction of mucous secretion
- reduction of capillary permeability and oedema formation.

Corticosteroids in lung disease inhibit the inflammatory late phase response to chemotactic agents released during the immediate response phase. They should be used regularly since maximum benefits are not obtained until 1–4 weeks after initiating treatment.

Clinical pharmacokinetics and toxicity of corticosteroids

Corticosteroids can be given by the inhaled route, orally or intravenously to treat asthma and COPD. There are currently three corticosteroids available for inhalation in a variety of devices:

- beclometasone
- budesonide
- fluticasone.

Prednisolone is the corticosteroid of choice for oral use whereas hydrocortisone is preferred for intravenous use. The inhaled route is preferred since when corticosteroids are used systemically the adverse effects encountered are detrimental to the patient and when used over a long period can result in the following side effects:

- osteoporosis
- weight gain
- increased body hair
- diabetes.

When taken by inhalation, only 10–25% of the drug is deposited in the respiratory tract, with the remainder being deposited on the back of the throat or swallowed. The drugs are well absorbed from the gastrointestinal tract and from the lungs. They are well distributed to all body tissues where they exert their effects.

The adverse effects of inhaled corticosteroids (Geddes 1992) are almost always as a consequence of using high doses over a long period of time. Local adverse effects include:

- hoarseness
- loss of voice (Selroos et al 1994)
- candidiasis.

These can be avoided by using large volume spacer devices when using a meter dosed inhaler and by rinsing the mouth after inhalation. It is worthwhile noting that once control of asthma is achieved, the dose of inhaled corticosteroids

Management of chronic asthma in adults and schoolchildren

- Avoidance of provoking factors where possible
- Patient's involvement and education
- Selection of best inhaler device
- Treatment stepped up as necessary to achieve good control
- Treatment stepped down if control of asthma good

Prescribe a peak flow meter and monitor response to treatment

Notes
- **Patients should start treatment at the step most appropriate to the initial severity. A rescue course of prednisolone may be needed at any time and at any step. The aim is to achieve early control of the condition and then to reduce treatment.**
- **Until growth is complete any child requiring beclomethasone or budesonide > 800 µg daily or fluticasone > 500 µg daily should be referred to a paediatrician with an interest in asthma.**

Step 1:

Occasional use of relief bronchodilators

Inhaled short acting β agonists "as required" for symptom relief are acceptable. If they are needed more than once daily move to step 2. Before altering a treatment step ensure that the patient is having the treatment and has a good inhaler technique. Address any fears.

Step 2:

Regular inhaled anti-inflammatory agents

Inhaled short acting β agonists as required
plus
beclomethasone or budesonide 100–400 µg twice daily or fluticasone 50–200 µg twice daily. Alternatively, use cromoglycate or nedocromil sodium, but if control is not achieved start inhaled steroids

Step 3:

High dose inhaled steroids or low dose inhaled steroids plus long acting inhaled β agonist bronchodilator

Inhaled short acting β agonists as required
plus either
beclomethasone or budesonide increased to 800–2000 µg daily or fluticasone 400–1000 µg daily via a large volume spacer
or
beclomethasone or budesonide 100–400 µg twice daily or fluticasone 50–200 µg twice daily plus salmeterol 50 µg twice daily. In a very small number of patients who experience side effects with high dose inhaled steroids, either the long acting inhaled β agonist option is used or a sustained release theophylline may be added to step 2 medication. Cromoglycate or nedocromil may also be tried.

Step 4:

High dose inhaled steroids and regular bronchodilators

Inhaled short acting β agonists as required with inhaled beclomethasone or budesonide 800–2000 µg daily or fluticasone 400–1000 µg daily via a large volume spacer
plus
a sequential therapeutic trial of one or more of
- inhaled long acting β agonists
- sustained release theophylline
- inhaled ipratropium or oxitropium
- long acting β agonist tablets
- high dose inhaled bronchodilators
- cromoglycate or nedocromil.

Step 5:

Addition of regular steroid tablets

Inhaled short acting β agonists as required with inhaled beclomethasone or budesonide 800–2000 µg daily or fluticasone 400–1000 µg daily via a large volume spacer and one or more of the long acting bronchodilators
plus
regular prednisolone tablets in a single daily dose

Stepping down:

Review treatment every three to six months. If control is achieved a stepwise reduction in treatment may be possible. In patients whose treatment was recently started at step 4 or 5 or included steroid tablets for gaining control of asthma this reduction may take place after a short interval. In other patients with chronic asthma a three to six month period of stability should be shown before slow stepwise reduction is undertaken.

Outcome of steps 1–3: control of asthma
- Minimal (ideally no) chronic symptoms, including nocturnal symptoms
- Minimal (infrequent) exacerbations
- Minimal need for relieving bronchodilators
- No limitations on activities including exercise
- Circadian variation in peak expiratory flow (PEF) < 20%
- PEF ≥ 80% of predicted or best
- Minimal (or no) adverse effects from medicine

Outcome of steps 4–5: best possible results
- Least possible symptoms
- Least possible need for relieving bronchodilators
- Least possible limitation of activity
- Least possible variation in PEF
- Best PEF
- Least adverse effects from medicine

NATIONAL **ASTHMA** CAMPAIGN
conquering asthma

Working for Healthier Lungs

in association with the General Practitioner in Asthma Group, the British Association of Accident and Emergency Medicine, the British Paediatric Respiratory Society and the Royal College of Paediatrics and Child Health

Adapted from poster designed by Business Design Group

Figure 5.1 British Thoracic Society asthma guidelines. Reproduced with permission from the British Medical Journal (British Thoracic Society 1997a).

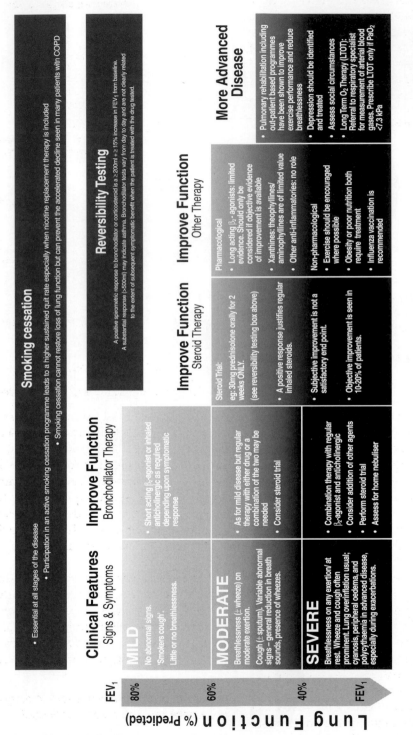

Smoking cessation

- Essential at all stages of the disease
- Participation in an active smoking cessation programme leads to a higher sustained quit rate especially when nicotine replacement therapy is included
- Smoking cessation cannot restore loss of lung function but can prevent the accelerated decline seen in many patients with COPD

Reversibility Testing

A positive spirometric response to bronchodilator or corticosteroid is a ≥200ml + ≥15% increase in FEV_1 from baseline.
A substantial response (>500ml) may indicate asthma. Bronchodilator tests vary from day to day and are not clearly related to the extent of subsequent symptomatic benefit when the patient is treated with the drug tested.

More Advanced Disease

- Pulmonary rehabilitation including out-patient based programmes have been shown to improve exercise performance and reduce breathlessness
- Depression should be identified and treated
- Assess social circumstances
- Long Term O_2 Therapy (LTOT): Referral to respiratory specialist for measurement of arterial blood gases. Prescribe LTOT only if PaO_2 <7.3 kPa

Improve Function
Other Therapy

Pharmacological
- Long acting β₂-agonists: limited evidence. Should only be considered if objective evidence of improvement is available
- Xanthines: theophyllines/aminophyllines are of limited value
- Other anti-inflammatories: no role

Non-pharmacological
- Exercise should be encouraged where possible
- Obesity or poor nutrition both require treatment
- Influenza vaccination is recommended

Improve Function
Steroid Therapy

Steroid Trial:
eg: 30mg prednisolone orally for 2 weeks ONLY.
(see reversibility testing box above)
- A positive response justifies regular inhaled steroids.
- Subjective improvement is not a satisfactory end point.
- Objective improvement is seen in 10–20% of patients.

Improve Function
Bronchodilator Therapy

- Short acting β₂-agonist or inhaled anticholinergic as required depending upon symptomatic response

- As for mild disease but regular therapy with either drug or a combination of the two may be needed
- Consider steroid trial

- Combination therapy with regular β₂-agonist and anticholinergic
- Consider addition of other agents
- Perform steroid trial
- Assess for home nebuliser

Clinical Features
Signs & Symptoms

MILD
No abnormal signs.
'Smokers cough'.
Little or no breathlessness.

MODERATE
Breathlessness (± wheeze) on moderate exertion.
Cough (± sputum). Variable abnormal signs – general reduction in breath sounds, presence of wheezes.

SEVERE
Breathlessness on any exertion/ at rest. Wheeze and cough often prominent. Lung overinflation usual; cyanosis, peripheral oedema, and polycythaemia in advanced disease, especially during exacerbations.

FEV_1
80%
60%
40%
FEV_1

Lung Function (% Predicted)

Figure 5.2 Summary of British Thoracic Society guidelines for the management of chronic obstructive pulmonary disease. Reproduced with permission from the British Medical Journal (British Thoracic Society 1997b).

should be reduced to as low a maintenance dose as possible (BTS 1997a). Systemic adverse effects from inhaled corticosteroids have been shown to be mainly as a consequence of the amount of drug deposited in the stomach and the potency of the drug (Boorsma et al 1996, Clark et al 1996, Pedersen & O'Byrne 1997).

Clinical use of bronchodilators and corticosteroids

Bronchodilators and corticosteroids have an important role to play in the management of both asthma and COPD. As well as understanding the actions and side effects of the drugs it is also necessary to understand at which stage in the disease process they should be introduced. The British Thoracic Society guidelines on asthma management (Fig. 5.1) and the management of COPD (Fig. 5.2) outline the stages when the different drugs should be introduced into the treatment of patients with asthma and COPD.

Leukotriene receptor antagonists

These represent a new class of drugs for the treatment of asthma. It is now well recognized that the airways in asthma show complex immunological activity. The cysteinyl leukotrienes LTC4, LTD4 and LTE4 are among the most important of the mediators in asthma (Chung 1999, Spector 1997). Leukotrienes are synthesized from arachidonic acid, a product of cell membrane metabolism (Fig. 5.3).

Montelukast and zafirlukast bind to Cyst LT1 receptors on airways cells and prevent the effects of the released cysteinyl leukotrienes, which are bronchoconstriction, plasma exudation, mucous secretion and possibly inflammation. They are licensed for the treatment of mild to moderate asthma (Chanarin & Johnston 1994, Sampson & Costello 1995). Clinical studies show a small positive effect on lung function (Drug and Therapeutics Bulletin 1998, Hendeles & Marshik 1997). A major advantage with this class is that the drugs are available in oral form which may aid adherence to treatment. Leukotriene antagonists are well tolerated (Spector 1997) with only gastrointestinal symptoms and headaches reported.

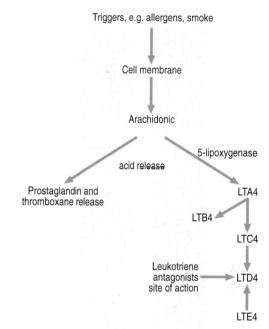

Figure 5.3   Pathway of leukotriene generation.

Agents for prophylaxis

Sodium cromoglycate and nedocromil sodium

These agents are not bronchodilators but can be used for the prophylaxis and prevention of asthma attacks. They are particularly useful in allergen induced and exercise induced asthma. Their mode of action is not entirely clear. They inhibit immediate type 1 hypersensitivity reactions to allergens including histamine release. They may also have a role in stabilizing mast cells, although this still has to be established. Both drugs also inhibit late phase reactions.

Nedocromil sodium is not a steroid but has antiinflammatory effects on the airways. Nedocromil prevents the activation and release of inflammatory mediators including histamine, leukotriene C4 from macrophages and mast cells, which are involved in causing inflammation in asthmatics.

Clinical pharmacokinetics and toxicity of sodium cromoglycate and nedocromil sodium

Both sodium cromoglycate and nedocromil sodium are poorly absorbed from the gastrointestinal tract. They are therefore administered as inhalations of aerosol droplets, nebulizers or dry powder. Peak plasma levels are achieved within 15 minutes of inhalation. Both drugs should be used regularly over a period of 3–4 weeks before full benefits are apparent. Sodium cromoglycate should be administered 4 times daily whereas nedocromil sodium only requires a twice daily administration once an effective maintenance dose is reached. The drugs are very well tolerated and adverse effects tend to be local, such as irritation of the throat.

Management of allergic rhinitis

Allergic rhinitis can be classified broadly as seasonal allergic rhinitis and perennial allergic rhinitis. These are characterized by:

- sneezing
- itchy eyes
- rhinorrhoea
- nasal congestion
- post-nasal catarrh
- nasal blockage.

Treatment consists of avoiding allergens and the use of pharmacological agents to control symptoms. In severe cases desensitization to the allergen may be necessary.

Oral antihistamines

Oral antihistamines are the commonest therapy and are effective against sneezing, itch and eye symptoms (Calderon-Zapata & Davies 1998, Youlten 1996). They have less influence on rhinorrhoea and are less effective for nasal blockage. They can be broadly categorized as sedating (first generation) and non-sedating (second generation) antihistamines. Sedating antihistamines, e.g. chlorpheniramine, tend to be less used nowadays mainly due to them causing drowsiness. The newer preparations such as cetirizine, loratadine, aztemizole and terfenadine are less sedating and cause less psychomotor impairment. Both terfenadine and aztemizole interact with a large number of drugs, potentially causing fatal arrhythmias. The new oral antihistamine fexofe-nadine, an active metabolite of terfenadine, lacks the adverse effects seen with terfenadine and aztemizole.

Topical corticosteroids

When symptoms are not relieved by antihistamines, small doses of topical corticosteroids are most effective. Their effects are primarily anti-inflammatory and they should be used regularly. Systemic absorption of corticosteroids administered nasally is extremely small and is not likely to be clinically significant. Topical corticosteroids administered nasally include:

- triamcinolone
- beclometasone
- fluticasone
- budesonide.

Other preparations

Azelastine (Rhinolast) is an antihistamine available as a nasal spray. It is less effective than nasal corticosteroids and is only useful in conditions where only nasal symptoms are present; some patients complain of a bitter taste in the mouth.

Sodium cromoglycate (Rynacrom) is effective at preventing rather than relieving acute symptoms. It should be used regularly during the hay fever season. It is less effective than corticosteroids or azelastine, but is the treatment of choice in children.

Ipratropium bromide nasal spray (Rinatec) is very effective in perennial vasomotor rhinitis where the main symptom is watery rhinorrhoea.

Cough suppressants

Coughing is a protective reflex. Its purpose is to keep the respiratory passages clear of mucus and foreign materials which may obstruct breathing. Treatment of cough should be aimed firstly at removing the triggers causing the cough and secondly at suppressing the cough rather than completely eliminating it. Demulcent and opioid preparations are the main group of drugs used for treatment (Knowles & Knowles 1998). Demulcent cough preparations contain soothing agents such as syrup which may relieve a dry irritating cough. Simple linctus is an inexpensive and harmless preparation. Low doses of opioid antitussives are also effective and do not tend to affect the respiratory centre. Antitussive syrups containing sugar should be used with caution in diabetics. In intractable cough associated with bronchial carcinoma, it may be necessary to use methadone linctus or morphine sulphate solution. These drugs may induce sputum retention, ventilatory failure and opioid dependence.

Nasal decongestants

Simple steam inhalation provides a cheap and effective means of relieving catarrh and congestion of the upper respiratory tract. Ephedrine and xylometazoline are sympathomimetics that can be used to relieve nasal congestion. They should not be used in the long term and it is recommended that treatment should not exceed 7 days as these drugs cause local irritations. After excessive use, tolerance occurs with diminished effects and rebound congestion. Pseudoephedrine administered orally may be considered at a dosage of 60 mg three to four times daily. The adverse effects of pseudoephedrine, due to the sympathomimetic effects, include dry mouth, anorexia, insomnia, anxiety, tremor, restlessness and palpitation, tachycardia and cold extremities.

Expectorants

Expectorants and mucolytics are usually without objective benefit and should not be used. Expectorants such as ammonium chloride and ipecacuanha claim to increase the volume of secretions and therefore facilitate clearance via mucociliary movement and coughing. Water is the best expectorant for prophylaxis or active treatment. Mucolytic agents such as oral carbocisteine and methyl cysteine hydrochloride work by reducing sputum viscosity and therefore facilitate expectoration. Long term benefits of these agents, in terms of improved lung function,

are yet to be demonstrated. The recommended treatment to assist with expectoration is:

- adequate fluid intake
- physiotherapy, including postural drainage
- sodium chloride 0.9% nebulized: 2.5–5 ml up to 2 hourly (nebulized over 10–15 minutes) but usually four times a day.

Drugs used in cystic fibrosis

In recent years several approaches have been adopted in order to improve lung function in cystic fibrosis (CF) patients. Dornase alfa alters the sputum viscosity. It was developed genetically to mimic the naturally occurring DNase enzyme which degrades DNA in the lung. The safety and efficacy of Dornase alfa is well documented (Aitken et al 1992, Hubbard et al 1992). Improvement in lung function, subjective scores and reduced frequency of respiratory infections (Fuchs et al 1994) have been reported. Reducing the inflammatory response is another approach. Prednisolone (Auerbach et al 1985, Eigen et al 1995), ibuprofen (Konstan et al 1995) and alpha-1 antitrypsin (McElvaney et al 1991) have all been tried as anti-inflammatory agents. New antibiotics have also been introduced. Preservative free tobramycin for nebulization (Ramsey et al 1999) and macrolide antibiotics are all thought to improve lung function (Jaffe et al 1998).

The ultimate treatment would, however, be to correct the gene defect. Several difficulties are present in the formulation of an effective delivery system for gene therapy (Ramsey 1996). Further research is required in order to develop the ideal system of delivery for an effective therapy.

Respiratory stimulant used for hypercapnic respiratory failure

Doxapram is the only respiratory stimulant that should be considered in the treatment of hypercapnic Type II respiratory failure in patients with COPD who are becoming drowsy or comatosed. Administration will often arouse a patient with marked CO_2 retention and it may then be possible, with low concentration oxygen therapy, physiotherapy and appropriate medical treatment, to avoid recourse to endotracheal intubation and intermittent positive pressure ventilation. Doxapram is effective only when given by intravenous injection or infusion. It is necessary to take frequent arterial blood gases to ensure the correct dose is used. It is difficult to keep patients on respiratory stimulants for more than 24–36 hours, as they often develop marked anxiety and sometimes hallucinations due to the stimulation of the central nervous system.

New developments

Intense research has led to a greater understanding of the underlying disease process of asthma. As the relevant mediators are identified, new ideas for drug development emerge. Phosphodiesterase inhibitors are among the next generation of anti-inflammatory drugs likely to be used for treating asthma (Elwood 1997). Research is already underway to identify the gene which might predispose to asthma (Hall 1997). The relevance of genetics, environmental factors (du Bois 1995) and a better understanding of the diseases together with new therapeutic approaches will certainly affect the management of respiratory disease in the future.

INHALER DEVICES
Selecting appropriate inhaler devices

A wide range of devices are available to allow drugs to be inhaled and exert their activity topically in the lungs. There are many different devices to deliver medication direct to the lungs, which include:

- metered dose inhaler (MDI)
- metered dose inhaler with spacer
- dry powder devices
- breath actuated devices
- nebulizers.

The prime responsibility of the healthcare professional is not only to diagnose the disease state, but also to ensure individual patients receive appropriate treatment. In respiratory disease this process involves selecting the correct inhaler device, i.e. the one that would offer maximum benefit to the patient.

Factors to be considered when choosing inhaler devices

In selecting the device, the healthcare professional should consider various factors. Patient factors should in practice be at the forefront of the decision making process. As regards the device itself, the consistency of the system is also important. Ideally the same device should be used for the different categories of drugs prescribed. This will minimize confusion and enable the practitioner to reduce the time taken to educate the patient. The ease with which a technique can be taught may also influence the practitioner when deciding on a delivery system. The delivery of the dose within the same device should also be constant. The effectiveness of a device during an acute attack is another factor to consider. Some dry powder devices may cause patients to experience more cough and worsen a situation, whereas metered dose inhalers could exacerbate the attack by means of the cold freon effect. On the other hand, metered dose inhalers attached to spacer devices are very effective at delivering large doses during an acute exacerbation. It is also important to consider the compatibility of inhaler devices with other devices, such as spacers, which may become a necessity at a later time. There is one other crucial factor which will affect the choice of system. The cost of the device may influence the practitioner who feels pressurized to minimize expenditure. Cost may unfortunately become the determining factor in selecting an inhaler device, although this should not be the only factor, as the patient should be the focus of the decision.

Patient factors influencing choice of devices

A number of factors should be considered when choosing an inhaler device for a patient. It is important to remember that if patients choose a device for themselves they are more likely to use it, thus improving adherence to the treatment. Since a large number of devices are available, it should be possible to tailor choice to individual need so that each patient may receive maximum benefit from the device used. In practice most patients are started on metered dose inhalers (Fig. 5.4) since they are the least expensive devices on the market.

For those who have difficulty coordinating actuation and breathing and for those receiving inhaled corticosteroids, the recommendation is to use the metered dose inhaler with a spacer device (Fig. 5.5).

Regardless of the inhaler device chosen, it is crucial to demonstrate to the patient the correct technique in order to use the device effectively. Although a metered dosed inhaler with or without a spacer is the most frequently prescribed inhaler device, it is important to consider factors that would make this choice inappropriate. There are many factors that can influence the choice of devices (Box 5.2).

The age of the patient will determine the type of device chosen by either the practitioner or the patients themselves. The elderly or the very young may not have the inspiration flow required to achieve adequate lung deposition with some of the devices. They may not be able to hold their breaths for long enough to achieve maximum effect. For these patients a pressurized metered dose inhaler is probably not the right device. The elderly may also have other problems such as arthritis, which can manifest as a lack of dexterity. For these patients with insufficient hand strength, actuation of the metered dose inhaler becomes difficult. When high doses of beta$_2$ agonists are used, hand tremor is often experienced, again leading to difficulty in

Metered dose inhaler (MDI)

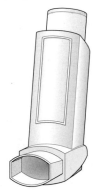

How to use
- Remove cap and shake inhaler
- Gently breathe out
- Make seal with lips around mouthpiece
- Press the canister at the start of inspiration and take a slow deep breath
- Hold breath for at least 10 seconds

Advantages
- Low cost
- Available in generic form
- Fits in a spacer device, allowing ease of use
- Not susceptible to moisture

Disadvantages
- Need to coordinate actuation and breathing
- No dose counter to identify when almost empty
- Low lung deposition
- Risk of oral candida due to oropharyngeal deposition of corticosteroids
- Cold-freon effect may impair inspiration

Figure 5.4   Metered dose inhaler (MDI).

Metered dose Inhaler (MDI) with spacer

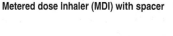
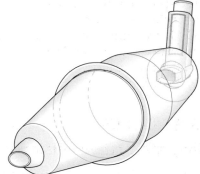

How to use
- Remove cap and shake inhaler and place into spacer
- Gently breathe out
- Make seal with lips around mouthpiece
- Press the canister once to release dose of drug
- Breathe in and out slowly and gently (tidal breathing) five times. This will make a clicking sound as the valve opens and closes

Advantages
- Eliminates the need to coordinate actuation and breathing
- Reduces oropharyngeal deposition
- Increases lung deposition
- Reduces the cold-freon effect
- One-way valve allows several breaths for one actuation

Disadvantages
- Bulky to carry around
- Needs to be cleaned regularly
- Complicates inhaler therapy

Figure 5.5   Metered dose inhaler (MDI) with spacer.

Breath-actuated devices – Easi-breathe and Autohaler

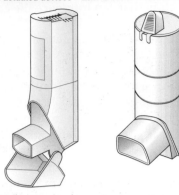

How to use
- Shake the inhaler and remove cap (with the Autohaler push lever up)
- Gently breathe out
- Hold the inhaler upright and do not occlude air holes
- Make seal with lips around mouthpiece
- Breathe in steadily through the mouthpiece
- Once inhaler is actuated take a deep breath
- Hold breath for at least 10 seconds
- Close the cap

Advantages
- Easy to use
- Coordination not required
- Not susceptible to moisture
- Low inspiration volume required

Disadvantages
- More expensive than MDI
- No dose counter
- The noise made when the dose is inhaled may disrupt breathing

Figure 5.6 Breath actuated devices – Easi-Breathe and Autohaler.

Case study 5.1

Dorothy, aged 71, has COPD and a tremor due to Parkinson's disease. She has been prescribed a metered dose inhaler with spacer to deliver her salbutamol and ipratropium bromide. She is becoming more breathless so attends her GP who discovers that she is only using her inhaled medication intermittently. She sees the practice nurse who assesses Dorothy's inhaler technique. Due to Dorothy's age and the presence of a tremor, she can not easily put the spacer together and does not have sufficient strength to depress the canister. Following discussion and demonstration of various placebo devices it was decided that a turbohaler with an aid to assist with twisting the inhaler would be most suitable and acceptable for Dorothy, together with combination therapy, consisting of a beta$_2$ agonist and an anticholinergic in the same inhaler, as Dorothy then only had to remember one inhaler rather than two. Dorothy felt she had been involved in the decision making regarding her health and started to use her medication regularly. She was followed up by the practice nurse.

Box 5.2 Factors influencing the choice of inlaler device

Patient factors
- Acceptance of the diagnosis
- Age
- Lifestyle
- Ease of use
- Inspiration flow rate
- Dexterity
- Taste
- Appearance of the device

Practitioner factors
- Cost
- Consistency of delivery
- Availability of various drugs in the same device
- Compatibility with other devices
- Easy to teach technique
- Effectiveness of the device

Dry powder device – Turbohaler

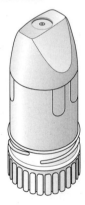

How to use
- Unscrew and remove cap
- Hold the device upright
- Twist the grip forwards then backwards. A click should be heard
- Gently breathe out
- Make seal with lips around mouthpiece
- Breathe in steadily and deeply through the mouthpiece
- Remove inhaler from mouth and hold breath for at least 10 seconds

Advantages
- Easy to use
- Very little taste in the mouth
- Has a marker to indicate when almost empty
- Low inspiration volume required
- High lung deposition
- Durable and less likely to break

Disadvantages
- More expensive than MDI
- Some patients feel that the shape is unacceptable
- No dose counter
- Likely to be affected by moisture

Figure 5.7 Dry powder device – Turbohaler.

Dry powder device – Accuhaler

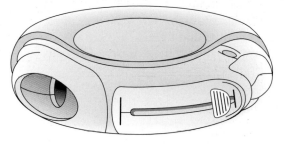

How to use
- Hold the outer casing with one hand while pushing the thumb grip away until a click is heard
- Hold the inhaler level
- Gently breathe out
- Make seal with lips around mouthpiece
- Breathe in steadily and deeply through the mouthpiece
- Remove inhaler from mouth and hold breath for at least 10 seconds

Advantages
- Easy to use
- Dose counter available
- Multiple doses available, therefore no need to refill
- Pleasant taste
- Moisture-proof

Disadvantages
- More expensive than MDI
- Some patients find the mouthpiece too small

Figure 5.8   Dry powder device – Accuhaler.

actuation. The elderly may also have poor eyesight leading to difficulty in reading the dose counter.

The lifestyle of the patient should be considered. Spacer devices may not be practical for those who have an active lifestyle requiring everyday travelling. Some patients may prefer devices that require a low maintenance and do not involve cleaning in order to fit in their daily routine. The appearance of the device is also important to the patient. The device should be compact, easy to carry around and easy to assemble and use.

Patients should feel at ease using their device and should not feel embarrassed by the shape of the device. Patients should be consulted regarding the taste that they sense from some of the devices. Some may wish for a taste sensation, which to them denotes a dose being delivered, whereas others may prefer not to experience any taste. Patients may also find that refilling of powder devices is not as easy as they think. It is not only the elderly or the very young who may

Dry powder device – Diskhaler

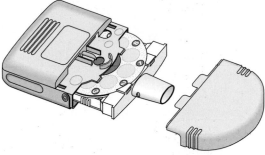

How to load
- Remove mouthpiece cover and then white tray by pulling it out gently and then squeezing ridges either side until it slides out
- Place foil disk on wheel and slide tray back. Slide disk in and out to rotate disk until highest number of blisters in disk is displayed

How to use
- Keep diskhaler level
- To pierce blister lift rear of lid up as far as it will go then close lid
- Hold diskhaler level and do not occlude air holes at side
- Gently breathe out
- Make seal with lips around mouthpiece
- Breathe in as deeply as possible through the mouthpiece
- Remove inhaler from mouth and hold breath for at least 10 seconds

Advantages
- Dose counter available
- Pleasant taste
- Moisture-proof

Disadvantages
- More expensive than MDI
- Need to refill when blisters are empty
- Can be awkward to refill
- Needs regular cleaning to avoid clogging with powder

Figure 5.9   Dry powder device – Diskhaler.

encounter this problem, but other patients may find that refilling is awkward. It is therefore imperative to consider all the factors when deciding on an inhaler device for a patient. Above all these, however, the practitioner must establish whether patients have accepted the diagnosis of their disease. All the factors discussed above are secondary to the fact that if the diagnosis is not accepted, then even if the ideal device is chosen, adherence to treatment is very unlikely.

In selecting the appropriate device for individual patients, practitioners must ensure that they themselves understand the principles involved in the use of these devices. An understanding of the advantages and disadvantages will also help practitioners to choose the right device.

Dry powder device – Clickhaler

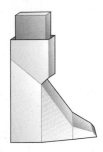

How to use
- Remove mouthpiece cover
- Shake the inhaler
- Hold the inhaler upright and press the dosing button down firmly
- Gently breathe out
- Make seal with lips around mouthpiece
- Breathe in steadily and deeply through the mouthpiece
- Remove inhaler from mouth and hold breath for at least 10 seconds

Advantages
- Low inspiration volume required
- Dose counter available
- Multiple doses available, therefore no need to refill
- Pleasant taste

Disadvantages
- More expensive than MDI
- Likely to be affected by moisture

Figure 5.10   Dry powder device – Clickhaler.

NEBULIZERS

Nebulizers are useful as they can provide a large dose of a drug in an aerosol form to the lungs. Nebulizers convert a drug in a liquid form into an aerosol or suspension with respirable particles of a size small enough to reach the bronchioles and alveoli in a fairly short period of time of 5–15 minutes. Nebulizers are important in the management of both acute and chronic respiratory disease and can be used to deliver bronchodilators, corticosteroids, antibiotics and dornase alpha.

Factors affecting efficiency of nebulizers

There are many factors affecting the efficiency of nebulizer therapy (BTS 1997c) which include:

- type of nebulizer
- driving gas and flow rate
- the design of the nebulizer chamber
- the fill volume
- residual volume
- the nebulization time
- characteristics of the drug, e.g. viscosity
- tapping of the nebuliser chamber.

Types of nebulizer

There are three main categories of nebulizers to deliver drugs to the lungs:

- jet nebulizer
- ultrasonic nebulizer
- adaptive aerosol delivery system.

The jet nebulizer is the most widely used device (Fig. 5.11). It consists of a reservoir that holds the drug for nebulization. Compressed gas (air or oxygen) is forced via a small hole, otherwise known as a venturi, in the nebulizer unit. The gas collides with the liquid solution and atomizes the solution into an aerosol form. Large droplets are selectively removed by colliding with baffles above the venturi and return to the reservoir while the finer mist of drug is released for inhalation. New advances such as spacer attachments and the addition of vents have increased the efficiency of jet nebulizers by making them breath actuated.

The ultrasonic nebulizer uses ultrasonic waves from a piezoelectric source passing through the liquid solution to generate aerosol droplets. The size of the droplets is inversely proportional to the frequency of the vibration used. Ultrasonic nebulizers are considered superior to jet nebulizers since they can nebulize larger volumes and are quieter. However, they tend to be more expensive and are less sturdy.

Adaptive aerosol delivery (Fig. 5.12) is an advance in nebulizer technology as the aim of the device is to deliver precise and reproducible doses of drug by adapting to the patient's individual breathing pattern. As the drug is delivered during inspiration only, a precise amount of drug is delivered efficiently to the airways and wastage during expiration is eliminated (Nikander 1997).

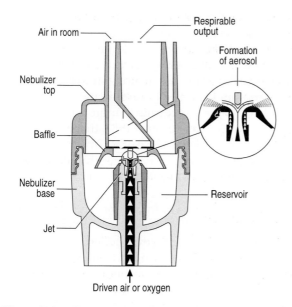

Figure 5.11   How a jet nebulizer works.

Driving gas and flow rates

A gas flow of 6–8 L/minute is required for jet nebulizers to provide 50% of the particles at a diameter of less than 5 microns. This is the size required for adequate drug deposition in the distal airways. Compressed air is most commonly used as the driving gas, unless oxygen is required and prescribed. Asthmatics who are hypoxic may nebulize bronchodilators using oxygen. Oxygen should not be used when nebulizing bronchodilator medications in patients with Type II respiratory failure, where there is a risk of carbon dioxide retention. Bronchodilators should then be nebulized using air. However, for these patients controlled oxygen should be administered via nasal cannulae at usual flow rate since bronchodilators, being weak vasodilators, can cause a fall in arterial saturation and worsening hypoxaemia.

Residual volume

This is the volume of solution left in the chamber when nebulization is complete. It is important to know this volume, since the fill volume required for drug delivery can then be deter-mined. Most nebulizers have a residual volume of 0.5–2.5 ml. A low residual volume allows a smaller fill volume.

Fill volume

In order to maximize the efficiency of the nebulizer, the drug chamber must be filled with a minimum volume of drug to enable a sufficient dose to be given. Most chambers require 2–4.5 ml depending on the residual volume. For residual volumes of less than 1 ml, the fill volume need not be more than 2.5 ml. For residual volumes of more than 1 ml, a fill volume of at least 4 ml is required in order to provide benefits to the patient.

Nebulization time

For bronchodilators, nebulization time should be 5–10 minutes. Longer nebulization time will decrease patient adherence to treatment (Smith 1986). Other drugs may require a longer time for nebulization to be completed in order to achieve a higher drug output. The end point of nebulization may be difficult to recognize. The general recommendation is to nebulize for an extra minute after 'spluttering' occurs. Tapping of the nebulizer towards the end of the nebulization time has been shown to increase the total volume of drug nebulized (Everard et al 1994).

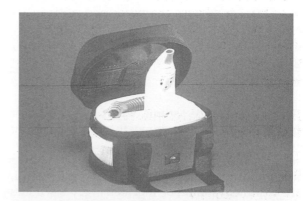

Figure 5.12   Adaptive aerosol delivery system.

Use of face masks or mouthpiece?

Wherever possible a mouthpiece is the preferred option as it provides better deposition of drug to the lungs and reduces the risk of adverse effects associated with some drug therapies. When nebulizing anticholinergics, it is recommended to use a mouthpiece rather than a mask, as it prevents the drug from coming into direct contact with the patients' eyes and causing acute angle closed glaucoma. The choice of one or the other should preferably be made by the patient, after discussion of potential problems. Face masks usually need to be tightly fitted onto the face. Patients may find them uncomfortable, not practical and socially unacceptable. Some patients may also experience drying of the skin around the nose. Face masks tend to be easier to use if the patient finds it tiring holding a mouthpiece.

Maintenance of equipment

Nebulizers should be cleaned on a regular basis. This is to reduce the risk of microorganisms growing in the residual fluid or the formation of crystals. For patients using their nebulizer daily, the nebulizer and mouthpiece or mask should be disassembled and washed at least once a day in warm water with a little detergent and dried with a soft tissue (Barnes et al 1987) or left to dry. The nebulizer should then be run empty for a few seconds prior to its next use.

Clinical uses of nebulizer treatment

Use of nebulizers in asthma

In asthma care nebulizers are used to deliver:

- bronchodilators
- corticosteroids
- anticholinergics.

In acute severe asthma when large doses of bronchodilators are required, the most convenient route is by nebulization, using oxygen as the driving gas. Salbutamol 5 mg or terbutaline 10 mg should be administered. If the response is good, the treatment should be repeated every 4–6 hours until peak expiratory flow (PEF) is more than 75% of predicted normal. Nebulized beta$_2$ agonists exert their effect within 10–15 minutes of inhaling the drug. Beta$_2$ agonists in large doses are more likely to cause adverse effects such as tremor and tachycardia. In acute severe asthma, nebulized ipratropium bromide in combination with nebulized beta$_2$ agonists results in more effective bronchodilation (O'Driscoll et al 1989) than when either agent is used alone. A dose of 500 micrograms is as effective as a 1 mg dose. The recommended dose is therefore 500 micrograms in acute severe asthma.

In chronic asthma or in patients with brittle asthma, nebulizer treatment is not always required to control symptoms. However, when severe airflow obstruction is present, high doses from inhalers may not be sufficient and benefits may arise when large nebulized doses are administered. In such cases, a formal assessment should be performed in order to determine suitability of drug administration via this route.

Nebulized corticosteroids are usually given to patients who require large doses of inhaled or oral therapy in the management of severe asthma. The recommended dose is 1–2 mg twice daily or higher in severe asthma until control is achieved. A lower maintenance dose can then be prescribed. Nebulized budesonide at a dose of up to 8 mg daily has also be used in steroid dependent patients in an attempt to reduce the oral dose (Otulana et al 1992). In chronic asthma, use of nebulized corticosteroids is controversial. Benefits must be balanced against the cost of the treatment and the complexity of the therapy for the patient. There is a need for randomized, placebo-controlled studies, showing positive results, before wide use is implemented. Budesonide solution can be mixed with solutions of 0.9% saline, salbutamol, terbutaline, sodium cromoglycate or ipratropium bromide. The most common adverse effect of nebulized corticosteroids is irritation of the throat, hoarseness and cough. A twice daily administration minimizes the incidence of these adverse effects. Facial skin irritation may occur in patients using face masks instead of mouthpieces when nebulizing the drugs. Patients should be advised to wash the face and rinse the mouth after administration in order to reduce the risk of oral candida.

Use of nebulizers in COPD

In COPD nebulizers are used to deliver:

- bronchodilators
- anticholinergics.

In severe exacerbation of COPD, nebulized anticholinergics together with a bronchodilator can be administered every 4–6 hours. Nebulized ipratropium bromide at therapeutic doses is not likely to cause many adverse effects. Patients may, however, complain of dry mouth. In the elderly patient, response to beta$_2$ agonists may be lower than in younger patients (Connolly et al 1995). It is therefore crucial to consider the use of ipratropium bromide as a bronchodilator. In practice, ipratropium bromide can be mixed with salbutamol in the nebulizer chamber prior to immediate administration.

Use of nebulizers in bronchiectasis and cystic fibrosis

In bronchiectasis and cystic fibrosis nebulizers are used to deliver:

- bronchodilators
- corticosteroids
- antibiotics
- dornase alfa
- sodium chloride.

The indications for use of nebulized bronchodilators and corticosteroids in patients with cystic fibrosis and bronchiectasis are essentially the same as in asthma.

Nebulized antibiotics are generally prescribed for patients with cystic fibrosis and bronchiectasis who become colonized with *Pseudomonas aeruginosa*. Repeated infections with the organism causes a reduction in pulmonary function and makes eradication difficult. Administering nebulized antibiotics at early stages of colonization has been shown to delay chronic colonization (Littlewood et al 1985). The antibiotics most commonly used for nebulization are:

- colistin
- tobramycin/TOBI
- gentamicin.

The choice of antibiotic must always be based on sputum culture and sensitivities. Nebulized antibiotics should be used for long term therapy as prophylaxis rather than for the treatment of acute infections. The most common adverse effect from nebulized antibiotics is bronchoconstriction. This can be minimized by nebulizing a beta$_2$ agonist prior to using the antibiotic. Mouthpieces should be used rather than face masks in order to maximize pulmonary deposition (Everard et al 1993). Systemic absorption of nebulized antibiotics is minimal and at high doses this therapy has been shown to be effective and safe (Ramsey et al 1993). There are also concerns for other individuals in the same environment where the antibiotics are nebulized (Littlewood et al 1993), therefore it is important that the nebulizer is filtered or vented.

The recommended dosage of dornase alfa is 2.5 mg daily and it should be nebulized using a jet nebulizer driven by compressed air. Ultrasonic nebulizers are unsuitable for use since they compromise the structure of the molecule. Dornase alfa also needs to be stored between 2 and 8°C due to sensitivity to heat and light. Timing of dornase alfa administration in relation to chest physiotherapy is also important. The recommendation is to administer the drug at least half an hour but preferably two hours after chest physiotherapy sessions. Dornase alfa is licensed only for cystic fibrosis (CF) patients with mild to moderate disease. The high yearly cost of the dornase alfa suggests that a trial period during which benefits are proven would provide a tool to select suitable patients (Bollert et al 1999).

Sodium chloride 0.9% and 3% nebulized can be useful in providing increased humidification to thick tenacious sputum as experienced by patients with cystic fibrosis and bronchiectasis. This is particularly useful prior to chest physiotherapy as it allows thinning of secretions and therefore easier sputum clearance.

Use of nebulizers in HIV/AIDS

In HIV/AIDS patients, nebulized pentamidine is used in the treatment or prophylaxis of *Pneumocystis carinii* pneumonia when other treatments have failed. The choice of a nebulizer and compressor, which can produce small droplets, is very important when pentamidine is used. Deposition in the alveoli is desired in order to provide both effective prophylaxis and to reduce bronchoconstriction.

MEDICATION ADHERENCE

The term 'patient compliance' has been widely used in the literature. Although very difficult to define, it usually refers to a behavioural state whereby the patient is expected to follow advice given by a healthcare professional. Medication adherence has been defined as the extent to which patients fulfil the intention of the pre-scriber in taking medication (McGavock et al 1996). Non-compliance is often viewed as the patient's responsibility, but it can be equally a failure of the relationship between patient and healthcare professional. Adherence is probably a more appropriate term as it better emphasizes the role of patients in negotiating their health-care. To take this concept a step further, the model of concordance has been suggested (Clark 1998, Sanghani 1998). Concordance involves a consultation between the patient and the health-care professional. It is about informing the patient of the disease state, the available treat-ment options and associated risks. The aim is to achieve a partnership whereby the relationship between the patient and the healthcare profes-sional is an open one and where the major thera-peutic decisions are made by the patient.

Factors that contribute to poor adherence

Several factors which contribute to poor adher-ence have been identified. These can be categor-ized under:

- medication and disease factors
- patient factors
- interaction between patient and healthcare professionals.

Medication and disease factors

There are many factors that impede adherence to medication, which include:

- dosage regimen greater than twice per day
- long duration of therapy
- complex treatment regimens
- adverse drug effects
- characteristics of formulation (i.e. taste, smell, size)
- container size.

Dosage regimens of once or twice daily have been shown to improve adherence (Pullar et al 1988), compared with three or four times daily regimens. There is little difference between a once daily and a twice daily regimen. In general, it is thought that patients are less likely to forget to take their medication if the daily dosage is reduced and the regimen is simplified. Adherence also becomes more difficult when the medication regimen becomes more complex and the number of medications to be taken increases (Murray et al 1986). A study in an elderly population confirmed this finding (Kroenke & Pinlhot 1990).

Another factor which is likely to contribute to poor adherence is the long duration of treatment of certain conditions. It is possible that some patients will stop treatment once they feel well (Sumartojo 1993), even though treatment should be continued, such as with inhaled corticosteroids for controlling asthma and anti-tuberculosis medi-cations. It is well known that adherence to anti-tuberculosis medications is poor (Menzies et al 1993), and that the duration of therapy is one of the many contributing factors.

Serious adverse drug effects can also affect adherence. In one study (Dixon et al 1957) assess-ing adherence to anti-tuberculosis drugs, the high incidence of nausea and diarrhoea resulted in more than 50% of the patients not taking their medication. Although medication side effects are mentioned as one of the factors, it appears that less serious adverse effects do not deter patients from taking their medication. Other medication related factors leading to poor adherence include the actual characteristics of the formulation. Patients' dislike of the taste, smell or size of the tablets or capsules can affect adherence.

Patients may also sometimes find that medica-tion containers are not to their liking. The size may not be convenient and some containers may

Case study 5.2

Ingred is a 39-year-old lady who lives in a two bedroom flat with her husband and four children. She had been diagnosed with smear positive tuberculosis and was started on anti-tuberculosis chemotherapy. She had been feeling unwell for about 5 weeks and although shocked by the diagnosis was pleased when told that she should start to feel better within a few weeks. It was emphasized that she needed to take her anti-tuberculosis drugs for 6 months. She was delighted that she was beginning to feel better within 2 weeks and able to play with her children again. She continued to comply fully with her drug regimen for the next 5 weeks, but then found that she was missing the occasional day of treatment. When she went to pick up her next prescription the pharmacist asked her if she was remembering to take her medication regularly as he had noticed that she should have run out of her medication a week ago. She explained that since she had started to feel well again she had found it difficult to remember to take her drugs. The pharmacist explained the importance of taking her drugs and completing the 6 month course and suggested she contact the TB nurse specialist. After this initial relapse and following further education and support, Ingred adhered to her treatment.

be difficult to open. In some instances, patients may empty the doses from the original container into a 'more convenient' container and thus lose the instructions on dosage regimens.

Patient factors

Poor adherence to medication can also result from a wide range of patient related factors. These can be broadly categorized as intentional and non-intentional lack of adherence. Non-intentional poor adherence may be as a result of poor communication between the patient and the healthcare professional, leading to the patient not understanding the instructions. Physical and mental disabilities and presence of cognitive defects can also negatively influence adherence. However, intentional poor adherence suggests a decision making process by the patient deliberately not to adhere to a treatment regimen. This attitude may in turn be brought about by several factors. According to the health belief model (McGavock et al 1996), patients are more likely to follow a course of treatment if they perceive their

illness as being serious and if the treatment will offer more advantages and be effective without resulting in adverse effects. The patient's knowledge and understanding of the disease and medication used, past experience with healthcare professionals, view of medicines as a whole, information obtained from the public and influence from friends and family are all contributing factors leading to poor adherence (Bender et al 1997).

Interaction between patient and other healthcare professionals

The relationship between the patient and the practitioner can be a primary determinant of adherence. Poor quality of information provided can lead to lack of trust within the relationship and can be due to:

- low rapport
- poor communication
- lack of time.

Box 5.3 Summary of factors contributing to non-adherence

Treatment and disease

- Long duration of treatments
- Adverse effects of medication
- High frequency of administration
- Complex regimens
- Cost of obtaining medication
- Characteristics of medication form
- Disruption to lifestyle
- Chronic conditions with no apparent symptoms

Patient

- Physical and mental status
- Poor understanding of disease and drugs
- Belief that condition is not serious
- Negative attitude towards treatments
- Lack of support from family and friends
- Health beliefs
- Cultural beliefs

Practitioner–patient relationship

- Lack of information
- Poor communication
- Poor inter-relationship
- Lack of trust

Box 5.4 Strategies for improving adherence

Increase patient commitment

- Self-administration in hospital (Lowe et al 1995)
- Involve patients in monitoring their conditions
- Set up an agreement with regard to medication taking

Provide information

- Educate about the disease and treatment
- Educate about adverse effects
- Provide written information
- Plan to cope with future complications

Increase motivation

- Involve other family members in treatment
- Discuss the consequences of missed doses
- Use negotiation
- Use persuasion

Simplify the treatment regimen

- Use once or twice daily regimens
- Change formulation to suit patient
- Minimize disruption to lifestyle
- Use compliance aids
- Use medication monitors, e.g. MEMS

Provide additional help

- Help to resolve personal, work problems
- Refer to other healthcare professionals for advice
- Set up telephone help lines

This can be further complicated by a lack of understanding of the patient's beliefs and perceptions which then results in a lack of trust in the suggested regimen. Poor adherence can therefore also be as a result of various simple or complex factors (Box 5.3).

Methods to improve medication adherence

A variety of methods (educational and behavioural) for improving adherence have been devised. Although several strategies are described (Box 5.4), the emphasis has been on educating the patient, changing the behaviour of non-adherent patients and simplifying the regimens used. The approach may be helpful, but it must also be recognized that a positive relationship between the patient and the healthcare professional can contribute to positive outcomes. Continuity of care and patient satisfaction can also determine the extent of adherence.

In order to improve adherence, the healthcare professional must earn the patients' trust. Only by doing so can issues such as non-adherence be discussed and improved. Healthcare professionals should provide information and thoroughly explain the diagnosis, treatment options, possible adverse effects and the reasons for various course actions. It is also important to listen to patients and to appreciate their viewpoint.

Educational strategies benefit those who do not adhere because they lack information, and those patients who have misconceptions about their treatments. In order to provide effective patient education and counselling, caregivers should develop their knowledge and skills to help them assess their patients' needs, attitudes and beliefs. The environment in which counselling takes place should allow for privacy, be comfortable and should encourage patients to increase their involvement and to voice their concerns about adherence (American Society of Health System Pharmacists 1997). Box 5.5 outlines the basic medication related information required by patients in order to promote adherence (George 1987, Herman et al 1978).

Self-management of medication

Patient education and self-management are of benefit to patients since they empower them to make decisions, may potentially improve care and ultimately result in improved patient outcomes. Self-management of medication is a

---

Box 5.5 Information to promote adherence required by patients

- The medication name, its use, expected benefits and action
- Directions for administration
- Duration of treatment
- Potential adverse effects
- Action to take to minimize the occurrence of adverse effects
- Interaction with other drugs/food
- Storage conditions
- How to obtain further supply
- Action to take when a dose is missed
- Self-monitoring plan

Your best (target) peak flow is

zone 1

Your asthma is under control if

- it does not disturb your sleep
- it does not restrict your usual activities

and

- your peak flow readings are above

action

continue your normal medicines

Your preventer is

You should normally take

_____ puffs/doses

_____ times every day (using a spacer), even when you are feeling well

Your reliever is

You should normally only take it when you are short of breath, coughing or wheezing, or before exercise

Your other medicines are

zone 2

Your doctor or nurse may decide not to use this zone

Your asthma is getting worse if

- you are needing to use your

_____ (reliever inhaler) more than usual

- you are waking at night with asthma symptoms

and

- your peak flow readings have fallen to

between _____ and _____

action

increase your usual medicines

- Increase your

_____ (preventer inhaler) to

- Continue to take your

_____ (reliever inhaler) to relieve your asthma symptoms

zone 3

Your asthma is severe if

- you are getting increasingly breathless
- you are needing to use your

_____ (reliever inhaler) every

_____ hours or more often

and

- your peak flow readings have fallen to

between _____ and _____

action

start a course of steroid tablets

- Take

_____ prednisolone (steroid) tablets

(strength _____ mg each) and then

- Discuss with your doctor how and when to stop taking the tablets

- Continue to take your

_____ (reliever and preventer inhalers) as prescribed

zone 4

It is a medical alert/emergency if

- your symptoms continue to get worse

and

- your peak flow readings have fallen to below

Do not be afraid of causing a fuss.
Your doctor will want to see you urgently.

action

get help immediately

- Telephone your doctor straightaway on

or call an ambulance

- Take

_____ prednisolone (steroid) tablets

(strength _____ mg each) immediately

- Continue to take your

_____ (reliever inhaler) as needed, or every five to ten minutes until the ambulance arrives

Figure 5.13   Asthma self-management plan. Reproduced with permission from the National Asthma Campaign.

component of the self-management plan. When implemented in the correct way, it allows patients to take control and adjust treatments depending on the severity of their disease. Self-management plans have been used very successfully with asthma patients. The National Asthma Campaign produce pre-printed self-management plans (Fig 5.13) that can be individualized for the patient. This requires education, support and agreement between the healthcare professional and the patient.

The use of medication to treat and control respiratory disease can be guided by clinical guidelines, but for it to be successful it is necessary to view medication in a more holistic way. Prescribing drugs is the beginning of the treatment process but without adequate education and support the patient is unlikely to benefit from the interventions.

REFERENCES

Aitken M L, Burke W, McDonald G et al 1992 Recombinant human DNase inhalation in normal subjects and patients with cystic fibrosis. Journal of the American Medical Association 267: 1947–1951

American Society of Health System Pharmacists 1997 ASHP guidelines on pharmacists-conducted patient education and counselling. American Journal of Health System Pharmacists 54: 431–434

Auerbach H S, Williams M, Kirkpatrick J A et al 1985 Alternate day prednisone reduces morbidity and improves pulmonary function in cystic fibrosis. Lancet 2: 686–688

Barnes K L, Rollo C, Holgate S T et al 1987 Bacterial contamination of home nebulisers. British Medical Journal 295: 812

Bender B, Milgrom H, Rand C 1997 Nonadherence in asthmatic patients: is there a solution to the problem? Annals of Allergy, Asthma and Immunology 79: 177–186

Bollert F G E, Paton J Y, Marshall T G et al 1999 Recombinant DNase in cystic fibrosis: a protocol for targeted introduction through n-of-1 trials. European Respiratory Journal 13: 107–113

Boorsma N, Andersson N, Larsson P, Ullman A 1996 Assessment of the relative systemic potency of inhaled fluticasone and budesonide. European Respiratory Journal 9: 1427–1432

British Thoracic Society 1997a The British guidelines on asthma management. Thorax 52 (suppl 1): S1–S21

British Thoracic Society 1997b Guidelines for the management of chronic obstructive pulmonary disease. Thorax 52 (suppl 5): S1–S28

British Thoracic Society 1997c Current best practice for nebuliser treatment. Thorax 52 (suppl 2): S1–S106

Calderon-Zapata M, Davies R 1998 Recommended treatment of allergic rhinitis. Prescriber 9(9): 47–72

Chanarin N, Johnston S L 1994 Leukotrienes as a target in asthma therapy. Drugs 47(1): 12–24

Chung K F 1999 Zafirlukast: a leukotriene antagonist for asthma. Prescriber 10(1): 30–38

Clark C 1998 Concordance is not a PC term. Pharmaceutical Practice March: 83

Clark D J, Grove A, Cargill R I, Lipworth B J 1996 Comparative adrenal suppression with inhaled budesonide and fluticasone propionate in adult asthmatic patients. Thorax 51: 262–266

Connolly M J, Crowley J J, Charan N, Nielson C P, Vestal R E 1995 Impaired bronchodilator response to albuterol in healthy elderly men and women. Chest 108: 401–406

Devoy M A B, Fuller R W, Palmer J B D 1995 Are there any detrimental effects of the use of inhaled long-acting beta$_2$ agonists in the treatment of asthma? Chest 107(4): 1116–1124

Dixon W M, Stradling P, Wooton I D P 1957 Outpatient PAS. Lancet ii: 871–872

Drug and Therapeutics Bulletin 1998 Montelukast and zafirlukast in asthma. 36: 65–68

Du Bois R M 1995 Respiratory medicine. British Medical Journal 310: 1594–1597

Eigen H R, Rosenstein B J, FitzSimmons S, Schidlow D V 1995 A multicenter study of alternate day prednisone therapy in patients with cystic fibrosis. Journal of Pediatrics 126: 515–523

Elwood W 1997 Phosphodiesterase inhibitors: the next generation. Inpharma 1111: 9–10

Everard M L, Hardy J G, Milner A D 1993 Comparison of nebulised aerosol deposition in the lungs of healthy adults following oral and nasal inhalation. Thorax 48: 1045–1046

Everard M L, Evans M, Milner A D 1994 Is tapping jet nebulisers worthwhile? Archives of Disease in Childhood 70: 538–539

Fuchs H J, Borowitz D S, Christiansen D H et al 1994 The effect of aerolised recombinant human DNase on respiratory exacerbations and pulmonary function in patients with CF. New England Journal of Medicine 331: 637–642

Geddes D M 1992 Inhaled corticosteroids: benefits and risks. Thorax 47: 401–407

George C F 1987 Telling patients about their medicines. British Medical Journal 294: 1566–1567

Hall I P 1997 The future of asthma. British Medical Journal 314: 45–49

Hendeles L, Marshik P L 1997 Zafirlukast for chronic asthma: convenient and generally safe, but is it effective? Annals of Pharmacotherapy 31: 1084–1086

Hendeles L, Iafrate R P, Weinberger M 1984 A clinical and pharmacokinetic basis for the selection and use of slow release theophylline products. Clinical Pharmacokinetics 9: 95–135

Herman F, Herxheimer A, Lionel N D W 1978 Package inserts for prescribed medicines: what minimum information do patients need? British Medical Journal 2: 1132–1135

Hubbard R C, McElvaney N G, Birrer P et al 1992 A preliminary study of aerolized recombinant human deoxyribonuclease 1 in the treatment of cystic fibrosis. New England Journal of Medicine 326: 812–815

Jaffe A, Francis J, Rosenthal M, Bush A 1998 Long term azithromycin may improve lung function in children with cystic fibrosis. Lancet 351: 420

Knowles G, Knowles V 1998 Guide to drug treatment of coughs and colds. Prescriber 9(17): 69–83

Konstan M, Byard P J, Huppel C L, Davis P B 1995 Effect of high dose ibuprofen in patients with cystic fibrosis. New England Journal of Medicine 332: 848–854

Kroenke K, Pinlhot E M 1990 Reducing polypharmacy in the elderly. A controlled trial of physician feedback. Journal of the American Geriatrics Society 38: 31–36

Littlewood J, Miller M G, Ghoneim A T, Ramsden C H 1985 Nebulised colomycin in early colonisation in cystic fibrosis. Lancet i: 865

Littlewood J M, Smye S W, Cunliffe H 1993 Aerosol antibiotic treatment in cystic fibrosis. Archives of Disease in Childhood 68: 788–792

Lowe C J, Raynor D K, Courtney E A et al 1995 Effects of self medication programme on knowledge of drugs and compliance with treatment in elderly patients. British Medical Journal 310: 1229–1231

McElvaney N G, Hubbard R C, Birrer P et al 1991 Aerosol alpha 1-antitrypsin treatment for cystic fibrosis. Lancet 337: 392–394

McGavock H, Britten N, Weinman J 1996 A review of the literature on drug adherence. Royal Pharmaceutical Society of Great Britain, London

Martin R J, Kraft M 1996 Nocturnal asthma: therapeutic considerations. Clinical Immunotherapy 6: 443–453

Menzies R, Rocher I, Vissandjee B 1993 Factors associated with compliance in treatment of tuberculosis. Tubercle and Lung Disease 74(1): 32–37

Murray M D, Darnell J, Weinberger M, Marz B L 1986 Factors contributing to medication non-compliance in elderly public housing tenants. Drug Intelligence and Clinical Pharmacy 20: 146–152

Nikander K 1997 Adaptive aerosol delivery: the principles. European Respiratory Review 7(51): 385–387

O'Driscoll B R, Taylor R J, Horsley M G et al 1989 Nebulised salbutamol with and without ipratropium bromide in acute airflow obstruction. Lancet i: 1418–1420

Otulana B A, Varma N, Bullock A, Higenbottam T 1992 High dose nebulised steroid in the treatment of chronic steroid-dependent asthma. Respiratory Medicine 86: 105–108

Pauwels R A, Lofdahl C G, Postma D S et al 1997 Effect of inhaled formoterol and budesonide on exacerbations of asthma. New England Journal of Medicine 337: 1405–1411

Pedersen S, O'Byrne P 1997 A comparison of the efficacy and safety of inhaled corticosteroids in asthma. Allergy 52 (suppl 39): 1–34

Pullar T, Birtwell A J, Wiles P J et al 1988 Use of a pharmacological indicator to compare compliance with tablets prescribed to be taken once, twice or three times daily. Clinical Pharmacology and Therapeutics 44: 540–545

Ramsey B W 1996 Management of pulmonary disease in patients with cystic fibrosis. New England Journal of Medicine 335: 179–188

Ramsey B W, Dorkin H L, Eisenberg J D et al 1993 Efficacy of aerosolised tobramycin in patients with cystic fibrosis. New England Journal of Medicine 328: 1740–1746

Ramsey B W, Pepe M S, Quan J M et al 1999 Intermittent administration of inhaled tobramycin in patients with cystic fibrosis. New Journal of Medicine 340(1): 23–30

Sampson A, Costello J 1995 Treatment guidelines for asthma – where will leukotriene receptor antagonists fit in? The Pharmaceutical Journal 255: 26–30

Sanghani P 1998 Comfortable with concordance? The Pharmaceutical Journal 261: 84

Selroos O, Backman R, Forsen K O et al 1994 Local side effects during 4 year treatment with inhaled corticosteroids – a comparison between pressurized metered-dose inhalers and Turbuhaler. Allergy 49(10): 888–890

Smith G 1986 A patient's view of cystic fibrosis. Journal of Adolescent Health Care 7: 134–138

Spector S L 1997 Leukotriene activity modulation in asthma. Drugs 54(3): 369–384

Sumartojo E 1993 When tuberculosis treatment fails. A social behavioural account of patient adherence. American Review of Respiratory Diseases 147(5): 1311–1320

Youlten L 1996 Hay fever: symptoms, signs and treatment. Prescriber 7(10): 43–66

6

Living with chronic respiratory illness and breathlessness

Carl Margereson

Respiratory disease is responsible for a great deal of chronic ill health in developed countries such as the UK. More people consult their GPs for respiratory problems than for any other group of diseases and the cost in terms of medical intervention and days off work, and to the employment prospects of the next generation as a consequence of time lost from school is correspondingly large (British Lung Foundation 1996). It is likely that the psychosocial and economic costs of respiratory illness will continue to rise, indeed will most likely escalate well into the 21st century.

In the last 30 years tremendous improvements have been seen in many areas of respiratory medicine and healthcare generally. Developments in diagnostics, pharmacological agents, bioengineering, dietetics, physiotherapy and surgical techniques in respiratory care, although not necessarily offering a cure, have been important in the management and improvement of symptoms. The continuing growth in respiratory nurse specialists both in hospital and in the community has meant that the specific needs of patients with respiratory illness may be met more effectively. However, more studies are needed to demonstrate the impact of respiratory nurse specialists on health outcome. Appropriate measures are needed not only in the area of disease progression but also in the area of quality of life.

Whilst these developments are to be welcomed, improved life expectancy for patients with respiratory illness has presented new problems and challenges. With more patients surviving longer, health professionals are likely to encounter more and more patients with respiratory difficulties in a variety of healthcare settings. Quality of life issues are of increasing concern for patients, health professionals and policy makers. Later we will explore policy implications concerning chronic respiratory illness. Initially however, it is to the impact of respiratory illness on individuals and their families that we turn.

An important aim of this chapter is to convey to the reader how chronic respiratory illness may impact on the patient in a number of complex ways. To do this a number of dimensions possibly contributing to the patient's 'illness experience' must be explored. The majority of patients with chronic respiratory illness enter the formal healthcare system only for brief periods during their lives. The rest of the time they must cope at home and how effective this coping is will depend on a host of different factors. Increasing recognition, therefore, is given to the importance of assisting patients to manage their illness more effectively and there is an increasing volume of literature exploring the concept of self-management.

THEORETICAL APPROACHES IN SELF-MANAGEMENT

Self-management has been defined as the performance of preventive or therapeutic healthcare activities, often in collaboration with healthcare professionals (Tobin et al 1986). A number of different disciplines have contributed in this area but it is health psychology and health education that perhaps provide most of the theoretical underpinning in self-management. An important aim in self-management is the adoption of behaviours by individuals which are health enhancing. Earlier theories in behavioural psychology placed great emphasis on classical and operant conditioning. Behavioural change, however, is more complex than once thought and the development of social learning theory recognizes that if behavioural change is to occur then individuals' beliefs and their social environment must also be taken into account. Research in social learning theory therefore stresses the importance

of cognitive processes and the environment in behavioural change.

Social learning theory encompasses:

- conditioning (e.g. classical and operant)
- social and environmental influences
- cognitions (e.g. beliefs, perceptions, attitudes).

All these may influence behavioural change.

Whilst social learning theory recognizes that there are three major dimensions involved in determining behaviour, a physiological dimension is lacking. Therefore a model for self-management of chronic illness was developed which included a fourth physiological dimension (Thoresen & Kirmil-Gray 1983). More recently, a similar framework has been used to demonstrate how these four dimensions in chronic illness may act as pathways possibly leading not only to behavioural changes but also to emotional and psychological difficulties (Cohen & Rodriguez 1995).

The above model is useful not only when considering the impact of chronic respiratory illness but also when assessing the patient's needs. All too often in healthcare settings the major focus is on the physiological dimension, usually in the method of symptom control. Although effective symptom control is, of course, important, failure to address the other three dimensions may well result in difficulties with coping and adaptation. Indeed, it is more than likely that psychosocial factors are more important than symptoms in determining how well the patient adjusts.

In exploring the impact of chronic respiratory illness this chapter will address the following dimensions:

- pathophysiology and symptoms
- behavioural responses
- cognitions
- social and environmental factors.

PATHOPHYSIOLOGY AND SYMPTOMS

There are many respiratory diseases which can result in chronic ill health but for the majority of patients varying degrees of breathlessness and fatigue will become troublesome as progressive respiratory impairment develops. As the processes of ventilation and oxygenation are disrupted and tissue hypoxia develops, certain pathophysiological manifestations of the disease will be seen:

- fatigue
- weakness
- activity intolerance
- breathlessness
- coughing
- possible changes in appearance
- sleep patterns may be disrupted
- hypoxia, hypercapnia and the use of medications may cause temporary states of confusion or delusion.

(Shekleton 1987)

Many of the above changes will be experienced by most patients at some point. However, in one study of patients with chronic respiratory disease 82% perceived breathlessness as a big problem in their daily lives (Williams 1990). Breathlessness and fatigue are directly linked to functional ability and as symptoms increase patients will find it increasingly difficult to carry out their normal activities of daily living. Measures of symptoms and lung function explain significant variance in level of functioning in patients with chronic obstructive pulmonary disease (COPD) who are oxygen dependent (Lee et al 1991), with symptoms a better predictor of functioning than lung function.

The first area to be explored in this section, therefore, will be breathlessness. An understanding of the mechanisms resulting in breathlessness will contribute to a more rational approach when considering interventions. As there is increasing evidence of significant psychosocial stress in the lives of some patients who are chronically ill, the second section will consider the relevance of the stress response in chronic illness. One suggestion offered here is that ongoing psychosocial stress may further compromise cardiorespiratory status in vulnerable patients. This highlights the importance of helping patients improve their coping ability, thus reducing psychosocial stress and the potentially harmful effects of the stress response.

Understanding breathlessness

Dyspnoea or breathlessness remains somewhat of an enigma as there is still a great deal we do not know about it. Although the terms dyspnoea and breathlessness are used interchangeably it has been suggested that breathlessness describes the phenomenon more accurately, particularly from the patient's perspective. These two terms will be used interchangeably here.

Breathlessness is a very subjective sensation and this makes research in this area very difficult to undertake. Much of the work in this area has been carried out by physiologists and, although progress has been made, the mechanisms resulting in breathlessness are still not fully understood. Where there is agreement, however, is in the recognition that dyspnoea is multidimensional in nature (McCord & Cronin-Stubbs 1992). The sensation of breathlessness and its interpretation and reporting by patients can be influenced by anger, depression, anxiety and cognitive impairment (Dales et al 1989). Fortunately, for many of us breathing is something we do not have to think about, but for many patients breathing becomes an uncomfortable and almost constant frightening struggle.

The psychophysical relationships possibly operating in dyspnoea have been extensively studied. Physiological mechanisms involve sensory receptors in the lung and chest wall, sensory input and processing of this sensory input by the central nervous system (Altose et al 1985). How the patient perceives and tolerates breathlessness is probably more to do with psychological rather than pathophysiological factors. Indeed, often there is very little correlation between objective measurements of lung function and perceived breathlessness.

Sensory receptors

A number of sensory receptors have been identified in the chest wall, airways and lung parenchyma. Chest wall receptors (e.g. in muscles and tendons) are able to detect changes in respiratory muscle length/tension relationship, alerting different areas in the central nervous system (cortex, cerebellum and medulla oblongata) to the moment to moment changes occurring. Also identified in the chest wall are nerve endings referred to as Type III and IV nociceptors which, in addition to sensing length/tension changes, can also fire as a result of chemical change such as increased lactate, K^+ ions and bradykinin (Frazier & Revellete 1991). These latter effects may be particularly important in chronic respiratory illness where there is a great increase in respiratory muscle activity with fatigue.

There are also three types of receptors in the lungs and airways: irritant, stretch and juxtacapillary (J) receptors. Each type is stimulated under different conditions. Irritant receptors in the airway epithelium are activated by noxious gases, dusts and in a number of lung diseases when chemical mediators are released. Not only do they increase minute volume but they also result in bronchoconstriction.

Stretch receptors are located in the smooth muscle of bronchi, for example, and have a minor role in normal breathing. They help to maintain tidal volume when breathing is stimulated. J receptors are found in the alveolar walls. These are stimulated when there is excess fluid in the alveoli and by inflammatory mediators such as histamine, bradykinin and prostaglandin. J receptors are probably activated, therefore, in pulmonary oedema, pneumonia and pulmonary embolism (Carrieri et al 1984).

The work of breathing

Energy needs to be expended during breathing for contraction of respiratory muscles in order to overcome several opposing forces during inspiration. Compliance work is necessary to counteract the normal inward elastic recoil of lung tissue (elastance). In health, lung and chest wall compliance is good and very little pressure change is needed to move air into the lungs. However, in some respiratory disorders the lungs become very stiff, resulting in poor compliance. In this situation much greater pressures are required for each tidal volume.

Another force that must be overcome during breathing is airway resistance. Most airway resistance is found in the larger upper airways where airflow is more turbulent. Although the terminal and respiratory bronchioles are smaller the total cross sectional area is greater, therefore resistance is lower than in the upper air passages. In obstructive disorders such as COPD and bronchial asthma airway narrowing occurs due to a number of factors. The resulting increased resistance will increase the work of breathing.

When the work of breathing is increased then the ventilatory load is increased and the body must respond to this by increasing both respiratory muscle tension and respiratory motor output (from the medulla oblongata) in order to maintain effective tidal volumes. When breathing is restricted in some way and/or the respiratory muscles are weakened, it is the increased effort (increased motor output) that contributes to the perception of breathlessness. The sensory impulses generated by the sensory receptors described earlier are transmitted by the vagus nerve and these are important in further increasing motor output and therefore the perception of breathlessness.

Increased respiratory effort

It appears, therefore, that the feeling of breathlessness depends on the degree of central motor (efferent) output, the intensity of the sensory (afferent) input from lung receptors and also activation of the central and peripheral chemoreceptors (as a result of changes in blood H^+ ions, PaO_2 and $PaCO_2$) (Chonan et al 1987, Redline et al 1991). Campbell et al (1980) also suggest that it is increased sensory input from respiratory muscles due to length/tension inappropriateness that results in breathlessness. In other words, the muscle shortening occurring in response to any given respiratory motor output is less than expected, resulting in an imbalance between motor output and the chest movement that is to be accomplished. The resulting increase in respiratory motor impulse output from the respiratory centre is responsible for the increasing sense of effort in breathlessness. With changes in blood chemistry due to hypoxaemia and hypercapnia, chemoreceptor activity will further increase the motor output to the respiratory muscles.

Box 6.1 Summary of the processes possibly contributing to the sensation of breathlessness

- Increased work of breathing (e.g. reduced compliance, increased airway resistance)
- Increased ventilatory load
- Inappropriate length/tension relationship of respiratory muscles
- Increased sensory input from chemoreceptors and lung receptors
- Increased motor output from medulla oblongata (i.e. increases the sense of effort)

Most respiratory diseases result in either a restrictive or an obstructive ventilatory pattern and these changes can increase the work of breathing considerably. The increased ventilatory load will increase the degree of muscular effort required to maintain the same tidal volumes. Both expiratory and inspiratory loads on the respiratory muscles may be increased (Keilty 1998). Accessory muscles are employed that not only increase energy expenditure but also increase the sensation of breathlessness.

Respiratory muscles in respiratory disease may be at a mechanical disadvantage and hyper-inflation in COPD, for example, will result in shortening of inspiratory muscle length and a decrease in the force of muscle contraction. Long term inactivity, poor nutrition, hypoxaemia and hypercapnia may lead to increasing muscle weakness and poor function. This can become life threatening during an acute crisis where force of contraction cannot respond to an increase in ventilatory demand. Ventilatory (pump) failure will result in poor gaseous exchange and deteriorating arterial blood gases with retention of carbon dioxide.

Increased knowledge regarding the altered pulmonary mechanics in respiratory disease enables a rational approach in the relief of dyspnoea and therefore an improvement in respiratory function generally. Because of the relationship between breathlessness and anxiety, interventions which alter perception may help patients to cope a little better with this distressing symptom. The use of cognitive–behavioural techniques, for example, may help to modify those cognitions, possibly decreasing breathlessness.

The stress response

The relationship between physical status and adjustment/quality of life is far from clear, with several authors suggesting that the link is weak. It is argued that although pathological processes in chronic respiratory disease interact with psychological and psychosocial factors as determinants of the individual's quality of life, psychosocial factors may be far more important than symptoms such as breathlessness (Griffith & Kronenberg 1991, Guyatt et al 1987, Kinsman et al 1983, Neill et al 1985, Salata & Berman 1981).

The reader may be wondering why the physiology of stress is being addressed at this point. Physiological, behavioural, cognitive and social factors may act independently or together in contributing to increased anxiety and stress. Distressing symptoms, complex treatments, loss of independence, and relationship, vocational and financial difficulties may all add to the patient's psychosocial stress. Some have argued that chronic illness itself is a major stressor. It is not surprising that for many patients with a chronic illness there is accompanying psychological disturbance.

Perceptions of symptoms and of vulnerability to disease contribute to the production of emotional reactions to illness (Leventhal & Patrick-Miller 1993). Ongoing psychosocial stress will result in physiological changes, which although normally adaptive in the short term, may be maladaptive if continued long term.

The physiology of stress

We have all experienced the 'fight or flight' stress response that is triggered when we are threatened and our survival is paramount. The resulting elevated levels of circulating catecholamines such as adrenaline (epinephrine) and noradrenaline prepare the body to cope with this increased challenge. Indeed, such a response, which is more often than not short lived, is actively sought by those seeking the 'adrenaline rush' from high-risk pursuits. These acute physiological changes are thought not to be damaging to our health long term. The stress response involves neuroendocrine physiological changes which are mediated through the hypothalamus, pituitary and adrenal glands. Sympathetic activation of the autonomic nervous system results in the release of noradrenaline from sympathetic nerves and adrenaline and noradrenaline from the adrenal medulla. Another important endocrine response, but slower acting than the sympathetic arousal, is the release of adrenocorticotrophic hormone (ACTH) from the anterior pituitary gland, which stimulates the release of cortisol, a glucocorticoid, from the adrenal cortex. All these somewhat complex changes were described by Selye (1956) who referred to the response as the 'general adaptation syndrome' (GAS).

The stress response described above may no longer be adaptive in chronic illness and may be detrimental in someone whose respiratory (and possibly cardiac) reserves are already compromised because of chronic respiratory illness. Raised circulating catecholamines may have a number of adverse effects. Oxygen demand will be increased further and this will lead to increased ventilatory effort. The effects of adrenaline on cardiac beta receptors will be to increase the heart rate and the contractility of the myocardium. This will increase pulmonary arterial blood flow and may contribute to $\dot{V}/\dot{Q}$ problems (e.g. right to left physiological shunt) with worsening hypoxaemia. In a patient with poor cardiac reserves increases in intravascular volume, myocardial oxygen demand, cardiac output and blood pressure may precipitate heart failure and pulmonary oedema.

With ongoing psychosocial stress there may be elevated levels of cortisol to counterbalance the body's defensive reactions to stress, thus a number of effects are seen (Munck et al 1984). Elevated cortisol can depress the immune response, particularly the numbers of T (helper) lymphocytes. The resulting reduced resistance may further increase the patient's vulnerability and contribute to recurrent infections. Unfortunately very little research has been undertaken exploring the effects of stress on pulmonary pathophysiology.

Failure to address issues relating to psychosocial stress will do nothing to increase the effi-

cacy of prescribed treatment programmes. It is suggested that understanding the patient's capacity for stress adaptation and intervening appropriately are central to effective care, especially from a nursing perspective (Kline Leidy et al 1990).

BEHAVIOURAL RESPONSES

Behavioural responses in chronic respiratory illness may be determined by physiological, cognitive and social factors and all these dimensions are to be addressed if patients are to be guided towards coping more effectively. Studies strongly suggest that the disruption of life caused by chronic illness is a constant source of stress. The coping strategies employed may therefore be important predictors of successful adjustment and it is therefore crucial that behaviours which are either potentially health damaging or health enhancing are monitored appropriately.

Symptom control is an important objective in the patient's treatment programme. As breathlessness and fatigue become more troublesome then functional impairment may result, with varying degrees of disability. The patient finds it more difficult to complete activities of daily living and independence may be affected. Assessment should involve all behavioural responses, which are attempts at coping, successfully or otherwise. Labelling patients as difficult or non-copers because of what may be seen as inappropriate behaviour should be avoided. Self-management involves many different individual behaviours and it is important to assess each rather than making a judgement on the perceived global picture (Eakin & Glasgow 1997).

Increasing difficulty with activities of daily living reminds patients of their increasing disability and can affect quality of life. Although the symptoms of breathlessness and fatigue are mild in the beginning, eventually household duties, work performance and leisure interests will be affeced. Profound breathlessness on exertion may limit the patient's activities dramatically and at times may be associated with panic and fear. Williams (1990) identified a 'vicious circle' in patients who are breathless that often leads them to avoid anx-

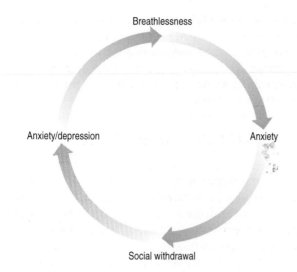

Figure 6.1 Breathlessness and anxiety cycle.

iety provoking situations, resulting in withdrawal from social interactions with others (Fig. 6.1).

Yet despite worsening symptoms some patients will cope surprisingly well and there is great variability in functional performance even between patients with similar symptoms and capacity. Moreover, pulmonary function tests are not very good predictors of functional ability (Jones et al 1989, Lee et al 1991), although symptoms are. It would seem prudent, therefore, to attempt to relieve distressing symptoms as much as possible.

A physiological exploration of stress has already been outlined. It is impossible, however, to consider stress without addressing coping. Research in this area recognizes that the individual's perception of a stressor is important. This transactional approach to stress is mainly credited to Lazarus & Folkman (1984) who suggest that coping in response to stress involves both primary and secondary appraisal. Primary appraisal involves determining whether or not the stressor is threatening. If the threat is real then secondary appraisal involves the utilization of various coping mechanisms that the individual has. Lazarus & Folkman see coping as either emotion focused or problem focused. In emotion focused coping there are attempts to modify the emotional impact of the stressor perhaps by

smoking, drinking excess alcohol, overeating or non-adherence to treatment. Similarly, a number of ego defence mechanisms may be employed such as denial, projection and regression. Emotion focused coping may help the patient in the short term but in the long term such strategies are maladaptive and will only lead to more difficulties such as poor control of symptoms.

Conversely, problem focused coping involves the utilization of skills to modify the source of the stressor. Such responses may involve problem-solving skills and additional skills needed for facilitating effective self-management. Health professionals must acquire the necessary specialist knowledge and skills to enable patients to develop behavioural responses that are more adaptive. Failure to achieve this may result in poor adherence manifested by poor symptom control, frequent hospitalization and overall reduction in quality of life. As control becomes more difficult, anxiety and depression may result in further inappropriate behavioural responses (Gregory & Smeltzer 1983). Emotional changes, particularly if sudden, may be especially problematic in respiratory illness, increasing the work and perception of breathing. Avoidance of such emotional states becomes crucial and the patient learns to live in an emotional 'straight jacket' (Dudley et al 1973). Inappropriate coping res-

Case study 6.1

Peter was a 57-year-old married man with cryptogenic fibrosing alveolitis, who continued to work despite being quite breathless even on gentle exertion. He worked as an accountant and his journey each day involved a round trip of over 100 miles. He blamed his illness on himself and had nothing but praise for the hospital. There was a punishing daily work schedule and cigarettes and alcohol seemed to help him through it. He admitted trying not to think about his illness and wanted life to carry on as normal.

Carrying on 'as normal' for Peter was not without cost. He had not re-evaluated his situation in light of his increasing symptoms and muddled through each day the best way he could. It is difficult to know why Peter behaved in this way but his responses were inappropriate and he did not seem to be coping too well with his illness. (Margereson 1998)

ponses may further increase the patient's difficulties and this is illustrated in Case study 6.1.

It is often difficult to ascertain whether psychological distress is a cause or a consequence of poor coping. It is acknowledged, however, that in patients with COPD depression, anxiety and selected psychiatric symptoms are common (Agle et al 1973, Borak et al 1991, Porzelius et al 1992). Psychological distress in COPD is associated with poor body image, increased loneliness, reduced social support, dissatisfaction with social support and negative self concept (Keele-Card et al 1993, Nicholas & Leuner 1992). This illustrates the somewhat complex interplay of all the dimensions being explored in this chapter.

It would appear that psychological difficulties are particularly prevalent in patients with COPD compared to other chronic illness groups. Other groups of patients with chronic respiratory illness do not seem to have the same degree of psychological problems. In a study of 240 patients with cystic fibrosis, perceived quality of life was similar to that in people with minor non-acute conditions (Congleton et al 1997). The fact that patients with cystic fibrosis have had a lifetime to adjust to the limitations imposed by the disease may be an important factor here. Interestingly, in this study the perceived quality of life in females with cystic fibrosis was better than that perceived by males. In another small study of 11 individuals with neuromuscular disorders requiring assisted ventilation, but cared for in the community, perceived quality of life was again high with most in the study not perceiving themselves as ill.

Whilst most studies of psychosocial adjustment have been performed in patients with COPD, generalizations must be avoided. Patients with chronic respiratory illness are not homogeneous and further studies are needed to explore the psychosocial impact of illness on other groups with different respiratory diseases. Similarly, there are likely to be differences in how various age groups experience and cope with chronic illness. Anticipated developmental changes are experienced by most people and these normative life transitions may be accompanied by additional health/illness stressors (Werner 1993). An awareness of these normal life transitions will prepare carers for pos-

sible problems which may come along as a result of perceived stressors such as changing roles and responsibilities. Most nursing frameworks, in considering the health/illness continuum, recognize the importance of a developmental perspective, e.g. the activities of living model (Roper et al 1996).

What is important is that health professionals are able to identify those patients who are experiencing psychological difficulties. Psychological distress predicts restricted activities of daily living and emotional/psychosocial factors are more predictive of functional capacity than are traditional physiological measurements (Beck et al 1988, Graydon & Ross 1995). Adjustment disorders occur in approximately one-quarter of general medical patients with anxiety and depressive disorders in a further 12–16% (Royal College of Physicians & Royal College of Psychiatrists 1995), yet psychological assessment is poorly addressed by health professionals. Given the current resource difficulties in the health service together with throughput in hospitals, it is hardly surprising that the psychosocial needs of patients are often unmet. However, it is important that those caring for patients with chronic illness are able to identify those most vulnerable so that appropriate intervention may be offered.

An inappropriate behavioural response as a consequence of poor coping may be difficulty in adherence by some patients to treatment regimens. This has been identified as a problem in most populations of patients with chronic illness. Non-adherence may occur not only with medication but with health promotion advice such as lifestyle changes, e.g. diet and exercise. Moreover, problems with non-adherence are more likely when regimens are long term and complex (Goodall & Halford 1991) as is often the case in respiratory illness. Lack of information may also be a factor as was the case with June in Case study 6.2. Although there are methodological difficulties in measuring non-adherence in patients, rates are estimated to be 30–60% (Dolce et al 1991, Kelloway et al 1994, O'Brien et al 1992).

Although non-adherence is a problem in chronic illness generally, the major focus in research has been on bronchial asthma. Despite an increase in asthma medication over the past 20 years, morbi-

Case study 6.2

June was a 58-year-old married woman who had been taking steroids long term. During a visit to the hospital her doctor reduced the steroid dose because of an improvement. June believed that this had been done because she was no longer responding to the treatment and for several months she worried a great deal about this.

Some time later June was watching a television programme about steroid therapy and this increased her anxiety considerably. She decided to cut the dose down herself over a 1 year period. During the next hospital appointment her test results showed that there had been a deterioration and though the doctors were puzzled she didn't say anything.

It was during an interview for research purposes that June disclosed this information. This illustrates how behavioural responses are driven by cognitions and how important it is to explore the patient's health beliefs. This may have avoided some of the distress which June must have suffered. (Margereson 1998)

dity and mortality remain alarmingly high. The development of more effective interventions to facilitate adherence may contribute to improved outcome in this group of patients. Factors promoting adherence are identified in Box 6.2.

The principles of self-management are relevant to all patients who are chronically ill and who are attempting to make the necessary adaptation. The use of self-management plans in some patient groups has been promising. Addressing the behavioural aspects of disease includes addressing actions that affect risk factors for disease development, psychobiological interactions in disease occurrence and behaviours useful in managing or controlling the course of the disease (Kohler et al 1996).

Giving information to patients with chronic respiratory illness is important in order to increase their knowledge regarding all aspects of their illness. Information must be tailored to each patient's specific needs but the use of diagrams and models is helpful in increasing awareness of the disorder. Partnership between patient and health worker is a significant factor in contributing towards the effectiveness of self-management. Patient education should be seen as an active process that is built upon open communication involving an integrative approach and joint development of a programme (Creticos 1994). Studies show that when patients are actively involved in the management of their asthma, for example, overall control is more effective (Clark et al 1994).

Health professionals caring for patients with chronic respiratory illness must be aware of the components that need to be addressed. Clark et al (1991), in a review of the literature on self-management, identified a number of common self-management behaviours across several chronic illness groups (Box 6.3).

Controlled studies measuring the effectiveness of self-management in asthma have demonstrated improved health outcomes, including reductions in morbidity and the use of resources. The use of written action plans seems to be particularly beneficial compared to programmes that don't use such plans. Self-monitoring and regular review are also important determinants of improved asthma con-

---

Box 6.2 Factors promoting adherence to treatment regimens

- Effective patient teaching
- Therapeutic relationship built on mutual respect
- Effective self-monitoring skills (e.g. symptoms)
- Exploring patients' health beliefs
- Use of self-management plans and/or contracts
- Realistic goal setting
- Effective problem solving skills
- Effective social support

Box 6.3 Self-management tasks

- Recognizing/responding to symptoms
- Monitoring physical indicators
- Controlling triggers to symptoms
- Using medication
- Managing acute episodes
- Maintaining nutrition and diet
- Maintaining adequate exercise/activity
- Giving up smoking
- Using stress reduction techniques
- Seeking information
- Adapting to work
- Managing relations with significant others
- Managing emotions and psychological responses

(Clark et al 1991)

trol. There have been a number of randomized controlled studies which have been able to show various benefits of such an approach in practice (Allen et al 1995, Cote et al 1997, Kotses et al 1996). These benefits have included:

- reduction in the number of patients requiring hospitalization
- reduction in the number of patients requiring unscheduled visits to doctors
- less use of Accident and Emergency department
- fewer days off work/school
- less nocturnal asthma.

The components of self-management programmes can vary and have involved one-to-one education, group sessions, self-monitoring, diary keeping (Allen et al 1995), nurse run clinics (Charlton et al 1990) and written action plans (Cote et al 1997). Lengths of programmes have varied from one hour to more than twelve hours for each patient over several weeks. It is difficult to identify which components have the greatest impact but education, self-monitoring and written action plans appear to be key areas which increase efficacy.

Time may be an important factor in the implementation of a comprehensive self-management programme. Wilson et al (1993) carried out a controlled trial of two forms of self-management education. Patients were randomly assigned to small group education or individual teaching and two controlled groups involving an information workbook or no formal asthma education. An interesting point in this study is that both small group and individual education were associated with significant benefits. The patients' understanding of their condition and its treatment, their motivation and their confidence were all increased. Not only this, but the group programme was easier to administer, better received by patients and educators and more cost-effective.

Self-management strategies may be of benefit in other groups of patients with chronic respiratory illness. Unfortunately there has been very little focus on the behavioural issues involved in other disorders such as COPD, interstitial lung disease and bronchiectasis. This is surprising

given that behavioural factors in the management of these disorders are just as important as in the disorders where self-management has shown positive outcomes. It is important that in focusing on specific groups other groups of patients with respiratory illness are not excluded and disadvantaged. Although some of these groups are smaller, the numbers involved are significant, and poor adjustment and symptom control will have an impact not only on the individual in terms of increased suffering but also on the health service in the way of escalating costs.

Pulmonary rehabilitation programmes have been shown to be of value for some patients with chronic respiratory illness, e.g. those with COPD. These programmes are widely available in North America, are multidisciplinary and include education, breathing training, dyspnoea management, lower extremity aerobic exercise training, psychosocial components and behavioural strategies to facilitate positive health behaviours. Comprehensive pulmonary rehabilitation programmes have been shown to improve dyspnoea associated with activities of daily living (O'Donnell et al 1995, Reardon et al 1994) and to improve quality of life (Goldstein et al 1994, Ries et al 1995). It is unfortunate that the development of pulmonary rehabilitation in Britain has been slow. However, it is argued that the NHS could provide short outpatient programmes with small costs and clear benefits (Singh et al 1998).

COGNITIONS

If health workers are to help patients cope more effectively the patients' cognitive processes cannot be ignored. Cognitions are the automatic thoughts, beliefs, assumptions, perceptions and expectations that form the individual's stream of consciousness, and the specific nature of cognitions may drive not only negative emotions, such as panic and fear, but also physiological responses, such as dyspnoea, and behavioural responses, which can either be adaptive or maladaptive (Littlefield 1995). The patients' cognitive processes, therefore, can contribute significantly in determining how their illness is experienced.

In most healthcare settings today time is at a premium. Yet it is vital that healthcare workers take time to get to know their patients. We can all identify situations in the past when poor communication with partners, friends and colleagues resulted in personal distress. We all have our view of the world and also our place in it. If only people could see our point of view! Our view, of course, is not the only view and may be very different from that of others. It is all too easy to make assumptions about patients and to make decisions based on how we see their situation. However, if we could just take a little time to listen to the patients' views we might be better placed to understand behaviour which at first hand seems totally inappropriate if not irrational.

Negative and irrational thoughts and beliefs may increase anxiety, depression and panic and the patient's personal interpretation of his situation and illness can have a major effect on coping ability and ultimate adaptation. Attempts have therefore been made to identify cognitive factors in a number of chronic illness groups. In COPD, for example, cognitive changes have been associated with affective disorders (Gift & McCrone 1993, McSweeney et al 1982, Prigatano et al 1984). Loss of control over one's activities and increased dependence on others, as in chronic respiratory illness, has been found to contribute to feelings of hopelessness, helplessness and loss of self-esteem (Taylor 1983).

Patients attempt to make sense of the onset of their illness, their treatment and life generally. Symptoms may be largely ignored initially, or accepted as an unavoidable sign of growing old or being unfit. There may not only be attempts to make sense of the period before diagnosis but also ongoing attempts at trying to understand the nature and unpredictable course of the illness. Often it is the perceived interference with vocational and physical activities that forces the patient to seek advice.

Many patients are able to offer possible explanations, not always accurate, as to why they developed respiratory problems, and such beliefs may influence treatment adherence. If there is self-blame, for example, there may be a great deal of guilt and the patient may feel that he does not deserve treatment. A search for meaning in chronic illness has been identified in a number of chronic illness groups. Scharloo & Kaptein (1997) identify five dimensions regarding the cognitive organization of illness experience in patients. These are as follows:

- Perceptions regarding the identity of the problem, involving labelling of the disease.
- Ideas about the causes of the problem.
- Ideas about possible consequences of the problem, both short and long term.
- Ideas and expectations about the duration and course of the disease.
- Ideas about cure or controllability.

(Scharloo & Kaptein 1997, p 105)

Being given a diagnosis is important for many patients, particularly after a long period of not knowing what is wrong, and is often a turning point in the process of being chronically ill. There may be relief about the diagnosis and the legit-

Case study 6.3

Pat was a 52-year-old woman with scleroderma and fibrosing alveolitis. Breathlessness and pain in her fingers were two distressing symptoms. As time went by these symptoms became worse and going out became something of an ordeal. The absence of visible signs of illness also created difficulties.

'You see, you can't see my illness. So [when you're] standing on the bus trying to hold on and getting breathless and feeling uptight all the time, people don't give you a seat because they can't see anything wrong with you. If they could see your problem then they would probably give you a seat. Instead you're on the underground pushing and shoving – and it's so tiring that in the end you just can't face going out.'

Not being able to go out as she would have liked also reduced her social circle. A source of embarrassment was the skin on her face which had changed because of the scleroderma and Pat had spent a great deal of money on expensive cosmetic creams. There was an opportunity for her to obtain a disability badge for her car and this would have increased her mobility and quality of life. However, because she needed to provide photographs she would not go through with it.

'I hate looking in the mirror. The scleroderma affects my face and it drives me nuts. I think my face is horrible. Look at these lines here around my mouth. I look dreadful. I won't have my picture taken with the family. I'd rather go to the dentist.' (Margereson 1998)

imizing of their illness may be important to them. A difficulty experienced by many with respiratory illness is that symptoms are often invisible and, with variable symptoms such dyspnoea, fatigue and pain, it may be difficult convincing others that their illness is real.

In the case study Pat experienced problems because others could not see anything wrong with her and this raises an interesting point. Visibility of disability in chronic illness often results in problems as patients see themselves as different. Indeed, visible signs set patients apart as different, thereby subjecting them to negative stereotypes and possible discrimination (O'Neill 1985). This can have an enormous social impact as attempts are made at 'normalizing' the situation, which can require a great deal of effort as the patient cannot afford to drop their guard. Yet problems can also arise through invisibility of disability where others may be less sensitive to the patient's needs. In the absence of visible signs, the patient is generally subjected to the expectations placed upon healthy individuals (Stephenson & Murphy 1986).

Whether disability is visible or invisible it is the patient's perception that is important. Often there are feelings of being different and this stigma may be particularly problematic in younger patients who don't want to feel or be seen as different from their peers. This may lead to failure to take prescribed medication and perform treatments such as postural drainage. There may be feelings of embarrassment and self-consciousness as a result of either worsening symptoms, such as cough and breathlessness, or side effects of treatment. Changes in appearance may be a source of distress and, to avoid situations where embarrassment is likely, social events may be avoided.

Various emotional and psychological problems may arise due to difficulties in adjusting to a changing body image. A number of factors may contribute to a change in how the patient perceives herself and this can result in a great deal of distress. As the illness progresses a number of losses may be incurred. These losses may occur over a period of time, gradually eroding the patient's self-concept. Losses relating to health, functional ability, relationships, occupation and leisure pursuits may all affect how the patient sees him/herself.

Significant in shaping our self-concept are the many roles we have in different areas of our lives. The constant feedback we receive from taking on roles such as parent, work colleague, lover and member of various social groups are all important in making us feel valued as individuals. Therefore changes in role functioning as a result of chronic illness may be a source of conflict. These role changes may also create difficulties for others in that their expectations of the person may not be met. It is not unusual for anger and/or resentment to be focused on a member of the family and occasionally on a member of the healthcare team (Lubkin 1990). Charmaz (1983) provides an excellent account of how 'loss of self' may be a form of suffering in the chronically ill. It is suggested that the experiences and meanings upon which patients built their former positive self-images are no longer available to them, and the accumulating loss of formerly sustaining self-images without the acquisition of new ones results in a diminished self-concept. Four major areas are identified as contributing to the crumbling away of the patient's former self-image:

- leading restricted lives
- experiencing social isolation
- being discredited
- burdening others.

Increasing symptoms, changing self-concept, role changes and poor communication between partners may all lead to difficulties with sexual intimacy. Loss of intimacy within a relationship may also contribute to the erosion of the patient's former self-concept and result in poor self-worth and self-esteem. Sexuality is an integral part of self-image and self-image is an integral part of how one functions in society (Monga & Lefebvre 1992), yet sexual intimacy as a basic human need is not very well addressed in practice, even though issues related to intimacy are an important area in the rehabilitative process.

Difficulties in expressing sexuality may occur in any group of respiratory patients. There are few research studies which have explored sexual behaviour and expression in patients with chronic respiratory illness. This is not to assume that sexual difficulties are not experienced in other groups, including those without disability, but we need to be aware of the concerns of specific groups and how these problems are or are not overcome. These findings will enable health workers to assist other patients who are experiencing similar difficulties. Sotile (1996) offers a useful guide for health professionals on how they can assist patients who are experiencing difficulties regarding sexuality as a result of chronic respiratory illness.

If sexuality is one taboo area as far as professionals are concerned, another area seems to be dying and death related issues. It is inevitable that at times throughout the course of their chronic illness patients will be made to confront their own mortality, something that many of us put off until much later in life when it is deemed more appropriate, although still uncomfortable. Quality of life, not only in living but also in dying, should be seen as an important aim by all health professionals. Often, however, issues around dying are addressed far too late when there is much left unresolved. Van der Maas et al (1991) argue that whilst the hours or days before death are important, the focus should be the weeks and months before death, so that this period of life becomes valuable and meaningful for patients and their families.

There is a delicate balance to be achieved between instilling hope and yet preparing the patient for what may be inevitable. It is recognized that patients' beliefs about their prognosis and their expectations about their future medical care can impact on their decisions, experience and, to a degree, health outcome. Hence professionals often attempt to foster hope which, it is thought, will strengthen the patient's will and help him/her cope. We do not know to what extent denial as a coping mechanism improves or reduces the patient's quality of dying. However, patients who overestimate their life expectancy or who think treatments are more effective than proven may simply put off the advance planning and preparation that they and their families need for the end of their lives (Institute of Medicine 1997).

Helping patients come to terms with their mortality is no easy task and there is no protocol available to make this easier. Many healthcare workers

are young, and caring for someone who is also young, maybe even a similar age, makes this a difficult area. Ongoing professional development is important and workshops should be available for staff to explore issues surrounding death so that personal insight is gained. An important aim should be for staff to feel confident and relaxed about discussing such sensitive issues. Patients will often seek 'permission' to explore these issues in an indirect way to determine the response of the professional and the last thing the patient should see is embarrassment.

Chronic illness suffered by one member of a family will have an impact on all other family members. In the case study Gordon's teenage son was finding it difficult to relate to his father and several explanations are possible. In addition to coping with the many changes of adolescence, he has had to cope with how his father's illness may have challenged the 'normal' father–son relationship. Gordon was very ill and the family had had to sit down together and talk about the implications of transplantation and the implications of not going through with this. This family was forced to re-evaluate aspects of their lives that they had previously taken for granted. Nothing was certain any more. Perspectives of family members may also differ. On the one hand patients may report feelings of burden, guilt, discomfort with growing dependence, or anger that others do not fully

 Case study 6.4

Gordon was 50 years old with fibrosing alveolitis and was married with three children, the youngest being 13 years old. He was oxygen dependent, virtually housebound and awaiting transplant.

'They've said there's a prospect that I may have to have a transplant which I'm not too happy about. The immunosuppressants didn't work so why should a transplant? The future doesn't seem too rosy at the moment but I'm getting used to the idea. I know that there's a chance that I might die sooner rather than later and although I used to get depressed about it I've accepted it. The dying doesn't worry me. If I'm going to get bad then I would rather it not drag on and on. It's our youngest I'm worried about. He's at a difficult age now. We try to get him to communicate but he's rebellious. But we'll work through it.' (Margereson 1998)

appreciate the extent of the illness, whilst on the other hand families may show a range of concerns about their own behaviours towards the patient and his or her efforts to manage the illness and adapt to its presence (Kerns 1995).

One area that has received a great deal of attention in the literature on chronic illness is the concept of control. Early work on health locus of control was undertaken by Rotter (1966) who distinguished between internal attribution, where events are perceived as being caused by the person himself, and external attribution, when the cause is perceived as outside the individual's control. Later work by Bandura (1977, 1989) attempted to explore the link between perceived control and health behaviour, articulating this association in terms of self-efficacy. Perceived self-efficacy involves the belief that

Case study 6.5

Christine was a 41-year-old with interstitial lung disease. She felt that a number of factors had contributed to her feelings of not coping well. First of all there were the steroids which she had been taking for some time. There was anger as she felt that insufficient time had been taken to explore the full implications of being on steroids.

'I had been told about some of the side effects but not everything. But the steroids changed my life completely, particularly my personality. I put on 2 stones. I retained water and if someone had put a pin in me I would have popped. It was awful. It made me so depressed and I wasn't happy with myself. I was angry with everyone. They (hospital staff) sit there and tell you that you should be taking this and taking that and then they say goodbye. They don't really care how the treatment invades your life. All they are concerned about is your lung problem. And that's what they want to try and cure, regardless of the effects on you.'

Her marriage break-up was a major factor in Christine coming off the steroids. She had not discussed this with her doctor. Aware of the consequences of stopping her steroids, she was prepared to take the risk. She was asked how she felt since coming off the steroids.

'I feel no worse. In fact I've started a basic aerobics class. Coming off the steroids has made me feel more human and I'm back in control of my life whereas before it was the tablets and the disease controlling me. Now I feel that I can control it and do what I want. I know he (doctor) will tell me off but I'm not going back on the steroids.' (Margereson 1998)

one will be able to perform a particular behaviour successfully (e.g. contribute to self-management), ultimately increasing motivation and health outcome.

A number of studies have found a positive association between perceived internal control and psychosocial adjustment (Jensen et al 1994, Schiaffano & Revenson 1992), although not all studies identified such a clear association. Difficulty in demonstrating an association in studies, however, is likely to be due to the methodology used, particularly the insensitivity of instruments used to measure the concept of control.

Perceived control over treatment and symptoms is more likely to result in positive mood and psychosocial adjustment. This finding has resulted in a dramatic rethink on the traditional relationship in healthcare encounters between patients and health professionals. Using a medical perspective and drawing on the work of Parsons (1951), health professionals have often placed patients in the 'sick' role, where they are expected to try and get well both by seeking help from expert professionals and by complying with treatment. Such a relationship between patient and health professional is not equal, with the patient adopting a more passive role.

Behaviour and cognitions are, therefore, inextricably linked. In assessing whether behavioural responses are appropriate or not in promoting health it is important to explore the patient's cognitions, which may be driving such responses.

SOCIAL AND ENVIRONMENTAL FACTORS

Social and environmental factors have always played a key role in contributing to health status. It was the public health movement throughout the 19th century that initiated the decline in infectious diseases such as consumption. Medical science, of course, contributed to this decline but its impact was seen much later (McKeown 1979). It is likely to be renewed efforts in the areas of public health and primary care that will result in the greatest success in tackling contemporary health problems, including many respiratory diseases. Report after report has clearly demonstrated the role of material deprivation incontributing to the worse health experience of those in the lower socioeconomic groups.

The focus in healthcare is often on the individual and indeed we have seen how behaviour can often be responsible for either enhancing or damaging health. However, the patient's social and physical environment, if not always responsible for the onset of disease, may be a key factor in precipitating and maintaining symptoms. Because factors in the patient's social and physical environment may act as cues to both cognitive processes and behavioural responses it may be possible to reduce symptoms by modification of the immediate environment. This is not to suggest, however, that the patient is always able to exert control over his environment.

It is useful at this point to consider some of the factors that might possibly precipitate the onset of respiratory symptoms.

Exposure to tobacco smoke is a major risk factor in the development of a number of diseases, including cardiovascular problems, lung cancer and COPD. Children are particularly susceptible to tobacco smoke, with a greater risk of developing respiratory problems. Although there has been a slight decline in the numbers smoking, the overall rate is still too high with a worrying rising trend in the young, particularly females.

The environment in which we live is changing more rapidly than perhaps at any other time in history and the lungs could well be described as a barometer responding to these changes. Most of us live in urban areas and the build up of pollutants in the atmosphere, both gaseous and particulate, may contribute to the development of respiratory disease or worsening of symptoms. A number of epidemiological studies have demonstrated the association between the prevalence of respiratory diseases and air pollution (Braun-Fahrlander et al 1992, Dockery et al 1989). Indoor pollutants have also been identified. Patients with respiratory illness are at risk of developing fur-

ther difficulties when pollution levels are high and may need advice regarding the monitoring of pollutant levels.

Social support

We do not always appreciate just how important our interactions are with others, both at home and at work, until they are no longer available. Humans are social beings and it is our interactions with others which promote feelings of being loved, cared for, appreciated and valued. Indeed, it has been recognized for some time that the support available to people through social networks is important in contributing to enhanced health status, and that limited access to social resources increases vulnerability to disease. (Berkman 1985, Berkman & Syme 1979, Broadhead et al 1983). When someone is faced with a number of stressors social support has been shown to act as an important moderator, promoting wellbeing and recovery. Social support therefore appears to be an important factor in psychosocial adjustment to illness.

Although social support has been identified as an important factor in chronic illness, it has been difficult for researchers to agree on a definition for measurement purposes. Friis & Taff (1986) define social support as the emotional and material resources available to an individual through relationships with others. This is clarified further by Amick & Ockene (1994) who identify five factors to be considered: emotional support, esteem support, sense of belonging, instrumental support and informational support.

It is difficult to identify precisely just how it is that social support contributes to health status the way it does. It is possible that social support has cognitive effects by improving self-esteem and perhaps behavioural effects by making it easier to adopt healthier lifestyles. Social support, for example, may be particularly important in helping patients to follow health promotion advice. Murray et al (1995) studied a large population of adult smokers with mild to moderate airway obstruction. Social support by an ex-smoking partner was the most significant predictor of successful cessation in men.

In chronic illness, as disability increases together with dependency on others, the patient's social network and hence social support may be affected in a number of ways. This may be as a result of relatives not being able, for various reasons, to give the support needed or as a result of interference with the patient's ability to participate as before in various social interactions. Relatives may not fully appreciate what the illness means to the patient and it is important that partners particularly are kept fully informed and involved in any decision making process. Creticos (1994) suggests that close family members have the most important role to play in ensuring the success of any educational programme by participating, encouraging, maintaining a positive attitude and providing the necessary positive feedback.

In patients with COPD Jensen et al (1994) showed that high risk patients with low social support were hospitalized significantly more frequently than low risk patients or high risk patients who were receiving increased social support. It is interesting that social support and life stress predicted the number of hospitalizations more accurately than did the patient's demographic characteristics, severity of illness or previous hospitalizations.

It must not be assumed, however, that members of an individual's social network, e.g. family, are best placed to provide the support that is necessary. It is the quality of any available support network which is important. Family members who are unable or unwilling to provide appropriate support may actually increase the individual's stress (Rook 1984).

With demographic changes resulting in people living much longer and possibly alone, together with the fact that chronic illness is more prevalent in the elderly, more effective policies will be needed to address the issue of social support. Currently this is not addressed adequately and patients are discharged back into the community where social support is often inadequate. This can only contribute

further to the patient's ongoing psychosocial stress.

MEASURING PSYCHOSOCIAL ADJUSTMENT

From the previous section it is clear that a number of complex factors may contribute to adjustment in chronic illness. The more successful adjustment is for patients, the more likely it is that overall quality of life will be perceived positively. Adjustment and quality of life have become important areas of study. How are we to know if a new treatment method is effective? Outcome measurement over recent years has become increasingly important. One reason for this is that with advances in medicine across many specialties there has been an increase in the numbers of patients living with a chronic illness. This has tremendous implications for health policy now and in the future. Given the realities of healthcare costs, not only in financial terms but also in emotional suffering, any evaluation of healthcare should include a user perspective, including quality of life.

There is often lack of clarity or consistency regarding the meaning and measurement of quality of life. According to Gill & Feinstein (1994), quality of life is a reflection of the way that patients perceive and react to their health status and to other non-medical aspects of their lives. Perceptions regarding quality of life may vary between individuals but most would include areas such as symptom control, functional status and emotional wellbeing, together with role performance, not only in the family but in social and vocational settings. Although quality of life is a complex concept, a number of instruments have been developed which incorporate some if not all of these areas.

It is difficult to identify a tool where there is agreement over appropriate quality of life domains that should be addressed in respiratory illness. Williams & Bury (1989) argue that an understanding of the quality of life outcomes in relation to patients with COPD is important in relation to the delivery of optimum care, yet because there is a lack of qualitative data about these patients, current scales remain problematic and unassessed (Williams & Bury 1989). There has been a great deal of literature over recent years exploring the psychosocial impact of COPD, particularly in the USA, and some of these problems have been overcome. However, more research needs to be undertaken to explore the experiences of patients with other respiratory problems.

EFFECTIVE POLICY

A number of studies over the last 20 years have identified a health gap between the different socio-economic groups, with those in the lower groups experiencing worse health (Townsend et al 1988). This was recently reiterated in an independent inquiry into inequalities in health (Acheson 1998). Life expectancy may be rising but this does not mean that the population is experiencing less morbidity and disability. Indeed, for many the additional years will mean living with a chronic illness, with respiratory disease an important cause in many cases.

When looking for possible reasons for social variations in health, factors at all levels of society must be considered, from the macropolitical and economic characteristics of a society through to individual factors such as lifestyle and genetic predisposition (Macintyre 1994). Similarly, attempts to formulate policies to improve the health of the population must involve a range of disciplines working together.

A useful place to start in any discussion regarding health policy is in the prevention of disease at the population level. Policies therefore need to tackle the root causes of ill health, and so poverty, education, employment, housing and the environment are all areas which must be targeted. As early as 1981 the World Health Assembly adopted a global strategy of 'Health for all by the year 2000' (HFA 2000) (World Health Organization 1981). The European HFA strategy identified targets and recognized the need for a new public health movement involving multi-sectoral collaboration, thus moving beyond the healthcare services. Many contemporary health problems were recognized as being social rather than simply individual problems.

Many now realize that medical care is only one dimension of healthcare and yet these terms are often used interchangeably. Much has been written about the 'medicalization' of our society and indeed many apparent social ills are dealt with inappropriately by the health service. Some have suggested that the medical profession and healthcare institutions have appeared to welcome this increased reliance on their services, regardless of the underlying causes of ill health (Hurowitz 1993).

There does, however, seem to be renewed interest in the development of policies which will address some of the wider social issues. The government recognizes that health professionals alone cannot be expected to improve the overall health of the population. The government paper *Saving lives – our healthier nation* (DOH 1999) sets out the importance of improving the health of the population as a whole by increasing the length of people's lives and the number of years people spend free from illness. The dangers of victim-blaming on the one hand and 'nanny state' social engineering on the other are recognized, and the need for individuals, families, local agencies and communities to work together is stressed. However, it is disappointing that the government has not made respiratory disease one of its key targets.

Even where individual lifestyle appears to be a major contributing factor, additional strategies, both fiscal and legislative, may be necessary in order to promote health. For example, problems related to smoking remain and without effective policies to reduce tobacco smoking the burden of smoking related diseases will continue for many years to come. Policies are needed which restrict smoking in public places and abolish tobacco advertising and promotion. It is known that an increase in the real price of tobacco would not only discourage young people from smoking but would also encourage established smokers to quit.

Effective polices to meet the ongoing needs of people with chronic respiratory illness are needed. These needs are likely to be best met by enabling and empowering individuals so they are able to remain at home where most would prefer to be. Appropriate models for healthcare delivery in chronic illness have not been utilized. The culture which pervades the NHS is one which focuses on the acute hospital sector. Chronic illness is not seen as challenging enough, with many nurses appearing not to value working with patients whose conditions are not amenable to cure (Nolan & Nolan 1995).

However, there is renewed interest in improving healthcare for patients with ongoing needs. The White Paper *The new NHS: modern and dependable* (DOH 1997) places primary care in the driving seat in deciding which local services are to be developed (see Chapter 13).

If individuals with chronic illness are better supported in the community, periods of hospitalization may be reduced. Given the throughput of patients in hospitals, it is rarely possible to meet long term needs effectively. Hospital discharge policy and practice may be driven rather by the need to empty beds (Wistow 1995). Indeed, it is argued that the political issues that drive throughput in hospitals and influence the speed of discharge are currently in opposition to the aims that underpin the community care reforms (Clark & Dyer 1998). The end result is that patients may be discharged following acute episodes ill equipped to cope effectively because of poor physical, social, financial and emotional resources.

No matter how successful health reforms are, legislation alone will not bring about the necessary changes. If social support is one of the major factors influencing quality of life, then changes outside the formal health and social services will also be necessary. Social relationships are of particular relevance for policy concerning community care. History reminds us of the influence of rapid change and sociologists have documented the earlier effects of industrialization and urbanization on social relationships, particularly the breakdown of social bonds and resulting alienation. We are once more experiencing a period of rapid change on almost every level and demo-graphic, social and economic changes may further transform social relationships, resulting in isolation. One thing is certain and that is that future community care policies cannot be based on images of 'the family' and the traditional village and working class neighbourhoods of yesteryear.

CONCLUSION

This book started with comment on how specialization in medicine, whilst bringing a number of benefits, is not without cost. For some specific illness groups additional funding provides opportunities for increased research activity and improvements in patient care facilities generally. Respiratory illness, however, does not have the same public and charity funding status as other illness groups. Respiratory disease is often perceived as unglamorous and lacking 'profile' as far as media coverage is concerned. Research into lung diseases attracts a small proportion of the funds available for medical research and government funding has been progressively withdrawn over the years. In 1985, with only 1% of government medical research funding available for lung disease, the British Lung Foundation was established (British Lung Foundation 1996).

Few of us will be fortunate enough to live our lives without suffering from some type of respiratory disorder. For many of those who do acquire a respiratory problem, this will probably be short lived. Yet more than 1 person in 10 suffers from a long term respiratory problem in Britain, sometimes resulting in significant disability. Respiratory disease therefore presents one of the greatest health challenges of the new millennium. Even where there is no cure, there is much that can be done to improve the patient's quality of life. Knowledge of the multidimensional nature of chronic respiratory illness and its psychosocial impact will hopefully enable health professionals to work with patients in helping them to manage their illness more effectively.

REFERENCES

Acheson D 1998 Independent inquiry into inequalities in health (The Acheson Report). The Stationery Office, London

Agle D P, Baum G L, Chester E H 1973 Multidisciplinary treatment of chronic pulmonary insufficiency. 1. Psychological aspects of rehabilitation. Psychosomatic Medicine 35: 41–49

Allen R M, Jones M P, Oldenburg P 1995 Randomised trial of a self-management programme for adults. Thorax 50: 731–738

Altose M D, Cherniack N S, Fishman A P 1985 Respiratory sensations and dyspnoea. Journal of Applied Physiology 58: 1051–1054

Amick T L, Ockene J K 1994 The role of social support in the modification of risk factors for cardiovascular disease. In: Shumaker.S A, Cajkowski S M (eds) Social support and cardiovascular disease. Plenum Press, New York

Bandura A 1977 Self efficacy: toward a unifying theory of behavioural change. Psychological Review 84: 191–215

Bandura A 1989 Perceived self efficacy in the exercise of personal agency. The Psychologist 2: 437–461

Beck J G, Scott S K, Teague R B 1988 Correlates of daily impairment in COPD. Rehabilitation Psychology 33: 77–84

Berkman L F 1985 The relationship of social networks and social support to morbidity and mortality. In: Cohen S, Syme S L (eds) Social support and health. Academic Press, Orlando

Berkman L F, Syme S L 1979 Social networks, host resistance and mortality: a nine year follow up study of Alameda County residents. American Journal of Epidemiology 109: 186–204

Borak J, Sliwinski P, Piasecki Z 1991 Psychological status of COPD patients on long term oxygen therapy. European Respiratory Journal 4: 59–62

Braun-Fahrlander C, Ackermann-Liebrich K, Schwartz J et al 1992 Air pollution and respiratory symptoms in pre-school children. American Review of Respiratory Disease 145: 42–47

British Lung Foundation 1996 The lung report. Lung disease: a shadow over the nation's health. British Lung Foundation, London

Broadhead W E, Kaplan B H, James S A et al 1983 The epidemiological evidence for a relationship between social support and health. American Journal of Epidemiology 117: 521–537

Campbell E J M, Gandevia S C, Killian K J 1980 Changes in the perception of inspiratory resistive loads during partial curarization. Journal of Applied Physiology 309: 93–100

Carrieri V K, Janson-Bjerklie S, Jacobs S 1984 The sensation of dyspnoea: a review. Clinical Review of Critical Care 13: 436–447

Charlton I, Broomfield J, Mullee M A 1990 Evaluation of peak flow and symptoms on self management plans for control of asthma in general practice. British Medical Journal 301: 1355–1359

Charmaz K 1983 Loss of self. A fundamental form of suffering in the chronically ill. Sociology of Health and Illness 5: 168–197

Chonan T, Mulholland M B, Cherniack N S 1987 Effects of voluntary constraining of thoracic displacement during hypercapnia. Journal of Applied Physiology 63: 1822–1828

Clark H, Dyer S 1998 Equipped for going home from hospital. Health Care in Later Life 3(1): 35–42

Clark N M, Becker M H, Janz N K et al 1991 Self management of chronic disease by older adults. Journal of Ageing and Health 3(1): 3027

Clark N M, Evans D, Zimmerman B J et al 1994 Patient and family management of asthma: theory-based techniques for the clinician. Journal of Asthma 31: 427–435

Cohen S, Rodriguez M 1995 Pathways linking affective disturbances and physical disorders. Health Psychology 14(5): 374–380

Congleton J, Hodson M E, Duncan-Skingle F 1997 Quality of life in adults with cystic fibrosis. European Respiratory Review 7(942): 74–76

Cote J, Cartier A, Robichaud P et al 1997 Influence on asthma morbidity of asthma education programs based on self management plans following treatment optimisation. American Journal of Respiratory and Critical Care Medicine 155: 1509–1514

Creticos P S 1994 Patient education in the United States. In: Johansson S G O (ed) Progress in allergy and clinical immunology. Hogrefe & Huber, Gottingen, vol 3, p 156

Dales R E, Spitzer W O, Schechter M T 1989 The influence of psychological status on respiratory symptom reporting. American Review of Respiratory Disease 139: 1459–1463

Department of Health 1997 The new NHS: modern and dependable. Cm3807. The Stationery Office, London

Department of Health 1999 Saving lives – our healthier nation. The Stationery Office, London

Dockery D W, Speicer F E, Frank E et al 1989 Effects of inhalable particles on respiratory health of children. American Review of Respiratory Disease 139: 587–594

Dolce J J, Crisp C, Manzella B et al 1991 Medication adherence patterns in chronic obstructive pulmonary disease. Chest 99: 837–841

Dudley D L, Wermuth C, Hague W 1973 Psychosocial aspects of care in the COPD patient. Heart & Lung 2(3): 389–393

Eakin E G, Glasgow R E 1997 The patient's perspective on the self-management of COPD. Journal of Health Psychology 2(2): 245–253

Frazier D T, Revellete W R 1991 Role of phrenic nerve afferents in the control of breathing. Journal of Applied Physiology 70: 49–56

Friis R, Taff G A 1986 Social support and social networks and coronary heart disease and rehabilitation. Journal of Cardiopulmonary Rehabilitation 6: 132–147

Gift A G, McCrone S H 1993 Depression in patients with COPD. Heart & Lung 22(4): 289–297

Gill T M, Feinstein A R 1994 A critical appraisal of the quality of quality of life measurements. Journal of the American Medical Association 272(8): 619–625

Goldstein R S, Gort E H, Stubbing D 1994 Randomised controlled trial of respiratory rehabilitation. Lancet 344: 1394–1397

Goodall T A, Halford W K 1991 Self management of diabetes mellitus: a critical review. Health Psychology 10: 1–8

Graydon J E, Ross E 1995 Influence of symptoms, lung function, mood and social support on level of functioning of patients with COPD. Research in Nursing and Health 18: 525–533

Gregory M D, Smeltzer M A 1983 Psychiatry. Essentials of clinical practice. Little Brown, Boston

Griffith D E, Kronenberg R S 1991 Psychological, neuropsychological and social aspects of COPD. In: Cerniack N S (ed) Chronic obstructive pulmonary disease. W B Saunders, Philadelphia

Guyatt G H, Townsend M, Berman L B, Pugsley S O 1987 Quality of life in patients with chronic airflow limitation. British Journal of Diseases of the Chest 81: 45–54

Hurowitz J C 1993 Sounding board. Toward a social policy for health. New England Journal of Medicine 329(2): 130–133

Institute of Medicine 1997 Approaching death: improving care at the end of life. National Academy Press, Washington DC

Jensen M P, Turner J A, Romano J M 1994 Correlates of improvement in multidisciplinary treatment of chronic pain. Journal of Consulting and Clinical Psychology 62: 172–179

Jones P W, Baveystock C M, Littlejohns P 1989 Relationships between general health measured with the sickness impact profile and respiratory symptoms, physiological measures and mood in patients with chronic airflow limitation. American Review of Respiratory Disease 140: 1538–1543

Keele-Card G, Foxhall M J, Barron C R 1993 Loneliness, depression and social support of patients with COPD and their spouses. Public Health Nursing 10: 245–251

Keilty S E J 1998 Physiotherapy and ventilatory management of patients admitted to critical care environments with acute exacerbation of chronic respiratory disease. Care of the Critically Ill 14(8): 275–278

Kelloway J S, Wyatt R A, Adlis S A 1994 Comparison of patients' compliance with prescribed oral and inhaled asthma medications. Archives of Internal Medicine 154: 1349–1352

Kerns R D 1995 Family assessment and intervention. In: Nicassio P M, Smith W (eds) Managing chronic illness. A biopsychosocial perspective. American Psychological Association, Washington DC, ch 6, p 207

Kinsman R A, Yaroush R A, Fernandez E et al 1983 Symptoms and experiences in chronic bronchitis and emphysema. Chest 83: 755–761

Kline Leidy N, Ozbolt J G, Swain M A P 1990 Psychophysiological processes of stress in chronic physical illness: a theoretical perspective. Journal of Advanced Nursing 15: 478–486

Kohler C L, Davies S L, Bailey W C 1996 Self management and other behavioural aspects of asthma. Current Opinion in Pulmonary Medicine 2(16): 16–22

Kotses H, Stout C, McConnoughty K et al 1996 Evaluation of individualised asthma self management programs. Journal of Asthma 33: 113–118

Lazarus R S, Folkman S 1984 Stress appraisal and coping. Springer, New York

Lee R N F, Graydon J E, Ross E 1991 Effects of psychological well being, physical status and social support on oxygen dependent COPD patients' level of functioning. Research in Nursing and Health 14: 323–328

Leventhal H, Patrick-Miller L 1993 Emotion and illness. The mind is in the body. In: Lewis M, Havisland J (eds) Handbook of emotions. Guildford, New York

Littlefield C 1995 Psychological treatment of patients with end stage pulmonary disease. Monaldi Archives of Chest Diseases 50(1): 58–61

Lubkin I 1990 Chronic illness. Impact and intervention. Jones Bartlett, London

McCord M, Cronin-Stubbs D 1992 Operationalising dyspnoea: focus on measurement. Heart & Lung 21: 167–179

Macintyre S 1994 Understanding the social patterning of health: the role of the social sciences. Journal of Public Health Medicine 16(1): 53–59

McKeown T 1979 The role of medicine. Dream, mirage or nemesis? Basil Blackwell, Oxford

McSweeney J A, Grant I, Heaton R K, Adams K M, Timms R M 1982 Life quality of patients with COPD. Archives of Internal Medicine 142: 473–478

Margereson C 1998 Psychosocial adjustment in patients with interstitial lung disease. Unpublished MSc dissertation, Middlesex University

Monga T N, Lefebvre K A 1992 Sexuality. An overview. Physical Medicine and Rehabilitation. State of the Art Reviews 9(2): 299–311

Munck A, Guyre P M, Holbrook N J 1984 Physiological functions of glucocorticoids in stress and their relation to pharmacological actions. Endocrine Reviews 5: 25–44

Murray R P, Johnston J J, Dolce J J et al 1995 Social support for smoking cessation and abstinence: the lung health study. Lung Health Study Research Group, Addictive Behaviour. Science 20: 159–170

Neill W A, Branch L G, Dejong G et al 1985 Cardiac disability: the impact of coronary heart disease in patients' daily activities. Archives of Internal Medicine 145: 1642–1647

Nicholas P K, Leuner J D 1992 Relationship between body image and chronic obstructive pulmonary disease. Applied Nursing Research 5: 83–88

Nolan M, Nolan J 1995 Responding to the challenge of chronic illness. British Journal of Nursing 4(3): 145–147

O'Brien M K, Petrie K, Raeburn J 1992 Adherence to medication regimens: updating a complex medical issue. Medical Care Review 49: 435–454

O'Donnell D E, McQuire M, Samis L 1995 The impact of exercise reconditioning on breathlessness in severe chronic airflow limitation. American Journal of Respiratory and Critical Care Medicine 152: 2005–2013

O'Neill J 1985 Five bodies. The human shape of modern society. Cornell University Press, Ithaca, New York

Parsons T 1951 The social system. Free Press, Illinois

Porzelius J, Vest M, Nochomovitz M 1992 Respiratory function, cognitions and panic in chronic obstructive pulmonary patients. Behaviour Research and Therapy 30: 75–77

Prigatano G P, Wright E C, Levin D 1984 Quality of life and its predictors in patients with mild hypoxaemia and chronic obstructive airways disease. Archives of Internal Medicine 144: 1613–1621

Reardon J, Awad E, Normandin E 1994 The effect of comprehensive outpatient pulmonary rehabilitation on dyspnoea. Chest 105: 1046–1052

Redline S, Gottfried S B, Altose M D 1991 Effects of changes in inspiratory muscle strength on the sensation of respiratory force. Journal of Applied Physiology 70: 240–245

Ries A L, Kaplan R M, Limberg T M 1995 Effects of pulmonary rehabilitation on physiological and psychosocial outcomes in patients with chronic obstructive pulmonary disease. Annals of Internal Medicine 122: 823–832

Rook K S 1984 The negative side of social interaction: impact on psychological well-being. Journal of Personality and Social Psychology 46: 1097–1108

Roper N, Logan W W, Tierney A J 1996 The elements of nursing. A model for nursing based on a model of living. Churchill Livingstone, London

Rotter J B 1966 Generalised expectancies for internal versus external control of reinforcement. Psychological Monographs 80(1): 1–28

Royal College of Physicians and Royal College of Psychiatrists 1995 The psychological care of medical patients. Royal College of Physicians and Royal College of Psychiatrists, London

Salata P A Berman L B 1981 Variables which distinguish good and poor function outcomes following respiratory rehabilitation. American Review of Respiratory Disease 123: 117

Scharloo M, Kaptein A 1997 Measurement of illness perceptions in patients with chronic somatic illness: a review. In: Petrie K J, Weinman J A (eds) Perceptions of health and illness. Harwood Academic Publishers, Reading, p 105

Schiaffano K M, Revenson T A 1992 The role of perceived efficacy, perceived control and causal attributions in adaptation to rheumatoid arthritis: distinguishing mediator from moderator effects. Personality and Social Psychology Bulletin 18: 709–718

Selye H 1956 The stress of life. McGraw Hill, New York

Shekleton M E 1987 Coping with chronic respiratory difficulty. Nursing Clinics of North America 22(3): 569–581

Singh S J, Smith D L, Hyland M E, Morgan M D L 1998 A short outpatient pulmonary rehabilitation programme: immediate and longer term effects on exercise performance and quality of life. Respiratory Medicine 92: 1146–1154

Sotile W M 1996 Psychosocial interventions for cardiopulmonary patients. A guide for health professionals. Human Kinetics, Leeds

Stephenson J S, Murphy D 1986 Existential grief. The special case of the chronically ill and disabled. Death Studies 10: 133–145

Taylor S E 1983 Adjustment to threatening events: a theory of cognitive adaptation. American Psychologist 38: 1161–1173

Thoresen C E, Kirmil-Gray K 1983 Self-management psychology and the treatment of childhood asthma. Journal of Allergy and Clinical Immunology 72: 596–606

Tobin D L, Russ V C, Reynolds K et al 1986 Self-management and social learning theory. In: Holroyd K A, Creer T L (eds) Self management of chronic disease. Handbook of clinical interventions and research. Academic Press, London, ch 2, p 29

Townsend P, Davidson N, Whitehead M 1988 Inequalities in health. Penguin, Harmondsworth

Van der Maas P J, van Delden J J M, Lijnenborg L, Looman C W N 1991 Euthanasia and other medical decisions concerning the end of life. Lancet 338: 669–674

Werner J S 1993 Stressors and health outcomes: synthesis of nursing research 1980–1990. In: Barnfather J S, Lyon B L (eds) Stress and coping: state of the science and implications for nursing theory, research and practice. Centre Nursing Press of Sigma Theta Tau, International. Indianapolis

Williams S J 1990 Chronic respiratory illness and disability: a critical review of the psychosocial literature. Social Science and Medicine 28: 791–803

Williams S J, Bury M R 1989 Impairment, disability and handicap in chronic respiratory illness. Social Science and Medicine 29: 609–616

Wilson S R, Scamagas P, German D F et al 1993 A controlled trial of two forms of self management education for adults with asthma. American Journal of Medicine 94(6): 564–576

Wistow G 1995 Aspirations and realities: community care at the crossroads. Health and Social Care in the Community 3: 227–240

World Health Organization 1981 Global strategy for health for all by the year 2000. WHO, Geneva

7

Oxygen therapy

Glenda Esmond   Christine Mikelsons

Oxygen therapy is used to correct hypoxaemia and prevent hypoxia. Hypoxaemia is a deficiency of oxygen in arterial blood whereas hypoxia is lack of oxygen in the tissues. Prevention of hypoxia is important as lack of oxygen to tissues will result in cell death. Hypoxaemia is a result of oxygenation and/or ventilatory failure, which form the physiological basis of respiratory failure, and can be caused by:

- intrinsic lung disease (i.e. asthma, chronic obstructive pulmonary disease (COPD), pneumonia, pulmonary embolism)
- neuromuscular diseases (i.e. muscular dystrophy, motor neurone disease)
- chest wall disorders (i.e. scoliosis, kyphoscoliosis)
- other causes including upper airway obstruction, adult respiratory distress syndrome (ARDS) and carbon monoxide inhalation.

Oxygen is a medication and should be prescribed according to clinical hypoxia and evidence of arterial hypoxaemia. In order to administer oxygen therapy safely it is necessary to understand:

- indications for oxygen therapy
- complications of oxygen therapy
- types of oxygen administration devices
- use of humidification
- home oxygen therapy – use of concentrators and portable oxygen
- patient education and problem solving.

INDICATIONS FOR OXYGEN THERAPY

The aims and uses of oxygen therapy are:

- to correct Type I respiratory failure (hypoxaemia only)
- to correct Type II respiratory failure (hypoxaemia and hypercapnia)
- palliative relief of shortness of breath.

Respiratory failure is the inability to maintain adequate oxygenation and/or adequate carbon dioxide elimination. Type I respiratory failure is recognized when the PaO_2 is less than 8 kPa and Type II respiratory failure is recognized when the PaO_2 is less than 8 kPa and the $PaCO_2$ is greater than 6 kPa (Table 7.1).

Use of oxygen therapy in Type I respiratory failure

In the presence of Type I respiratory failure oxygen therapy must be prescribed at a level that will correct hypoxaemia (PaO_2 > 8 kPa/SaO_2 > 90%). For example, a patient with asthma or pulmonary embolism may require 60–100% oxygen initially to prevent hypoxia, until specific disease management is initiated and becomes effective. Oxygen saturation monitoring is sufficient in this group for reassessment purposes, providing arterial blood gas results have shown no rise in the level of arterial carbon dioxide on initial assessment.

Use of oxygen therapy in Type II respiratory failure

Patients who have Type II respiratory failure may have developed sensitivity to falling oxygen levels in the blood. This is the opposite in normal subjects who display sensitivity to rising levels of carbon dioxide and will adjust the rate of respiration in order to try to normalize this situation should it arise (e.g. Kussmaul breathing). In Type II failure the respiratory centre no longer displays this response to raised carbon dioxide levels. The peripheral chemoreceptors then become important in stimulating breathing and respond to falling of oxygen levels. This therefore means that providing an artificial source of oxygen to the body in the form of oxygen therapy carries with it the danger of loss of hypoxic drive of the respiratory centre and the risk of inducing hypercapnia. This rise in carbon dioxide, if untreated, causes narcosis, disorientation and ultimately death due to respiratory acidosis.

Titration of oxygen therapy in the presence of Type II respiratory failure must be made in response to arterial blood gas results (Bateman & Leech 1998). In these patients initial treatment is with low percentage oxygen (24–28%) which can be progressively increased on the basis of repeated arterial blood gases. It may be necessary to accept partial correction of hypoxaemia in order that hypercapnia is not exacerbated, but again this can only be decided in response to arterial blood gas results and clinical assessment.

Oxygen for palliation

The use of oxygen for palliation, for example in the terminal stages of lung cancer which causes

Table 7.1 Definition of Type I and Type II respiratory failure

Arterial blood gas values	Normal	Type I respiratory failure	Type II respiratory failure
pH	7.35–7.45	7.35–7.45	7.35–7.45 or < 7.35
PaO_2	12–14 kPa	< 8 kPa	< 8 kPa
$PaCO_2$	4.6–6.0 kPa	4.6–6.0 kPa	> 6 kPa
SaO_2	95%+	< 92%	< 92%

distressing shortness of breath, may be considered. Some patients describe a subjective benefit in their breathlessness from using oxygen during this time and it is usual to prescribe its use in this form as short burst therapy, to be used as and when patients feel they would benefit from using it.

Acute assessment of patients for oxygen therapy

Assessment of patients using oxygen therapy should be based on clinical assessment (Box 7.1) and includes arterial blood gas monitoring.

In order to assess the patient's condition accurately it is necessary to use an arterial sample of blood to obtain levels of the partial pressures of oxygen and carbon dioxide. The arterial sample used could be taken either from an artery or from the ear lobe. The patient should have an arterial blood gas taken breathing room air, wherever possible, having spent at least 30 minutes off any supplemental oxygen. The patient should then spend

---

Box 7.1 Assessment of patients for oxygen therapy in the acute setting will include the following

History of present condition

- Previous medical history
- Subjective assessment: what is the patient complaining of?

Objective assessment

- Cough +/– productive
- Haemoptysis
- Shortness of breath
- Smoking history
- Family history of respiratory disease
- Respiratory rate
- Heart rate/blood pressure
- Cyanosis
- Clubbing
- Plethora
- Ankle oedema
- Audible chest sounds
- Chest X-ray (CXR) – hyperinflated, cardiomegaly
- Arterial blood gases
- SpO_2
- Polycythaemia
- Haematocrit
- White cell count
- Lung function tests
- Drug history

Case study 7.1

Paul, aged 33 years, suffers from asthma and was admitted with an acute asthma attack. He was cyanosed, tachycardic, hypotensive and was sitting upright fighting to get a breath. There was an audible wheeze and his SpO_2 measured on the oximeter was 87%. He was immediately given 60% oxygen using a fixed performance oxygen mask and his SpO_2 increased to 93%. He was administered nebulized salbutamol via oxygen, intravenous aminophylline and intravenous hydrocortisone. Due to the presence of cyanosis and his diagnosis of asthma, oxygen was given prior to arterial blood gas measurements. His arterial blood gases were performed on 60% oxygen which showed correction of hypoxaemia (PaO_2 9.2 kPa) with no signs of hypercapnia (PaO_2 5.5 kPa). As his bronchoconstriction responded to treatment his SpO_2 increased to 99%, his wheeze decreased and there was no cyanosis present. His flow rate of oxygen was reduced to 35% giving him an SpO_2 of 96%. He continued to be monitored using oximetry as his initial arterial blood gases excluded carbon dioxide retention.

at least 30 minutes on supplemental oxygen before a further blood gas is taken, so that a comparison of PaO_2 and $PaCO_2$ on and off the oxygen can be made. Monitoring oxygen therapy in the acute setting is recommended (Bateman & Leech 1998) and should involve the following:

- Arterial blood gases should be performed before commencing oxygen therapy (if possible).
- Arterial blood gases should be measured or oximetry performed (only if CO_2 retention has been excluded) within 2 hours of starting oxygen therapy.
- Hypoxaemic patients at risk of arrhythmias should be monitored continuously by oximetry.
- Patients with Type II respiratory failure should have arterial blood gases recorded more frequently to assess $PaCO_2$, and SpO_2 should be monitored continuously by oximetry until the patient is stable.
- In the acute stage response should be assessed daily by arterial blood gases and/or oximetry and oxygen adjusted accordingly.

Arterial sampling from a radial or a femoral artery can be painful especially when performed by inexperienced hands and, if possible, sampling from the earlobe is the method of choice (Pitkin et al 1994). This involves taking a sample of arterial blood using a scalpel to place a small nick in the earlobe. The sample is drawn using a fine bore capillary tube and is then analysed in a blood gas analysis machine.

COMPLICATIONS OF OXYGEN THERAPY

Oxygen is classified as a drug and as with any drug it is necessary to have knowledge of the treatment being administered as well as any side effects. The main problems associated with oxygen therapy are:

- retention of carbon dioxide
- mucosal drying and mucociliary dysfunction
- dehydration of respiratory secretions and subsequent sputum retention.

In addition to the side effects oxygen also presents potential hazards which include:

- fire
- oxygen toxicity.

Fire can occur as oxygen is a combustible gas. Facial burns and deaths of patients who smoke when using oxygen have occurred.

Oxygen toxicity can occur if high concentrations of oxygen (> 60%) are given for more than 48 hours continuously. Alveolar membrane damage can occur progressing to adult respiratory distress syndrome (Bateman & Leech 1998).

ADMINISTRATION OF OXYGEN

The delivery of oxygen to the patient is dependent on a number of factors that include the type of system used to deliver the oxygen and the patient's rate and depth of respiration. The choice of system will be determined by the degree to which it is necessary to deliver accurate levels of oxygen therapy. There are two categories of oxygen delivery devices:

- fixed performance devices
- variable performance devices.

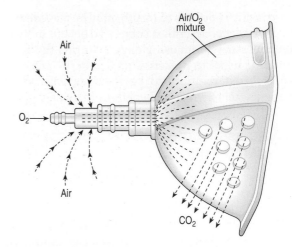

Figure 7.1 Fixed performance oxygen device.

Fixed performance devices

Fixed performance devices include in the delivery circuit a venturi adaptor that supplies oxygen to the patient and allows for mixing of the oxygen with air drawn into the system through holes in the adaptor (Fig. 7.1). The adaptors come with varying sized holes that allow a range of percentages of oxygen to be delivered. This, together with the fact that the masks in this system are large enough to allow further oxygen and air mixing and the large holes in the mask allow removal of carbon dioxide, means that patients receive a percentage of oxygen that is independent of their rate or depth of respiration.

Fixed flow devices should be used in cases where it is important to deliver an accurate percentage of oxygen to the patient in Type II acute respiratory failure.

Variable performance devices

Variable performance devices include nasal cannulae (Fig. 7.2a), Hudson delivery systems (Fig. 7.2b) and any system that does not incorporate a venturi adaptor. These devices deliver a percentage of oxygen that depends on the rate and depth of the patient's respiration. They are suitable for patients who do not require accurate percentages

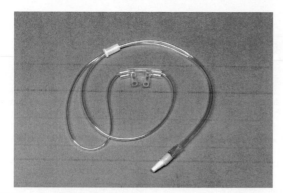

Figure 7.2a Variable performance nasal cannulae.

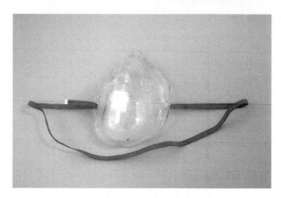

Figure 7.2b Variable performance oxygen mask.

of oxygen to be delivered, such as those with Type I respiratory failure, for postoperative surgical patients in the absence of Type II failure and for patients with stable chronic Type II respiratory failure.

Sometimes in the case of Type II failure it may be necessary to adopt a flexible regimen for the patient, for example where it is desirable that a patient receives supplemental oxygen using a fixed performance mask but he finds it difficult to eat and drink with it on. In this situation it would be appropriate to use nasal cannulae when eating and drinking. It should be noted that the flow rates of the two types of delivery system are not interchangeable (Sykes et al 1976), for example 2 L of oxygen delivered from nasal cannulae will not give the same percentage of oxygen as 2 L from a Venturi system (Box 7.2).

Box 7.2 Flow rates used for different oxygen devices

Fixed performance devices

- Venturi mask
  - 2 L/min 24%
  - 4 L/min 28%
  - 8 L/min 35%
  - 15 L/min 60%

Variable performance devices

- Nasal cannulae
  - 1 L/min 24%
  - 2 L/min 28%
  - 3 L/min 32%
  - 4 L/min 36%
- Hudson mask
  - 1–4 L/min not advised
  - 5–6 L/min 40%
  - 6–7 L/min 50%
- Intersurgical mask
  - 2 L/min 28%
  - 4 L/min 40%
  - 6 L/min 53%

Humidified oxygen system

- Respiflow or Aquapak
  - 5 L/min 28%
  - 8 L/min 35%
  - 10 L/min 40%

Principles of humidification

When oxygen is delivered at low flow rates of 1–2 L per minute and in the absence of respiratory tract infections the nasopharynx provides adequate humidification. In some instances it may be necessary to humidify the supplemental oxygen delivered to the patient to prevent:

- mucosal drying
- mucociliary dysfunction
- dehydration of respiratory secretions
- sputum retention.

Patients using oxygen therapy require individual assessment; however, the general indications to humidify oxygen are:

- high flow rates (> 2 L/min)
- respiratory infections
- nasal discomfort and/or dryness
- tracheostomy.

If oxygen is delivered with inadequate humidification, complications can occur (Fell & Boehm 1998) and can include:

- atelectasis (lung collapse)
- increased risk of infections
- pain from dry secretions
- blocking of tracheostomy tubes leading to respiratory arrest.

The practice of humidifying nasal cannulae should also be discouraged as it is impossible to humidify through narrow bore tubing (Campbell et al 1988). The 'bubble-through' type humidifiers that consist of a stream of gas bubbled through a water container do not provide adequate humidification and their use should be discouraged.

Humidification systems must provide a mist of the correct particle size in order to deliver a therapeutic aerosol. The majority of the particles should be in the range of 0.5–1.0 microns in order to reach the peripheral airways of the lungs (Newman & Clarke 1983). There are a number of systems available which allow the delivery of 28–60% humidified oxygen (Fig. 7.3).

In order to deliver humidified oxygen at 24% it is necessary to run the humidifier off an air supply and entrain oxygen at 2 L via an adaptor (Gunawardena et al 1984) (Fig. 7.4). This should

Case study 7.2

Jamie is a 28-year-old who has cystic fibrosis and was admitted with an acute infective exacerbation. He required 28% oxygen to correct his hypoxaemia. His sputum was thick and dark green and currently growing Pseudomonas aeruginosa. He was commenced on intravenous antibiotics and was having chest physiotherapy twice a day. Although he only required low flow oxygen, the decision to commence him on humidified oxygen was based on the presence of infection and the difficulty he was having in adequately clearing his sputum. After 5 days his sputum was less tenacious and lighter in colour. Jamie requested getting a break from wearing the oxygen mask, particularly when his friends came to visit him. It was decided after discussion with Jamie that he would use the humidification overnight and intermittently during the day, and that when he had friends and at mealtimes he would use 2 L/min of oxygen via nasal cannulae. Jamie felt he was part of the decision making process and felt his feelings had been considered.

only be indicated in the presence of Type II respiratory failure where the patient demonstrates increased hypercapnia in the presence of higher percentages of oxygen therapy.

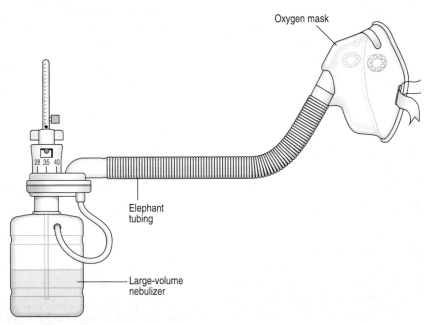

Oxygen mask

Elephant tubing

Large-volume nebulizer

Figure 7.3 Humidified oxygen system.

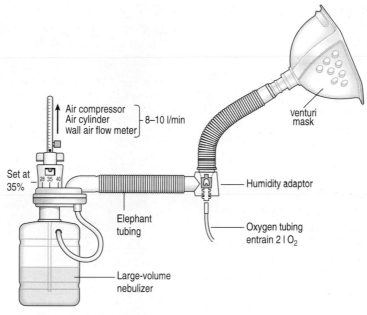

Figure 7.4 24% Humidified oxygen system.

Summary

- In the acute setting fixed performance devices should be used whenever possible
- Flexibility of oxygen device may be necessary to increase compliance with oxygen therapy (e.g. fixed performance device plus intermittent use of nasal cannulae)
- All patients should be assessed for inclusion of humidification
- Ensure humidification delivers a therapeutic aerosol (0.5–1 micron) using an effective delivery system

LONG TERM OXYGEN THERAPY – USE OF CONCENTRATORS AND PORTABLE OXYGEN

Assessment for long term oxygen therapy

The prescription of long term oxygen therapy for use at home was formalized as a result of two randomized controlled trials published in the early 1980s, both of which demonstrated that patients with hypoxaemic COPD who used long term oxygen therapy for at least 15 hours a day showed improved survival rates (Medical Research Council Working Party (MRC) 1981, Nocturnal Oxygen Therapy Trial Group (NOTT) 1980) (Fig. 7.5).

Chronic hypoxaemia caused by any of the respiratory diseases, such as COPD and cystic fibrosis, can cause:

- raised pulmonary artery pressures
- secondary polycythaemia

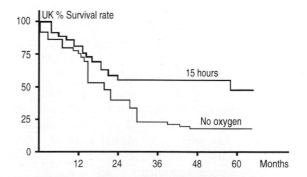

Figure 7.5 Survival rate with and without supplementary oxygen. Reproduced with permission from Medical Research Council Working Party 1981.

- psychological disturbances such as mood changes
- sleep disturbances.

The mechanism of action of long term oxygen therapy in patients with chronic respiratory disease remains unclear. However, it is known that its use affects a number of parameters that could contribute to its confirmed effect of improved survival. The results of the MRC (1981) and the NOTT (1980) studies showed that, in addition to increasing survival, long term oxygen therapy:

- reduced the symptoms of cor pulmonale
- gave a neuropsychological benefit
- improved quality of sleep
- helped to prevent cardiac arrhythmias
- reduced secondary polycythaemia.

A domiciliary oxygen concentrator service was therefore set up in the UK in 1985 (Department of Health and Social Security 1985) as a result of these studies and since that time increasing numbers of patients have been treated at home with oxygen concentrators (Fig. 7.6).

On a practical level, the provision of a concentrator as opposed to cylinders for the delivery of oxygen has many benefits:

- it frees the patient from relying on the delivery of the cylinders
- it allows the patient to be more mobile around the home
- it eliminates the need for storage of numerous cylinders.

Long term oxygen therapy may be prescribed for the treatment of a variety of pulmonary conditions including COPD, cystic fibrosis, interstitial lung disease, neuromuscular/skeletal disorders, pulmonary hypertension and palliation in lung cancer. Long term oxygen therapy delivered by an oxygen concentrator has been shown to be well accepted and tolerated by the majority of patients (Dilworth 1990, Restrick et al 1993). However, patients need education and support to overcome reported problems which include:

- noise of machine/sleep disturbance
- restricted movement

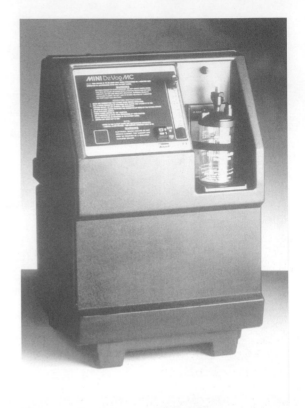

Figure 7.6 Oxygen concentrator. Reproduced with permission of Sunrise Medical Ltd.

- nasal discomfort
- ear discomfort
- embarrassment.

Oxygen concentrators are more economic than cylinders for long term use at home. The provision of concentrators is cost-effective when compared to the provision of cylinders as each cylinder only lasts 8 hours when set at 2 L/min. It was originally considered only to be cost-effective to provide a concentrator if patients were using 2 L/min oxygen for 15 hours a day. However, it is now considered to be cost-effective to prescribe a concentrator if a patient is using 2 L/min oxygen for 8 hours a day. Guidelines have been produced by the Royal College of Physicians (1999) which set out criteria for prescribing long term oxygen therapy (Box 7.3).

Box 7.3 Indications for prescribing long term oxygen therapy

- $PaO_2 < 7.3$ kPa during a period of stability of 4 weeks
- PaO_2 between 7.3 and 8 kPa on air during a period of stability of 4 weeks or more together with
  - secondary polycythaemia
  - nocturnal hypoxaemia (i.e. SaO_2 below 90% for at least 1/3 of the night)
  - peripheral oedema
  - pulmonary hypertension
- Palliation to relieve breathlessness
- Frequent use of cylinders (> 8 hours per day)

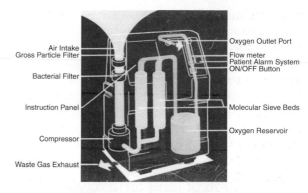

Figure 7.7 How an oxygen concentrator works.

The assessment for long term oxygen therapy should include the following:

- diagnosis
- optimization of the medical management of the condition causing hypoxaemia
- assessment should be made whilst the patient is in a stable phase of the disease, not during an acute exacerbation
- the condition should have been in a stable state for at least 4 weeks
- two arterial blood gases should be taken not less than 3 weeks apart during stable phase.

Principles of the oxygen concentrator

The oxygen concentrator is a device for the delivery of low flow oxygen and consists of a compressor powered by electricity. It stands about 60 cm in height and draws in room air that is then passed through bacterial filters and a molecular sieve bed. These sieve beds contain zeolite, which has an affinity with nitrogen when under pressure, and work by removing gases and 'concentrating' oxygen that is delivered through a flow meter at the front of the concentrator (Fig. 7.7).

The resultant effect is an increased concentration of low flow oxygen, between 0.5 and 4 L. The percentage of oxygen delivered is 95% accurate at 1 and 2 L/min but becomes less accurate above 3 L/min (Table 7.2). If more than 3 L/min is required, two concentrators in series should be prescribed.

Interfaces for use with oxygen concentrators

The oxygen can be delivered to the patient by either nasal cannulae or face mask. Nasal cannulae are probably the interface of choice as they allow the patient to eat, drink and communicate easily whilst remaining on the oxygen. The use of a face mask with an oxygen concentrator may prove more difficult for the patient but it could still be used, for example, if the patient experienced irritation from the prongs of the nasal cannulae. As described earlier, the choice of oxygen mask includes either a fixed or a variable performance device, depending on the accuracy of the delivery of oxygen that is required. In the stable chronic phase of respiratory disease, variable performance devices are usually sufficiently accurate for most patients.

It is possible to prescribe a humidifier for use with the concentrator. However, as has been stated previously, it is not possible to deliver a therapeutic aerosol through small bore tubing and the presence of such a humidifier could also present an infection control hazard. It is

Table 7.2 Percentage accuracy of oxygen concentrators	
1 L/min	95% +/− 3%
2 L/min	95% +/− 3%
3 L/min	92% +/− 3%
4 L/min	80% +/− 3%

probably more sensible to prescribe nebulized saline using a jet nebulizer for use at regular intervals in the presence of tenacious secretions. However, it is not possible to run a nebulizer from a concentrator because the concentrator provides a low flow output that is insufficient to drive a nebulizer, therefore an air compressor needs to be provided to drive the nebulizer.

Organization of long term oxygen therapy

Oxygen concentrators are prescribable on a regional tendering basis, with three companies supplying different regions in the UK: British Oxygen Company (BOC), DeVilbiss Healthcare and Oxygen Therapy Company Ltd. The concentrator and accessories should be prescribed on form FP10 by the patient's GP. The number of hours per day, the flow rate that the patient requires and provision for a back up cylinder should be set out on the prescription. The prescriber then phones the oxygen concentrator company and requests installation of the concentrator.

Patients should be informed that the supplier will contact them to make arrangements for the installation of the concentrator within 4 working days and that the person installing the concentrator will ask for the prescription. The oxygen concentrator will be installed by a trained engineer from the supplying company, who will discuss with the patient the best location for the concentrator. This is usually in the hallway or spare bedroom so that the patient is not disturbed by any noise from the concentrator. Oxygen is piped through oxygen tubing, which is usually secured to skirting boards to ensure that the patient does not trip over it, to two outlets, usually the sitting room and the bedroom. The engineer will allow a maximum of 50 ft of tubing from each point to enable the patient to be as mobile as possible.

The provider of the oxygen concentrator is required to:

- service the concentrator every 3 months
- supply additional accessories if required

- read the meter every 3 months and reimburse the cost of the electricity the machine has used
- provide the patient with emergency telephone numbers
- provide a 24-hour breakdown service.

Patients who have been newly started on domiciliary oxygen should have a formal follow-up by a healthcare practitioner (Restrick et al 1993, Royal College of Physicians 1999) that should include:

- oxygen saturation (SpO_2) measurement to ensure that oxygen therapy is correcting hypoxaemia
- addressing psychological and social concerns and issues that may prevent the patient complying with the oxygen therapy
- monitoring of the patient's condition and observation for signs of deterioration (e.g. peripheral oedema)
- assessing if continued domiciliary oxygen is required.

The patient should be given written information, be taught about the use of oxygen at home and be told the reason for prescription. Many patients will have a poor understanding both about how their bodies work and about what the oxygen is expected to do for them. It is essential that the patient's worries and concerns about the use of oxygen are addressed in order to ensure that the oxygen therapy is used both safely and effectively (see Case study 7.3).

PORTABLE OXYGEN

Indications for prescribing portable oxygen therapy

The Royal College of Physicians (1999) report on provision of domiciliary oxygen therapy suggests that patients with the following diagnoses should be considered for portable oxygen therapy:

- patients with COPD with long term oxygen therapy
- patients with COPD without long term oxygen therapy but who show oxygen desaturation on

Case study 7.3

Arthur is a 73-year-old gentleman who lives with his wife in a 2 bedroom ground floor flat. He was diagnosed with COPD 12 years ago. At his outpatient appointment 4 weeks after being discharged home following admission to hospital with an acute exacerbation of his COPD, he had spirometry and arterial blood gases performed on air. The results were FEV_1 1.2 L, FVC 1.7 L, PaO_2 7.1 kPa, $PaCO_2$ 5.8 kPa, SaO_2 88%. He was advised that he would require long term oxygen therapy for 15 hours per day at 2 L/min. He was referred to the respiratory nurse specialist who explained what long term oxygen therapy was and what benefits Arthur could expect. Arthur and his wife were given time to ask questions and given an information booklet regarding installation of the oxygen concentrator and ongoing care. Arthur's main concern was how he would fit in the 15 hours. The respiratory nurse went through his typical day with him and then they decided when he would use the oxygen. He decided to use the oxygen from about 8pm as he usually watched television until he went to bed, then use it all night. He usually got up around 7am but felt he would benefit from using it first thing in the morning as he often got breathless whilst washing and dressing. He felt that being free from his oxygen in the afternoon and early evening would still allow him to go to his social club and allow him and his wife to visit their daughter and 2-year-old grandchild. The respiratory nurse liaised with Arthur's GP who provided a prescription for an oxygen concentrator (2 L oxygen 15 hours per day) and a back up cylinder. Arthur's wife collected the prescription, which she gave to the engineer who installed the oxygen concentrator 4 days later. The respiratory nurse did a home visit 2 weeks later to find that Arthur was getting on very well using the oxygen therapy and that his SpO_2 using pulse oximetry was 94% on 2 L/min oxygen via nasal cannulae, indicating correction of hypoxaemia. The respiratory nurse sent a letter to the GP and wrote in the hospital notes regarding her finding from the home visit.

sary, for example where patients have had difficulty coming to terms with their need to use portable oxygen at an earlier stage of their disease. In most, but not all, cases these patients will already have an oxygen concentrator at home. The formal test for portable oxygen therapy involves:

- demonstrating a fall in oxygen saturation on walking
- patients achieving an improved walking distance and/or
- improvement in sensation of breathlessness when using oxygen.

Who is portable oxygen appropriate for?

It is important that the purpose for which the portable oxygen is prescribed is fully established with the patient, namely for use when walking or on exercise, in order to minimize oxygen desaturation. The healthcare professional involved with the supply of portable oxygen should explain the use of the cylinder before entering into testing the patient so that the patient fully appreciates what is involved in having a cylinder. Lock et al (1991) highlighted the low compliance of patients who have portable oxygen at home so it is vital that steps are taken to ensure maximal adherence. Explanation should include a detailed discussion about how much the patient goes out of doors, and over what period of time, in order to ascertain how useful the cylinder will be to the

exercise, improved levels of exercise with oxygen and who are motivated to use portable oxygen
- patients with interstitial lung disease, e.g. fibrosing alveolitis
- patients with cystic fibrosis
- patients with neuromuscular/skeletal disorders.

The decision to prescribe portable oxygen should usually be made following formal assessment of the benefit to be gained by the patient. In some cases a formal assessment may be unneces-

Box 7.4   Points to cover with patients who are about to be assessed for portable oxygen

- Ask patients about how much they go out to find out what the potential use of the cylinder might be
- Ask how long the trips last, as the capacity of the cylinder is limited
- Show patients how the oxygen will be delivered to them, e.g. nasal cannulae or mask, and discuss how they will cope with this in public
- Discuss what is involved in refilling the portable cylinder at home
- Ascertain if patients are going to be safe and capable of managing the refilling of the cylinder

patient. The mechanism of delivery of the oxygen from the cylinder to the patient should be demonstrated so that the patient has time to appreciate and understand what is expected of them if a portable cylinder is prescribed.

Assessment for portable oxygen

The assessment procedure for portable oxygen should be explained fully to the patient. The patient should not take bronchodilators prior to or during the assessment. Adequate time in which to do the assessment should be allowed as the patient should rest for 30 minutes between walks. The assessment involves the patient doing a walking test. This could either be the six minute walking test or the shuttle walking test. There are advantages and disadvantages in the use of both tests.

Six minute walking test

The six minute walking test (Butland et al 1982) involves the patient walking for six minutes having been instructed to walk as if late for an appointment. Patients should feel that they could not have walked any further at the end of the test but may stop at any given time for a rest. During the walk a record is made of the distance walked, oxygen saturation, heart rate, and the time spent resting during the walk. An estimation of the degree of breathlessness should be made by using, for example, the visual analogue score for breathlessness (Fig. 7.8) before and immediately after the walk and during recovery time to give an indication of the patient's subjective response to supplemental oxygen.

The time taken for the patient to recover should also be noted, by recording the time taken

for oxygen saturation and heart rate to return to normal. The patient should perform a baseline walk on air, a walk using 2 L of oxygen and a further walk using 2 L of air from a portable air cylinder. The walk with the air cylinder will give an idea of the placebo effect of using a cylinder. If there is insufficient correction of oxygen desaturation using 2 L of oxygen it may be necessary to perform a further walk using 4 L. One of the major disadvantages of using the six minute walking test is that three practice walks are required to ensure reproducibility, with the distance walked increasing with each of the first three walks due to the learning effect; i.e. the patient will walk further with each of the first three walks because he or she is learning how to do the test. It is also an effort dependent test, dependent on how hard the patient pushes him/herself.

Shuttle walking test

The shuttle walking test (Singh et al 1992) is an incremental, externally paced test that involves the patient walking around two cones set 10 m apart, turning around each cone in time to bleeps from a cassette tape. The advantages of this test are that only one practice walk is required for reproducibility and that the test is paced by bleeps from a cassette as opposed to the patient's effort. The disadvantage is that the test does not assess endurance but maximal effort, and in some cases this may not prove to be the most appropriate test. Recordings of distance walked, oxygen saturation and heart rate during the walk, and scores for breathlessness should still be made as with the six minute walk and the walks performed as described above. It is necessary to allow the patient to rest for 30 minutes between walks.

The results of the walking test need to be analysed to determine if portable oxygen therapy would benefit the patient. Criteria for suitability for portable oxygen therapy have been devised (Lock et al 1991) and include:

- a fall in SpO_2 of at least 4% on exercise below 90% on a baseline walk breathing room air and

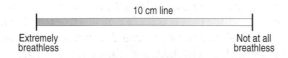

Figure 7.8   Visual analogue scale for breathlessness.

- a 10% increase in walking distance or
- a 10% improvement in visual analogue score.

The criteria are based on comparing results using portable oxygen compared to an air cylinder.

Prescribing portable oxygen for use at home

Having performed the walking test and obtained a positive result the patient should be issued with a portable cylinder (Fig. 7.9). The standard portable cylinder has a filling capacity of 230 L of compressed oxygen, weighs 2.3 kg and will last 1.5 hours set at 2 L or 45 minutes set at 4 L.

The provision of an AF cylinder should be made by the prescriber via the patient's GP. This large cylinder will provide the means by which the patient will fill the small cylinder at home and once the large cylinder becomes empty a full one will be supplied by the patient's local pharmacy. The AF cylinder will be provided without a flow head to allow filling of the small cylinder. If the patient already has a spare cylinder for use in the event of failure of the oxygen concentrator, this cylinder should not be used to fill the portable cylinder.

Instructions on filling the portable cylinder

Patients should be instructed in the filling of the portable cylinder, shown how to do it and warned of the dangers of the use of oxygen in the home. They should be provided with written instructions and given a contact number to use in an emergency or in the event of failure of the cylinder.

Those healthcare professionals who have responsibility for teaching the filling of portable cylinders should themselves be approved to do so. The Medicines Act (1968) states that doctors and pharmacists are able to fill and therefore teach the filling of such cylinders, as decanting of gases constitutes dispensing a drug. However, it may be possible, by gaining approval from the hospital's Medicines Committee, to set up a system of approving other healthcare professionals to offer this service.

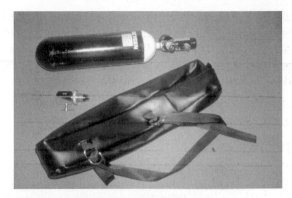

Figure 7.9   Portable oxygen cylinder.

Alternatives to portable oxygen therapy

PD cylinder

In some cases, for example where patients need a cylinder but not for the purposes of mobilizing or exercise, it may be appropriate for them to be prescribed a PD cylinder. This cylinder has a bulky carrying handle and is too heavy for a patient to carry independently but is ideal for short trips out in a wheelchair. Again the cylinder has a small capacity and will only supply oxygen for limited periods but is available on an FP10 prescription from the patient's GP.

Oxygen conserving devices

Oxygen conserving devices were originally made to conserve small volumes of oxygen in a reservoir created in the tubing just before the prongs on nasal cannulae (Moore-Gillon et al 1985).

More recently, oxygen conserving devices have been developed as an adjunct to the portable oxygen cylinder in order to maximize the use of the oxygen (Garrod et al 1999). They work by pulsing the dose of oxygen on inspiration only and allowing variable levels of oxygen to be supplied. This is achieved by selecting how frequently a breath triggers a pulse of oxygen (35 ml per breath) which could be every breath, or every second, third or fourth breath. In this way the total amount of oxygen consumed is reduced so that the cylinder will last 3–4 times longer than a portable cylinder (Fig. 7.10). It is important to assess the patient on the chosen setting prior to issuing the cylinder to ensure that the delivery of oxygen is sufficient to meet the needs of the patient when mobilizing, as the delivery of the oxygen will be dependent on the patient's rate of respiration.

Liquid oxygen

The use of liquid oxygen in a portable cylinder has been developed more recently for portable oxygen delivery. The system involves the supply of a large tank of liquid oxygen to the patient's home from which the smaller cylinder is filled (Fig. 7.11). The liquid oxygen is kept at a temperature of −240°F and a vaporizer converts the liquid oxygen to a gas on use.

This system offers the advantage that the cylinders last much longer than the compressed gas variety, supplying 8 hours of oxygen at 2 L/min. However, the cost of liquid oxygen is

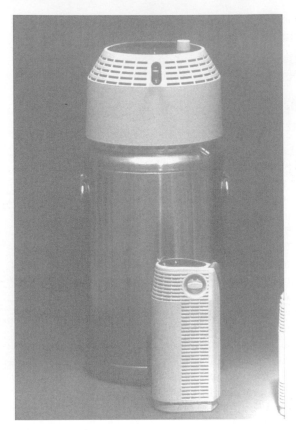

Figure 7.11 Liquid oxygen delivery system.

far greater than that of compressed oxygen. In addition, liquid oxygen evaporates quickly if it is not used, thus requiring the portable cylinder to be refilled even if it has not been used (Lock et al 1992).

Transtracheal oxygen

Transtracheal oxygen was developed in the USA as an alternative system to delivering oxygen via nasal cannulae or mask in patients requiring long term oxygen therapy. This system involves a surgical procedure to site a cannula into the patient's trachea through which oxygen is delivered directly to the lungs, which can greatly reduce the flow rate required by the patient and therefore allow greater mobility. A secondary advantage is that cosmetically this system eliminates

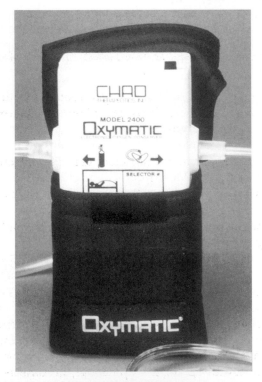

Figure 7.10 Oxygen conserving device.

the need for nasal cannulae or mask and thus could help to maximize patient adherence. However, in practice complications arose out of the use of these devices. Difficulties were experienced concerning the maintenance of a patent catheter and the catheter requiring attention once inserted (Kampelmacher et al 1997).

Summary

- Domiciliary oxygen therapy should be prescribed according to the guidelines
- Patients receiving long term oxygen therapy should be followed up and reassessed to ensure correction of hypoxaemia
- There should be liaison between primary and secondary care in relation to patients on long term oxygen therapy
- Patients who appear to be suitable for portable oxygen should be assessed
- Patients receiving long term oxygen therapy should be provided with education and support

---

PATIENT EDUCATION AND PROBLEM SOLVING

Assessment of patient knowledge and skill

It is vital that patients receive as much instruction and education about the use of long term oxygen therapy as they require in order to ensure the safe and effective use of oxygen at home. This will clearly vary from patient to patient and it will be the responsibility of the healthcare professional to ascertain in each individual case that there is an adequate level of knowledge and understanding about the use of oxygen. The patient should receive advice that includes the following:

- information about the disease process
- education about reasons for and benefits of using oxygen therapy
- safety measures that need to be observed when using oxygen
- types of devices available to use with oxygen therapy (i.e. nasal cannulae and masks)
- contact numbers for advice and support.

Information about the disease process

The patient should be educated about the disease process and about why oxygen therapy works, in order to maximize adherence to oxygen therapy at home. The more informed patients feel, the more they are likely to cope with changes in their condition and with what is expected of them. Education about the disease process should include an awareness of the symptoms of their disease, how to identify when their chest may be getting worse, what to do about it and how to maximize their functional capacity whilst using oxygen at home.

Education about reasons for and benefits of using oxygen therapy

Patients should be educated about why they have been prescribed oxygen therapy for use at home and what the benefits are of using the oxygen therapy. They should be advised about:

- safe use of oxygen
- number of hours
- number of litres per minute.

Safety measures that need to be observed when using oxygen

The patient should be taught about the safety measures that must be observed when using oxygen. These include:

- no smoking or naked flames near the oxygen supply
- no grease or oil near the source of oxygen as they support combustion
- not altering the setting of the oxygen without prior instruction from a healthcare professional.

The patient must fully understand the implications and the likely effects of increasing the dosage of oxygen, in order to prevent accidental use of high levels of oxygen. Patients should know what to do in the event of a deterioration in their condition, for example if they become more drowsy, or develop headaches.

Types of devices available to use with oxygen therapy

Teaching the patient about the different types of interface available for use with oxygen therapy will increase patient choice and adherence to treatment. Many find that the interface of choice is nasal cannulae as these allow the patient to communicate and eat and drink without difficulty.

Contact numbers for advice and support

Patients should be given the name of a healthcare professional to contact should they run into any difficulties with using their oxygen, as well as emergency telephone numbers in case of equipment breakdown. Patients should also have regular follow up and reassessment to ensure that hypoxaemia continues to be corrected.

Addressing questions patients may ask

Healthcare professionals who are dealing with patients who require oxygen should be prepared to advise and answer questions.

It is important that the learning needs of the healthcare professionals responsible for advising patients about the use of oxygen are met and that they themselves are knowledgeable and experienced in dealing with problems concerning the use of oxygen. This may require a programme of education to be in place that addresses all of the appropriate issues with the staff concerned.

Box 7.5   Questions patients frequently ask

- How is it decided how much oxygen I require?
- Will I become addicted to oxygen?
- How many years will I need it for?
- How does the concentrator work?
- Is enough oxygen left in the room for my family to breathe?
- Is the concentrated oxygen clean enough for me to breathe?
- Can I cook whilst I am on my oxygen?
- What do I do if visitors want to smoke?

Summary

The person receiving oxygen therapy should be able to:

- State the reason why they require oxygen therapy
- State safety measures when using oxygen
- State flow rate and hours per day oxygen therapy is required
- Demonstrate the use of oxygen equipment and the use of oxygen devices
- State how to avoid dry mouth and nasal congestion
- Decide best position for oxygen equipment in the home
- State who to contact in case of medical and equipment problems

TRAVEL

British Oxygen Company (BOC) recommends that patients carrying a portable oxygen cylinder in a car should carry a 'transport emergency card' that they will supply. This card has details on it regarding the safety measures required in an emergency, for example fire or accident. BOC also issues a 'vehicle safety card' that gives advice about the safe carriage of oxygen cylinders in private cars. The company recommends that patients with oxygen at home inform their household contents insurer and that those transporting portable oxygen cylinders in their cars inform their car insurers.

For patients going on holiday in the UK by car, it is possible to take the oxygen concentrator with them. Alternatively, it may be necessary to organize the provision of oxygen cylinders via a local GP. Most rail and coach companies will make arrangements for patients who require oxygen cylinders when travelling and most shipping companies will allow travel with a concentrator. For short stays abroad it may be necessary to organize the provision of oxygen cylinders via the local pharmacist, but this is probably best done in advance and via the booking agent.

Airline travel

Long haul flight travel is known to cause oxygen desaturation, in some cases down to 8 kPa, due to reduced cabin pressure. In normal travellers this is thought not to cause any difficulties. However, a reduction in arterial oxygenation of this magnitude in patients who are already hypoxaemic places them at risk. Studies have shown that a group of COPD patients experienced falls in arterial oxygen levels down to 6 kPa at 7000 feet (Schwartz et al 1984). The British Thoracic Society (2000) have produced guidelines for managing passengers with lung disease planning air travel. A pre-flight assessment is recommended that includes:

- history and examination
- previous flying experience
- spirometry
- arterial blood gases/SpO_2.

Schwartz et al (1984) suggest that the best predictor of in-flight hypoxaemia is pre-flight PaO_2. Assessment and advice regarding in-flight oxygen should be given to respiratory patients intending to take a flight (Table 7.3).

In some cases the airline concerned will make a charge for the cost of the provision of the oxygen. If necessary, it is possible to test patients at sub-atmospheric levels of oxygen in the laboratory by subjecting them to 15% oxygen and taking an arterial blood gas at that level (Cramer et al 1996). Again it is advisable for patients who are oxygen

Table 7.3 Guide to need for in-flight supplemental oxygen

Assessment SpO_2	In-flight oxygen requirements
SpO_2 > 95%	No oxygen
SpO_2 92–95%	No oxygen
SpO_2 92–95% and additional risk factors (i.e. cardiac disease)	May need oxygen (further assessment required)
SpO_2 < 92%	In-flight oxygen required
Uses long term oxygen therapy	May need increased flow rate

dependent to arrange holiday insurance if travelling abroad.

CONCLUSION

Oxygen therapy can be used for a wide range of acute and chronic respiratory conditions. To ensure that healthcare professionals are able to provide high quality care and support for patients using oxygen therapy it is vital that they have adequate education and knowledge to deal with patient problems.

REFERENCES

Bateman N T, Leech R M 1998 ABC of oxygen: acute oxygen therapy. British Medical Journal 317: 798–801

British Thoracic Society 2000 Managing passengers with lung disease planning air travel. British Thoracic Society Standards of Care. British Thoracic Society, London

Butland R J A, Pang J, Gross E R et al 1982 Two-, six-, and twelve-minute walking tests in respiratory disease. British Medical Journal 284: 1607–1608

Campbell E J, Baker D, Crites-Silver P 1988 Subjective effects of humidification of oxygen for delivery by nasal cannula. Chest 93(2): 289–293

Cramer D, Ward S, Geddes D 1996 Assessment of oxygen supplementation during air travel. Thorax 51: 202–203

Department of Health and Social Security 1985 Introduction of oxygen concentrators to the domiciliary oxygen service. Health notice: HN (FP) (85) (35)

Dilworth J P 1990 Acceptability of oxygen concentrators: the patient's view. British Journal of General Practice. October, 415–417

Fell H, Boehm M 1998 Easing the discomfort of oxygen therapy. Nursing Times 94(38): 56–58

Garrod R, Bestall J C, Paul E, Wedzicha J A 1999 Evaluation of pulsed dose oxygen delivery during exercise in patients with severe chronic obstructive pulmonary disease. Thorax 54: 242–244

Gunawardena K A, Patel B, Campbell I A et al 1984 Oxygen as a driving gas for nebulisers: safe or dangerous? British Medical Journal 288: 272–274

Kampelmacher M J, Deenstra M, Van Kesteren R G et al 1997 Transtracheal oxygen therapy: an effective safe alternative to nasal oxygen administration. European Respiratory Journal 10: 828–833

Lock S H, Paul E A, Rudd R M, Wedzicha J A 1991 Portable oxygen therapy: assessment and usage. Respiratory Medicine 85: 407–412

Lock S H, Blower G, Prynne M, Wedzicha J A 1992 Comparison of liquid and gaseous oxygen for domiciliary portable use. Thorax 47: 98–100

Medical Research Council Working Party 1981 Long term domiciliary oxygen therapy in chronic hypoxic cor pulmonale complicating chronic bronchitis and emphysema. Lancet i: 681–686

Moore-Gillon J C, George R J D, Geddes D M 1985 An oxygen conserving nasal cannula. Thorax 40: 817–819

Newman S P, Clarke S W 1983 Therapeutic aerosols 1: physical and practical considerations. Thorax 38: 881–886

Nocturnal Oxygen Therapy Trial Group 1980 Continuous or nocturnal oxygen therapy in hypoxaemic chronic obstructive lung disease. Annals of Internal Medicine 93: 391–398

Pitkin A D, Roberts C M, Wedzicha J A 1994 Arterialised earlobe blood gas analysis: an under used technique. Thorax 49: 364–366

Restrick L J, Paul W A, Braid G M, Cullinan P et al 1993 Assessment and follow up of patients prescribed long term oxygen treatment. Thorax 48(7): 7708–7713

Royal College of Physicians 1999 Domiciliary oxygen therapy services: clinical guidelines and advice for prescribers. Royal College of Physicians, London

Schwartz J S, Bencowitz H Z, Moser K M 1984 Air travel hypoxaemia with chronic obstructive pulmonary disease. Annals of Internal Medicine 100: 473–477

Singh S J, Morgan M D L, Scott S et al 1992 The development of the shuttle walking test of disability in patients with chronic airways obstruction. Thorax 47: 1019–1024

Sykes M K, McNicol M W, Campbell E J M 1976 Respiratory failure, 2nd edn. Blackwell Scientific Publications, Oxford, pp 142–146

USEFUL ADDRESSES

British Oxygen Company (BOC)
PO Box 6
Priestley Road
Worsley
Manchester M28 2UT
(Contracted to provide oxygen concentrators)

DeVilbis (Sunrise Medical Ltd)
High Street
Wollaston
West Midlands DY8 4PS
(Contracted to provide oxygen concentrators)

Life Support (Europe) Ltd
19 Cartmel Drive
Dunstable
Bedfordshire LU6 3PT
(Supplies oxymatics)

Mallincrodt Nellcor Puritan Bennett
10 London Road
Bicester
Oxfordshire OX6 0JX
(Produces liquid oxygen system)

Oxygen Therapy Company Ltd
Shearwater House
Ocean Way
Cardiff CF24 5TF
(Contracted to provide oxygen concentrators)

Sabre Safety Ltd
Matterson House
Ash Road
Aldershot
Hampshire GU12 4DE
(Supplies portable cylinders)

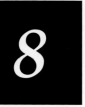

8

Respiratory support techniques

Christine Mikelsons   *Glenda Esmond*

Respiratory support techniques include those
modalities which are capable of supporting
gaseous exchange without the use of invasive
measures such as endotracheal intubation,
thereby treating underlying diseases which
result in Type I or Type II respiratory failure
(Table 8.1).

The treatment of Type I respiratory failure will
centre around:

- oxygen therapy
- maximizing medication such as
  bronchodilators, corticosteroids, antibiotics
  and diuretics
- +/− continuous positive airway pressure
  (CPAP).

The treatment of Type II respiratory failure may
involve:

- oxygen therapy
- maximizing medication such as
  bronchodilators, corticosteroids, antibiotics
  and diuretics
- respiratory stimulants in the form of
  intravenous doxapram
- non-invasive ventilation

Table 8.1 Definition of Type I and Type II respiratory failure

Arterial blood gas values	Normal	Type I respiratory failure	Type II respiratory failure
pH	7.35–7.45	7.35–7.45	7.35–7.45 (compensated) or < 7.35 (respiratory acidosis)
PaO_2	12–14 kPa	< 8 kPa	< 8 kPa
$PaCO_2$	4.6–6.0 kPa	4.6–6.0 kPa	> 6 kPa
SaO_2	95% +	< 92%	< 92%

- intubation and intermittent positive pressure ventilation (IPPV).

In the presence of Type II respiratory failure, with an uncorrected respiratory acidosis (pH < 7.35), there is a poor prognostic outcome for the patient. When considering the range of options available to provide any type of non-invasive respiratory support, it is essential that the patient is fully assessed prior to starting the therapeutic intervention. It is equally important that the mode of action of the intervention is fully understood and applied appropriately. This is important because the types of respiratory support vary in their functional capacities and as a result should not be considered to be interchangeable in their use; for example, CPAP should not be substituted for non-invasive ventilation, or high flow CPAP substituted for CPAP from a machine supplying compressed air.

NON-INVASIVE VENTILATION

The term non-invasive ventilation applies to ventilatory support delivered via a non-invasive interface, such as a nasal mask, full face mask or nasal pillows. Non-invasive ventilation (NIV) may also be referred to as non-invasive positive pressure ventilation (NIPPV).

Long term use of domiciliary non-invasive ventilatory support has been demonstrated to be effective in the treatment of Type II respiratory failure as a result of restrictive diseases such as neuromuscular diseases, kyphoscoliosis and thoracoplasty, and obstructive diseases such as chronic obstructive pulmonary disease (COPD). It has also been shown to have a place in the treatment of certain groups of patients in the acute setting, for example in weaning from intubation and in acute respiratory failure caused by chronic lung disease.

The use of non-invasive ventilation should be confined to those patients in Type II respiratory failure who require ventilatory support. This method of ventilation involves the use of a non-invasive interface through which ventilatory support can be given and as a technique it confers the advantage of not requiring endotracheal intubation, thereby helping to avoid associated problems (Antonelli et al 1998). The incidence of pneumonia in patients ventilated via an endotracheal tube has been shown to increase by 1% per day (Hotchkiss & Marini 1998). Indeed, Estes & Meduri (1995) found that endotracheal intubation was the most important predisposing factor for the incidence of pneumonia associated with ventilation.

As a technique it can also be used with those for whom intubation and ventilation may not be indicated due to their associated risks and the likely poor outcome of weaning, as in some patients with COPD. It also offers an alternative method of ventilation to be considered with patients for whom intermittent non-invasive ventilation may be appropriate, for example when used palliatively to reduce distressing breathlessness. However, it is important that clear aims of treatment are identified to ensure that the use of non-invasive ventilation rather than intermittent positive pressure ventilation (IPPV) is indicated, since an inappropriate choice or a delay in starting treatment could result in increased risk of patient mortality. Little evidence exists to support the use of non-invasive ventilation in an acute asthma attack (Hotchkiss & Marini 1998). Moreover, its use could prove fatal if a patient in worsening hypercapnic respiratory failure due to status asthmaticus were to be denied further intervention such as treatment with IPPV.

Box 8.1   Advantages of non-invasive ventilation

- Avoids intubation
- Has a sensitive trigger to help decrease the work of breathing
- Provides adequate oxygenation and clearance of carbon dioxide
- Allows for hydration and chest clearance
- Improves quality of sleep
- Allows patients to communicate
- Allows patients to eat and drink when off the machine
- Relatively inexpensive

Physiological evidence to support the use of non-invasive ventilation

There are four main physiological theories to support the use of non-invasive ventilation:

- Fatigued respiratory muscles are 'rested' (Braun & Marino 1984).
- Control of nocturnal hypoventilation is of prime importance in reversing chronic ventilatory failure and is thought to restore chemosensitivity of the respiratory centre (Elliott et al 1991).
- Ventilatory load is reduced as a result of improvements in lung compliance and improved levels of arterial $PaCO_2$ which relate to reduced gas trapping and residual volume (Elliott et al 1991).
- Changes in arterial blood gas tensions when non-invasive ventilation is used overnight are maintained during spontaneous breathing during the day and lead to improved sleep quality and reduced sensation of breathlessness.

Elliott (1999) suggests that the probable mechanism of action for non-invasive ventilation is a combination of resting the respiratory muscles, controlling nocturnal hypoventilation and improving quality of sleep with each component playing a greater or lesser role at different stages of the disease and in different individuals. Correction of hypoventilation during sleep by the use of non-invasive ventilation can be demonstrated using polysomnographic sleep studies (Fig. 8.1a, 8.1b).

The importance of this lies in the fact that patients with Type II respiratory failure are at most risk of slipping into worsening respiratory

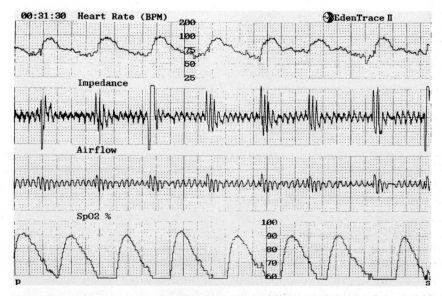

Figure 8.1a   Polysomnographic sleep study showing deranged heart rate, chest wall movement (impedance), airflow and oxygen saturation levels (SpO_2) in a patient with Type II respiratory failure on room air.

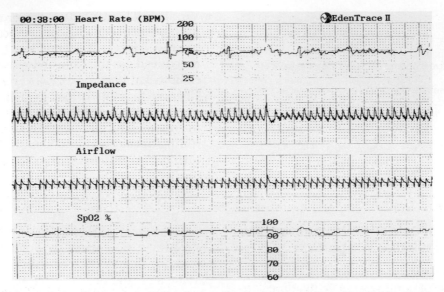

Figure 8.1b Polysomnographic sleep study showing correlation of heart rate, chest wall movement (impedance), airflow and oxygen saturation levels (SpO_2) in a patient using non-invasive ventilation.

failure during sleep. In those with normal respiratory drive, sleep will result in a variety of physiological changes which will not produce any detrimental side effects. These changes may include a reduction in postural muscle tone, increased upper airway resistance and a reduction in ventilatory drive and response to hypoxaemia and hypercapnia. Douglas et al (1982) found that this could result in a fall in ventilation of the order of 10–15% during sleep. In addition, there may be a fall in ventilation by as much as 40% during the rapid eye movement (REM) phase of sleep when diaphragmatic function assumes the main role in ventilation. The onset of nocturnal respiratory failure may begin during REM sleep, caused by hypoventilation during that phase, and may go unnoticed. Progression of the underlying disease leads to sleep disturbance in non-REM sleep. This results in deteriorating arterial blood gases, early morning headaches and daytime sleepiness. The onset of nocturnal respiratory failure may take years to develop and may therefore be confused with a deterioration in the patient's underlying respiratory condition (Piper & Ellis 1998). The use of nocturnal non-invasive ventilation has been demonstrated to control noctural hypoventilation.

Acute use

Weaning from intubation

In addition to preventing the need for endotracheal intubation, non-invasive ventilation can also assist in weaning intubated patients with underlying respiratory disease. These patients may have weak respiratory muscles which may

---

Box 8.2 Use of non-invasive ventilation

Acute use
- Weaning from intubation
- Acute respiratory failure in chronic lung disease

Restrictive pulmonary diseases
- Neuromuscular and chest wall diseases
  - Duchenne muscular dystrophy
  - dystrophia myotonica
  - poliomyelitis
  - kyphoscoliosis
  - thoracoplasty

Progressive neuromuscular disease
- Motor neurone disease

Obstructive pulmonary diseases
- COPD
- Bronchiectasis
- Cystic fibrosis

have been exacerbated by prolonged intubation and ventilation. This can make the process of weaning difficult and slow and staged efforts may be required before the process is successful. Brochard et al (1994) compared the use of pressure support, synchronized intermittent mandatory ventilation and T-piece trials as methods of weaning patients from intubated ventilation and found that the use of pressure support ventilation reduced both the length of time spent weaning and the time spent in the intensive care unit.

Two studies have looked at the use of non-invasive ventilation in the weaning of patients from IPPV. Both studies included patients with a variety of conditions including chest wall diseases, neuromuscular diseases and postoperative complications. Udwadia et al (1992) found that the use of non-invasive ventilation reduced the time spent on the ventilator and reduced the length of hospital stay as a result (Fig. 8.2). Restrick et al (1993) found significant improve-

ments in PaO_2 and $PaCO_2$ where non-invasive ventilation was used in weaning from full ventilation.

Successful weaning of a patient from IPPV via endotracheal tube or tracheostomy requires a team approach in setting appropriate goals and an agreed plan of action for the weaning process so that the care of the patient is coordinated. It is important that the patient's condition is optimized and that he is alert, oriented and off all sedating agents. It is also important that the patient remains in the intensive care unit for a period of time after extubation to avoid potential crises should his/her condition deteriorate suddenly.

Acute respiratory failure in chronic lung disease

The use of non-invasive ventilation in patients with acute respiratory failure as a result of chronic lung disease is now well documented. Three large randomized controlled trials support its use in acute respiratory failure due to COPD (Bott et al 1993, Brochard et al 1995, Kramer et al 1995). The benefits of non-invasive ventilation in patients with acute respiratory failure are:

- a significant reduction in the need for intubation in the non-invasive group
- a significant reduction in mean hospital stay and in-hospital mortality
- significant improvements in pH, PaO_2 and $PaCO_2$ post non-invasive ventilation (Fig. 8.3).

Ambrosino et al (1995) looked at predictors of success in the use of non-invasive ventilation in acute respiratory failure due to COPD treated with non-invasive ventilation. Success or failure was determined by survival or need to intubate. Unsuccessful episodes of treatment with non-invasive ventilation were associated with:

- pneumonia
- low body mass index (BMI)
- severe level of neurological deterioration
- inability to comply with ventilation

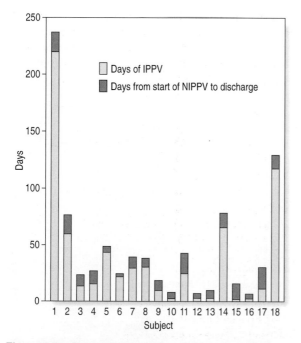

Figure 8.2 Bar graph of number of days on ventilation (IPPV) and number of days from the start of nasal ventilation (NIPPV) until discharge. Reproduced with permission from Udwadia et al 1992.

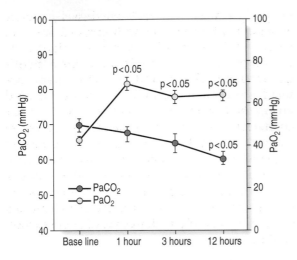

Figure 8.3 Mean values for PaO_2 and $PaCO_2$ during the first 12 hours of non-invasive ventilation (p values are for comparison with baseline values). Reproduced with permission from Brochard et al 1995. Copyright 1995 Massachusetts Medical Society. All rights reserved.

- severely deranged baseline pH and $PaCO_2$.

In summary, the following criteria are important when using non-invasive ventilation for acute respiratory failure:

- Respiratory acidosis is an important prognostic factor.
- Early correction of acidosis will decrease mortality.
- Non-invasive ventilation significantly improves gaseous exchange, respiratory acidosis, rates of intubation, hospital stay and mortality compared to standard therapy.
- The early use of non-invasive ventilation in the progression of respiratory failure is important for maximum effectiveness (Wedzicha 1996).

Long term use

There is now a wealth of evidence to support the long term domiciliary use of non-invasive ventilation in chronic respiratory failure due to both restrictive and obstructive respiratory diseases. Restrictive respiratory diseases are those which result in reductions in both forced expi-

ratory volume in 1 second (FEV_1) and forced vital capacity (FVC), giving a near normal ratio of FEV_1/FVC. This group therefore includes those diseases which impede chest wall movement due to reduced muscle function, such as the neuromuscular diseases and those which restrict lung capacity due to chest wall deformity. The obstructive respiratory diseases are those which result in reduced lung function caused by destruction of the lung tissues leading to gas trapping. This group includes diseases such as COPD, bronchiectasis and cystic fibrosis. These changes result in a reduced FEV_1/FVC ratio, as although both values are reduced, FEV_1 is reduced by the greater amount (American Thoracic Society 1986).

Over a 5 year period Simonds & Elliott (1995) studied patients with a variety of diseases who were using non-invasive ventilation, in order to compare its continued use in each group (Fig. 8.4). The use of non-invasive ventilation was equated with survival, since the reason for stopping non-invasive ventilation in most cases was death.

The results identified that those patients with restrictive diseases fared better than those with obstructive diseases. Patients with post-polio-

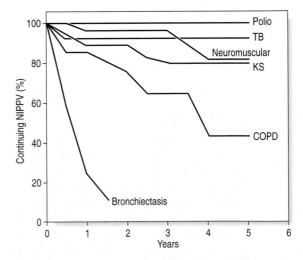

Figure 8.4 Probability of continuing non-invasive ventilation (polio = poliomyelitis; TB = tuberculosis; KS = kyphoscoliosis). Reproduced with permission from Simonds & Elliott 1995.

myelitis, post-tuberculosis, neuromuscular diseases and scoliosis have a chance of continuing with non-invasive ventilation at 5 years of 100%, 94%, 81% and 79% respectively, and those with COPD and bronchiectasis having a 43% chance and a less than 20% chance respectively.

Restrictive pulmonary diseases

Neuromuscular and chest wall diseases

Studies support the use of non-invasive ventilation in patients with Duchenne muscular dystrophy, dystrophia myotonica and poliomyelitis (Ellis et al 1987, Leger et al 1989). Here the problem is one of muscle weakness as a result of neuromuscular disease leading to poor respiratory effort.

In patients with kyphoscoliosis and post-tuberculosis thoracoplasty the chest wall deformity will limit the extent of their respiratory effort but this can in part be corrected by non-invasive ventilation (Ellis et al 1988, Kerby et al 1987).

In summary, the evidence supporting the use of non-invasive ventilation in these groups shows:

- improved daytime arterial blood gases
- decreased symptoms of hypoventilation
- improved quality of sleep.

Progressive neuromuscular disease

Motor neurone disease

The use of non-invasive ventilation in motor neurone disease (MND) as palliation for symptomatic ventilatory failure is now becoming more widely recognized in the UK (Polkey et al 1999). It may be appropriate for use with terminally ill patients where a degree of flexibility and patient choice about the use of the machine may be of paramount importance (Borasio & Voltz 1998). Cazzolli & Oppenheimer (1996), working in the USA, advocate offering non-invasive ventilation and tracheostomy to patients with bul-

bar palsy at an early stage in the disease, as there is some evidence showing improved survival levels in this group. However, this option needs careful consideration in relation to the patient's quality of life. The respiratory problems encountered by patients with MND centre around progressive chest wall weakness and bulbar palsy. In the later stages of the disease, secretion aspiration may become more troublesome as patients become less able to swallow or expectorate their secretions due to poor tidal volumes and therefore poor cough, and carers should be taught how to help the patient clear secretions effectively, possibly with the use of home suction equipment.

Obstructive pulmonary diseases

COPD

Evidence supports the long term use of non-invasive ventilation in selected patients with COPD with proven improvements in arterial blood gases and quality of sleep. Indications for initiating the use of non-invasive ventilation are when the symptoms of nocturnal hypoventilation and daytime hypercapnia develop. However, the optimal time for starting ventilation is still unclear. Of note is the reduced survival rate for those patients with COPD receiving non-invasive ventilation compared to the neuromuscular and chest wall disease groups, demonstrated by two studies (Leger et al 1994, Simonds & Elliott 1995). The recommendations for the instigation of non-invasive ventilation in patients with COPD are that it should be started early in the natural history of the disease where there is documented nocturnal hypercapnia that is reversed by non-invasive ventilation (Meecham-Jones et al 1995).

Cystic fibrosis and bronchiectasis

Simonds & Elliott (1995) showed that patients with bronchiectasis using domiciliary non-invasive ventilation had the poorest chance of continuing non-invasive ventilation of all of the disease groups. Two other studies showed that non-invasive ventilation did not improve arterial blood gas results in this group but both showed decreased hospitalizations whilst using it (Benhamou et al 1997, Gacouin et al 1996).

The use of non-invasive ventilation in patients with cystic fibrosis has been recommended as a bridge to transplantation (Hill et al 1998, Hodson et al 1991). It may also be a useful adjunct to treatment when patients are receiving maximal therapy in an acute exacerbation of the disease (Piper et al 1992). However, clear aims for treatment should be identified when using non-invasive ventilation in patients with cystic fibrosis, for example for reversal of an acute episode or for palliation of breathlessness, with clearly identified outcome measures. It is important to introduce an element of patient choice about its use and to allow patients to determine their usage themselves, with the possibility of stopping should it no longer give benefit.

ASSESSING THE NEED FOR VENTILATORY SUPPORT

Clinical indications for non-invasive ventilation may vary depending on whether it is for use in the acute situation, in weaning or for long term use at home (Box 8.3).

When assessing the patient for non-invasive ventilation it is important to consider both the factors for consideration before commencing non-invasive ventilation and the contraindications to its use (Box 8.4).

The assessment of the patient for ventilatory support in the acute setting should be thorough and careful. Patients who are being considered for this kind of support will be unwell and all patients will be in Type II respiratory failure. The referral to the anaesthetic team for assessment, intubation and ventilation should not be delayed when this is indicated. It may be necessary to consider an early referral for an anaesthetic opinion if the patient is being treated on the ward rather than on the intensive care or

---

Box 8.3 Clinical indications for the use of non-invasive ventilation

Acute use
- History of deteriorating blood gases (acidotic pH, hypoxaemia, hypercapnia)
- Increased breathlessness
- Sputum retention
- History of chronic lung disease

Weaning
- History of difficulties in weaning in the presence of underlying pulmonary disease in postoperative patients
- Failed weaning attempts due to fatigue and breathlessness

Acute on chronic
- History of deteriorating arterial blood gases
- Cyanosis
- Dyspnoea
- Tachycardia
- Sputum retention
- Confusion
- Hypercapnic flap
- Morning headache
- Cor pulmonale
- Ankle swelling

Box 8.4 Assessing the patient for non-invasive ventilation

Factors for consideration before commencing non-invasive ventilation
- Inability to correct oxygen levels due to hypercapnia
- Ability to cooperate with treatment
- Normal or near normal bulbar function
- Haemodynamic stability
- Ability to clear bronchial secretions

Contraindications to the use of non-invasive ventilation
- Undrained pneumothorax
- Extensive bullae
- Severe epistaxis
- Cardiovascular instability
- Pneumoencephalus
- Allergy to mask material
- Risk of aspiration when using full face mask in patient who is vomiting

---

high dependency unit (ICU/HDU) to ensure timely treatment.

A thorough assessment should be made by all members of the healthcare team and all existing medical interventions should be optimized prior to initiating the use of non-invasive ventilation. This technique should not be used instead of other therapeutic interventions and the assessment should include all systems of the body (Box 8.5).

Before instituting non-invasive ventilation a pre-treatment arterial blood gas should be taken. This can be taken either on room air or on supplementary oxygen, provided that a record is made of what the patient was breathing to aid future assessment. The patient should then have repeat arterial blood gases taken 1 hour after successful use of non-invasive ventilation and the two results compared for changes.

Studies in the use of non-invasive ventilation for the treatment of Type II respiratory failure due to COPD have demonstrated that where there is respiratory acidosis (decreased pH) which is not corrected by ventilation the prognosis for the patient's survival is poor (Ambrosino et al 1995). Therefore treatment with non-invasive ventilation should be aimed at the correction of respiratory acidosis and reduction of the partial pressure of carbon dioxide in the blood.

NON-INVASIVE VENTILATORS

The types of machine available for the delivery of non-invasive ventilation have a variety of modes of operation (Box 8.6). Generally the machines fall into one of two categories:

- pressure pre-set
- volume pre-set machines.

Each machine will have slightly differing features and it is important to understand these parameters in order to deliver effective ventilation.

Assist mode

Assist mode allows the patient to trigger the breaths supplied by the machine. Examples of

---

Box 8.5 Additional points to consider when assessing a patient for non-invasive ventilation

- Respiratory status
  - pre-existing disease process: what are baseline arterial blood gases?
  - overwhelming sputum retention will prevent adequate ventilation
  - respiratory breathing pattern (rate, rhythm)
  - sleep study/oximetry results
  - apnoea
- Neurological status
  - level of consciousness
  - level of ability to cooperate and communicate
  - unilateral weakness: will the patient manage to apply the non-invasive ventilation independently?
- Cardiovascular status
  - cor pulmonale: optimize medical management
  - fluid overload/renal failure
- Gastrointestinal status
  - constipation inhibits diaphragmatic function: particularly important in patients with low lung volumes
  - pain inhibits chest wall movement
- Infective processes
  - chest infection
  - septicaemia
- Drug therapy
  - oxygen therapy
  - steroids
  - doxapram
  - review type of pain relief and exclude opioids
  - antibiotic therapy
  - theophylline therapy
  - nebulized drug therapy
  - consider anxiolytics, e.g. haloperidol

Box 8.6 Features of non-invasive ventilators

- Assist mode
- Assist/control mode
- Control mode
- Expiratory positive airway pressure (EPAP)
- Pressure characteristics
- Trigger and response time
- Alarms
- Proportional assist ventilation (PAV)

---

machines with this mode are BiPAP S (Respironics Inc, USA), VPAP II (Resmed (UK) Ltd), Breas 401 (Breas Medical AB, Sweden).

Assist/control mode

Assist/control mode allows for patient triggering with the addition of a controlled back up rate which can be set in the event of a patient hypoventilating. Some machines will only cycle when the patient does not breathe (BiPAP ST30, VPAP II ST), others will cycle alongside patient breaths (Breas 401).

Control mode

Patients will receive all pre-set ventilator breaths regardless of how much breathing they do.

Expiratory positive airway pressure (EPAP)

EPAP should be set at between 2 and 6 cm H_2O. EPAP helps to eliminate $PaCO_2$ by giving a longer time for gaseous exchange and it is also thought that in COPD it may offset the inspiratory threshold load caused by the patient's intrinsic positive end expiratory pressure (PEEPi). PEEPi occurs in the presence of severe COPD. It is thought to increase the patient's work of breathing by increasing the inspiratory threshold load as a result of premature airway closure and air trapping. PEEPi has to be overcome in order for pressure and flow change to occur and it is thought that EPAP can do this by reducing the pressure change required (Elliott & Simonds 1995).

Pressure characteristics

The ease of delivery of either pressure or volume to the patient will be dependent on the pressure characteristics of the machine used. Each type of machine has its own type of pressure characteristics and in some machines this can be altered by using a ramp feature which allows the speed of delivery of the breath to be varied (Fig. 8.5).

The pressure characteristics will determine the speed of delivery of the breath from the machine. The importance of this lies in the fact that if a machine achieves a quick rise in pressure and the patient has high airway pressures and non-compliant lungs, efficient ventilation may not be achieved. In this case a machine delivering a slow rise may be more efficient in ventilating the patient. Turbulence in the tubing may also increase airway pressure which may cause an increase in bronchospasm.

Trigger and response time

Most non-invasive ventilators have a sensitive trigger enabling a quick response time in delivery of the breath to the patient. If the trigger is not sensitive enough the patient has to struggle for a triggered breath, thereby increasing the work of breathing. This will result in further fatigue which is clearly undesirable. Some machines allow for the setting of trigger sensitivity (Monnal DCC, Taema, France; Breas 501, Breas Medical AB, Sweden).

Alarms

Some machines have built-in alarms registering low and high airway pressures and leak. Alarms should be set appropriately according to the clinical need of the patient. Patients in hospital should be provided with a means of communicating whilst on the machine to encourage adherence and give peace of mind.

Proportional assist ventilation (PAV)

Proportional assist ventilation allows the pressure delivered to the patient to vary proportionately according to how much effort the patient makes throughout each breath and from breath to breath. The machine monitors the patient's respiratory rate and volume and varies the delivered pressure accordingly. This allows the patient to retain control over his breathing and therefore helps to prevent over ventilation, maximizing patient comfort, reducing peak airway pressure required for ventilation and preserving the patient's own reflexes (Younes 1992).

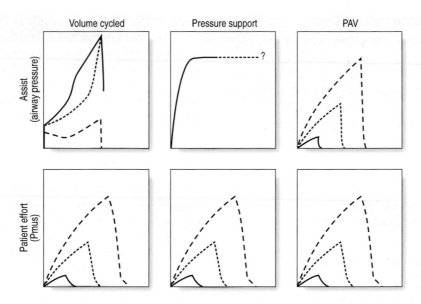

Figure 8.5 Comparison of modes: volume cycled, pressure support and proportional assist ventilation. Reproduced with permission from Respironics Inc, USA.

Pressure versus volume

The type of machine is identified by looking at the parameters which are displayed on the machine. It is important to synchronize the machine with the patient to optimize ventilation and patient comfort and it is therefore important to have assessed which machine will most easily meet the needs of the patient. In COPD or chest wall disorder patients in the chronic state no advantage is conferred by the use of a pressure or a volume machine, but volume pre-set machines were shown to increase minute ventilation (Elliott et al 1994, Meecham-Jones & Wedzicha 1993).

However, when treating acutely ill patients in hospital there are some differences in performance between pressure and volume machines which require consideration. Pressure pre-set machines work by delivering a pre-set pressure, either by time or flow cycling, at the point when expiration occurs. This means that this type of machine copes well with small leaks in the circuit and compensates for them. However, in the presence of high airway pressures the pre-set pressure may be achieved regardless of whether the volume delivered is sufficient to achieve good gaseous exchange in the patient.

Pre-set volume machines

Pre-set volume machines will deliver a fixed tidal or minute volume before cycling into expiration. In this type of machine the volume is delivered regardless of pulmonary characteristics such as airway pressure. This confers the advantage of providing adequate ventilation in the presence of high airway pressures. However, these machines cope poorly with leaks in the circuit and in most cases a low pressure alarm will identify the presence of leak. For this reason pre-set volume machines are capable of delivering efficient ventilation in the presence of high arterial carbon dioxide levels and poorly compliant lung tissue, and may be the machine of choice for these patients (Table 8.2).

Simonds & Elliott (1991) found that patients were less well controlled on pressure support if they required higher inflation pressures (> 25 cm H_2O) and that, in this situation, they were likely to have severe airflow obstruction, poor lung compliance or poor chest wall compliance. These

Table 8.2 Types of machines

Machine	BiPAP ST30	Breas 401	VPAP ST	Breas 501	Monnal DCC	Puritan Bennett LP10	Puritan Bennett Achieva
Type of machine	pressure	pressure	pressure	volume	volume	volume	pressure and volume
Cycling	flow/time	pressure	flow	volume	volume	volume	pressure or volume
Variable trigger sensitivity	yes but machine controlled	✓	×	✓	✓	✓	yes; either flow or pressure
Respiratory rate: fixed rate or back up	back up, fixed in timed mode	fixed and back up	back up	fixed and back up	fixed and back up	fixed and back up	fixed and back up
Ramp	×	✓	✓	×	×	×	✓
PEEP	✓	×	✓	×	✓	×	✓
Battery back up	×	✓	×	✓	✓	✓	✓
Alarms	×	✓	✓	✓	✓	✓	✓

✓ = present
× = absent

patients may therefore benefit from volume pre-set systems.

When using volume pre-set non-invasive ventilators the rule of thumb used to ventilate patients is:

$$1.5 \times 10 \text{ ml/kg (body weight)}$$
$$\text{e.g. } 1.5 \times 10 \times 70 \text{ kg} = 1050 \text{ ml tidal volume}$$

This may sound excessive when compared to the guide used to estimate tidal volume when ventilating using an endotracheal tube, which is 10 ml/kg, but it accounts for the losses in circuitry and upper airway tract deadspace and leaks. As has been stated earlier, the success of ventilation lies in the correction of deranged arterial blood gases and, in particular, the correction of an acidotic pH.

Pressure pre-set ventilators

Bilevel positive airway pressure machines, such as the VPAP and BiPAP (Fig. 8.6), allow for the setting of inspiratory and expiratory positive airway pressures which are delivered in response to the patient triggering the machine, with some machines allowing for the setting of a back up breath rate when the machine is set to the 'spontaneous/timed' mode, which will only be activated in the event that the patient does not trigger a breath him/herself. In the 'timed' mode the patient receives the pre-set breath rate from the machine and cannot trigger breaths him/herself.

Patients usually have a starting inspiratory positive airway pressure (IPAP) of greater than 14 cm H_2O up to a maximum of 30 cm H_2O. This starting pressure can be titrated against the arterial blood gases. If patients are unable to tolerate therapeutic levels initially, it is wise to lower the starting pressure to allow them to get used to it. However, it is not advisable to leave patients on a low IPAP for an extended period of time as there is a danger of re-breathing and exacerbating already high levels of carbon dioxide.

A pressure pre-set machine such as the Breas 401 (Fig. 8.7) allows for the setting of an inspiratory pressure to a maximum of 40 mbar, a respiratory rate and a trigger sensitivity.

This machine can be used in the 'pressure support' mode, which means that each patient breath is assisted by a pre-set level of pressure, and in addition it allows the setting of 'expiratory sense' which gives a degree of control over how long the patient is spending in expiration. In the 'pressure control' mode a back up rate of breaths can be pre-set, which will allow patients to take their own breaths and will then provide a back up breath should this not happen. This mode also allows for

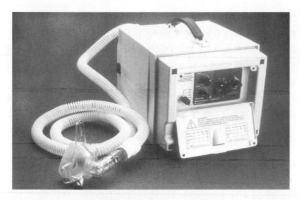

Figure 8.6 Bilevel positive airway pressure. Reproduced with permission from Medic-Aid Ltd.

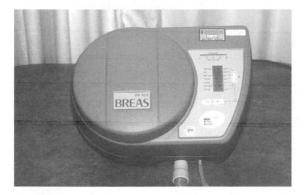

Figure 8.7 Breas 401.

the setting of inspiratory time, which gives a degree of control over the patient's ratio of inspiration to expiration (I:E ratio). The display will also show a reading of the estimated expiratory volume. There is a facility called the plateau which enables the setting of a variable ramp, from a square wave pattern to a slow rise in inspiration. This machine therefore offers a flexible approach to ventilatory support by virtue of the fact that it can provide both pressure support and assist control modes. It can also be powered by an external battery (24 v DC) supply if necessary. Some machines come with alarms fitted as standard.

Volume pre-set ventilators

These machines allow for the pre-setting of tidal volume or minute volume. They may also allow for the setting of respiratory rate, I:E ratio, PEEP, trigger sensitivity and low and high pressure alarms. They therefore have the advantage of supplying a fixed volume, which can prove useful in ventilating patients with a high respiratory rate and small tidal volumes for whom pre-set pressure ventilation proves fruitless due to its inability to increase tidal volumes. Examples of these machines are the Monnal DCC and the Breas 501. In addition these models also have a battery back-up. The Breas 501 is portable and will fit on the back of a wheelchair (Fig. 8.8).

SETTING A PATIENT UP ON NON-INVASIVE VENTILATION

When commencing a patient on non-invasive ventilation it is advisable to complete the following checklist:

- Complete a multidisciplinary assessment of the patient, identifying the need for non-invasive ventilation.
- Do baseline arterial blood gases.
- Assemble the required equipment.
- Ensure the patient is in a comfortable and supported position.
- Explain the aims of treatment and how the machine will feel.
- Allow patients to feel the air delivered from the machine on their hand to increase awareness.
- Entrain oxygen.

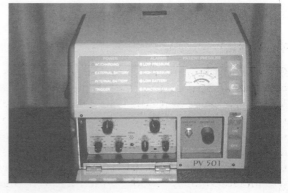

Figure 8.8 Breas 501.

- Allow patients to hold the mask over their nose/face themselves for the first few breaths so that they can remove the mask quickly if required.
- Reassure the patient about how the machine will feel.
- Ensure the mouth is closed if a nasal mask is used.
- Try to maintain a calm environment to give the patient confidence.
- Apply headgear so that there are no air leaks around the mask.
- Use an oximeter to monitor progress – this does not replace the need for arterial blood gases.
- Inform patients how long they are expected to keep the machine on for.
- Give the patient a means of communicating and summoning assistance.
- There should be a multidisciplinary assessment to decide on the plan of treatment, i.e. how long the patient should remain on the machine.
- Where possible allow the patient to have periods off the ventilator for eating and drinking, depending on how acutely ill he is.
- Monitor the stability of the patient on and off the ventilator.
- Remind the patient not to eat or drink whilst on the machine.

Oxygen entrainment should be titrated against the arterial blood gases and in most cases will be between 1 and 3 L/min if the patient is hypercapnic. Oxygen can be entrained at one of the ports on the mask, via a T-piece with an entertainment port, or, in some cases, by an entrainment port at the back of the non-invasive ventilator.

Repeat arterial blood gases should be taken after an hour on non-invasive ventilation in order to assess the effects of the treatment and to ensure that the treatment is not detrimental to the patient. Once repeat arterial blood gases have been taken, the patient should be reviewed in the light of the results. It may be necessary to alter ventilation if the results obtained were not those expected (Table 8.3).

If possible it is best to make one alteration to settings at a time, to enable identification of a problem. The arterial blood gases should be re-checked if the ventilator settings are changed, or if the machine is changed.

A plan of treatment should be agreed with the multidisciplinary team which may involve patients using the machine for the whole of the first 24–48 hours if they are acutely unwell. Once patients have become more stable, usage of the machine can be decreased by extending the periods spent off the machine. It is important that adequate monitoring is carried out at this stage. Patients should be encouraged to use the machine at night until a decision about whether

Table 8.3 Altering ventilation in relation to arterial blood gas results

Arterial blood gas result	Action
pH & $PaCO_2$ unchanged	increase ventilation by increasing respiratory rate, tidal volume, pressure, or change of machine
$PaCO_2$ increased	decrease fraction of inspired oxygen and/or increase ventilation
PaO_2 unchanged or decreased	increase fraction of inspired oxygen and/or increase ventilation

 Case study 8.1

Donald, aged 58 years, has smoked since the age of 23 years. He stopped smoking 2 years ago when he became breathless when walking on the flat. He has COPD and has been on long term oxygen therapy (LTOT) 15 hours per day at 2 L/min via nasal cannulae for the past 18 months. He was admitted to hospital with an acute exacerbation of his COPD. On admission on 28% oxygen his arterial blood gases were: pH 7.29; PaO_2 7.01 kPa; $PaCO_2$ 11.57 kPa. Due to his inability to correct his PaO_2 without retaining $PaCO_2$, it was decided to commence non-invasive ventilation using a BiPAP S with settings of: IPAP 16 cm H_2O; EPAP 4 cm H_2O; 1 L/min O_2.

His arterial blood gases on non-invasive ventilation were: pH 7.37; PaO_2 11.89 kPa; $PaCO_2$ 7.80 kPa.

Donald was in hospital for 8 days and discharged home with long term oxygen therapy at home but without a non-invasive ventilator.

or not they are to go home with it is taken. If they are not going home with the machine, its use should be discontinued a few days prior to discharge to ensure that the patients' condition does not deteriorate once they have stopped its use. If patients are to go home with the machine, the few days prior to discharge are useful for encouraging independent use of the machine. This will allow patients to become competent and to gain confidence using non-invasive ventilation.

Interfaces

There is now a wide variety of interfaces for applying non-invasive ventilation to the patient. The initial choice of interface will depend on a variety of factors, as shown in Table 8.4. The interface of choice should be sized and fitted according to the manufacturer's instructions using the recommended headgear for each interface.

Nasal masks

Nasal masks are user friendly, leaving the patient's mouth free which helps to decrease any feelings of claustrophobia (Figs 8.9, 8.10).

Table 8.4   Choice of interface

Problem	Solution
Patient never used non-invasive ventilation before	Start with nasal mask
Patient is mouth breathing	Try face mask
Nasal and face masks leak	Can the machine overcome a small degree of leak, i.e. is it a pre-set pressure machine?
Nasal patency	Try mouthpiece (not for long periods of time)
Claustrophobia	Try nasal pillows (Adams circuit); Monarch mini-mask
Expertise	Ensure staff are fully trained in use of the interface
Availability	Ensure stock is accessible and reordered
Cost	Ensure service is appropriately resourced

The nasal mask should allow for a comfortable, leak free fit around the patient's nose as the presence of large leaks will detrimentally affect the ventilatory capacity of the machine. It is worth remembering that pre-set pressure machines will cope with a small degree of leak. Overtightening should be avoided as this could contribute to the development of pressure sores. Eye leaks should be eliminated to minimize the risk of conjunctivitis. The patient should be reminded to keep the mouth closed when using a nasal mask to prevent the loss of gas and therefore of ventilatory support. Chin straps are available to minimize large leak problems through the mouth when the patient is using a nasal mask.

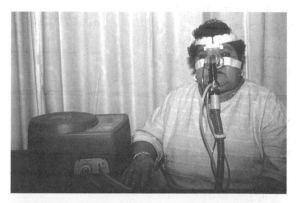

Figure 8.9   Patient receiving non-invasive ventilation via a nasal mask. Reproduced with permission from The London Chest Hospital.

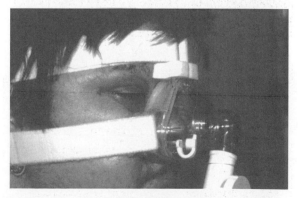

Figure 8.10   Close up of patient receiving non-invasive ventilation via a nasal mask. Reproduced with permission from The London Chest Hospital.

Face masks

Face masks (Fig. 8.11) may be the interface of choice where a patient continues to have mouth sealing difficulties using a nasal mask with a chin strap.

Face masks should be used with caution if a patient is vomiting, due to the risk of aspiration.

Alternative interfaces

- Monarch mini-mask (Fig. 8.12)
- Simplicity mask (Respironics Inc, USA)
- Nasal pillows (Adams circuit, Mallincrodt Puritan Bennett UK Ltd)
- Mouthpieces
- Sefam moulded masks (Sefam, France)

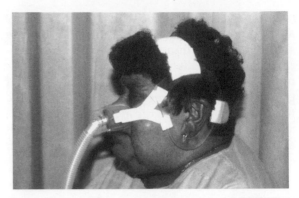

Figure 8.12 Patient receiving non-invasive ventilation via a Monarch mini-mask. Reproduced with permission from The London Chest Hospital.

In the presence of pressure sores it may be necessary to switch to using a device which will avoid pressure over the bridge of the nose altogether, by choosing an alternative interface such as nasal pillows (Adams circuit), a Monarch mini-mask or a Simplicity mask. These devices apply the incoming pressure directly to the nares. They can also be useful in alleviating claustrophobia caused by wearing a nasal or face mask. The Sefam system allows moulding of a nasal mask on an individual patient basis. It is possible to use this type of ventilation through a mouthpiece and this method has been used for patients with neuromuscular disease in the USA (Bach et al 1987). However, it is not recommended for patients to sleep using ventilation through a mouthpiece.

Circuit

It is important to use the circuit recommended by the manufacturer and to ensure that the correct exhalation valve is used in the circuit, according to the manufacturer's guidelines.

TROUBLESHOOTING AND PROBLEM SOLVING

The problem-solving aspect of non-invasive ventilation is of utmost importance since it is the ability and skill of the team caring for the patient that will determine how successfully the

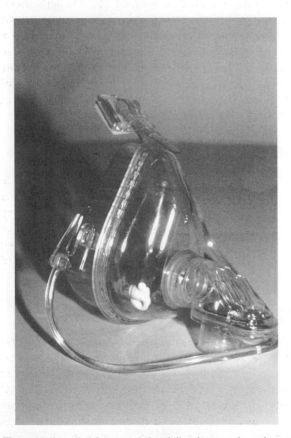

Figure 8.11 Full face mask for delivering non-invasive ventilation.

> **Box 8.7** Areas of particular concern
>
> - Patient reports insufficient ventilatory support from the machine
> - Transient hypoxaemia
> - Sputum retention
> - Mask leaks
> - Skin trauma
> - Nasal stuffiness/rhinitis
> - Nutrition
> - Abdominal discomfort

patient is ventilated. It is therefore important that all members of the team are able to contribute to the problem-solving process in order to ensure that the patient is not denied an opportunity for treatment.

Patient reports insufficient ventilatory support from the machine

If the patient's condition is deteriorating it may feel as if the machine is not keeping up as the patient struggles for breath. In real terms the maximal rate of delivery of breaths from the ventilator will be between 30 and 40 breaths per minute and may not keep up with the patient's increased demand. This can be quite distressing for the patient who may report that the machine is no longer working correctly. It is essential, in this situation, to ensure that the machine is checked for mechanical failure, to assess the patient for signs of deterioration and to reassure the patient in order to re-establish confidence in using the machine.

Transient hypoxaemia

It is essential that patients are adequately monitored whilst they are on non-invasive ventilation to ensure that they are being effectively ventilated and also that they are safe. It is also essential that the patient is safe to have time off the ventilator, that at such times adequate monitoring takes place and that the patient is given supplemental oxygen, where prescribed, when not on the machine. Initially it may be necessary to limit the time spent off the machine until the patient's con-

dition is stabilized, with greater periods spent off the machine as the patient's condition improves. The aim of treatment will depend on whether the patient will need to use the machine in the long term at home.

Sputum retention

Sputum retention may be effectively addressed by the use of humidification. For patients with large volume sputum production who are receiving ventilation, for example those with bronchiectasis or cystic fibrosis, it is advisable to humidify the ventilation that the patient receives so that secretions are not made more tenacious due to the passage of dry air over the airways. It may also be useful to supply humidification in the presence of rhinitis. Fisher & Paykel systems (Fisher & Paykel Healthcare Ltd, UK) are recommended for use with non-invasive ventilators; the HC100 is suitable for general use with a nasal or face mask and the heated wire version is recommended for use with tracheostomized patients as it overcomes the problem of condensation in the tubing and monitors temperature via a thermometer at the patient end of the circuit.

Mask leaks

It is important that mask fitting is done with care as a poorly fitting mask will result in inadequate ventilation. The mask should fit comfortably with minimal leaks and should not obstruct the nares. Mask fitting gauges are available for fitting some mask types but on the whole observation of the patient is all that is required.

Skin trauma

Some patients requiring non-invasive ventilation will have friable skin due to steroid therapy or poor nutritional status and it is vital in these patients that adequate attention is paid to facial skin care, particularly around vulnerable areas such as the bridge of the nose. Once the skin has broken down it may become impossible to continue to ventilate using a mask, which requires continued pressure over the affected area. It is therefore good practice to address any areas of skin which look vulnerable as soon as they show signs of prolonged reddening or irritation on wearing the mask. This could take the form of applying a strip of Granuflex (Convatec Ltd, UK) or Spenco dermal pad (Spenco Medical (UK) Ltd) to the affected area so that it sits between the mask and the patient's skin. An alternative which could be considered is the use of a moulded silastic mask prosthesis using a proprietary preparation, Otoform K2 (PC Werth Ltd, UK), which is a silicone impressioning product moulded to the correct shape to provide a prosthesis which fits over the bridge of the nose between the face and the mask, thereby protecting the vulnerable area (Meecham-Jones et al 1994). In patients with an allergic reaction to silicone, self-adhesive towelling can be used to line the mask. It may be appropriate to use an alternative type of device such as nasal pillows or Monarch mini-mask.

Nasal stuffiness/rhinitis

Some patients suffer from rhinitis in response to wearing the device, which is thought to occur because the air pressure generated results in drying and inflammation of the nasal mucosa. The use of a corticosteroid nasal spray to reduce nasal mucosal inflammation or the use of a humidifier in the circuit may relieve this problem (e.g. Fisher & Paykel HC100).

Nutrition

It is essential that attention is paid to patients' nutrition whilst they are receiving non-invasive ventilation. If patients require long periods on the machine it may be necessary to start feeding them nasogastrically. This should be done via a small bore nasogastric tube to minimize the degree of leak caused by the presence of the tube. The aim of treatment should be to restore 'normality' as soon as possible for the patient, i.e. to allow periods off the machine for eating, drinking and talking to relatives and healthcare professionals as soon as the patient's clinical condition will allow.

Abdominal discomfort

Some patients swallow a lot of air during ventilation. In some cases instruction about how to relax on the machine will alleviate the problem. Alternatively, it may be necessary to try peppermint water, carbonated drinks or charcoal biscuits. Patients who are small in stature, have chest wall deformity and are constipated may need laxatives in order to maximize diaphragmatic movement and therefore ventilation.

Table 8.5 summarizes problems and possible solutions.

PATIENT EDUCATION

Although the techniques employed to deliver non-invasive ventilation are not difficult, it is necessary to apply them in a skilled manner in order to ensure that patients receive ventilatory support that is effective. It is the ability to ensure maximal adherence, comfort and confidence in the patient that will enable healthcare professionals to apply this therapy successfully. To achieve this patients should have the procedure explained to them and should be allowed to try the machine themselves before having the headgear attached. Patients should understand why the machine is being used and what is expected of its use. They should be told not to eat or drink whilst on the machine.

Clear guidelines should be given about what is expected of the patient in terms of length of use of the machine and whether the patient should be taken off the machine for nebulizers. The aim is to stabilize the patient initially, which may mean using the machine continuously for 24 hours a day at first and then decreasing use gradually thereafter. This may mean decreasing usage during the day but maintaining it at night to alleviate the problems caused by nocturnal hypoventilation. If patients are not going home with a machine then they should be weaned off its use. This is done by reducing the number of hours it is used in the day, maintaining overnight use initially and then weaning the patient off the machine altogether.

Table 8.5 Problems and solutions

Problem	Possible cause	Solution
Mask leak	1. Is the mask sized and fitted correctly? 2. Is the patient mouth breathing?	1. Refit mask 2a) Try chin strap 2b) Consider using face mask N.B. Pre-set pressure ventilators will overcome a small degree of leak
Oxygen saturation level is falling	1. Is the patient's condition deteriorating? 2. Is there a technical fault?	1. If so, inform medical staff 2a) Check oxygen supply 2b) Check oximeter probe is on finger 2c) Check circuit connections
Redness over the bridge of the nose	1. Is the headgear too tight? 2. Is the mask fitted correctly? 3. Irritation or allergic reaction to mask?	1. & 2. Refit mask and headgear 3. Line the mask with self-adhesive towelling
Pressure sore over the bridge of the nose	1. Is the mask fitted correctly?	1a) Try Granuflex or Spenco dermal pad 1b) Try a mould placed between the mask and the skin, e.g. Otoform 1c) Consider alternatives, e.g. nasal pillows (Adams circuit), or Monarch mini-mask (Respironics)
Rhinitis/nasal congestion	1. Nasal irritation caused by air flow	1a) Try nasal sprays, e.g. Beconase or Flixonase 1b) Humidify air flow using Fisher & Paykel system
Dryness of throat and nose	1. Airflow too dry	1. Humidify air as above
Sinus or ear pain	1. Sinus or middle ear infection	1. Inform medical staff

If patients are candidates for long term use of the machine at home it is important that they become independent in its use for the last few days of their inpatient stay, ensuring that any difficulties can be sorted out prior to discharge home. It is also a good idea to teach any relatives or carers about the machinery and its use to maximize patients' ability to cope at home. It is advisable to provide patients going home with the machine with written information, including pictures of how the circuit fits together and the settings of the machine, in order to help them should they experience difficulties once they get home. It is worth reiterating advice regarding the use of oxygen therapy and nebulizers at home as patients may erroneously assume that a new addition to treatment will replace existing treatments. Patients must be educated about the care of the equipment, changing of filters, how to clean the mask and how and where to entrain an oxygen supply. It is also important to provide a contact phone number for use in emergencies at home so that help can be obtained quickly and easily, and patients should be advised to contact the helpline in the event of their condition worsening, so that advice about the course of action to be taken can be given in the event of machine or mask failure.

CHOOSING A MACHINE AND DELIVERING A SERVICE

There are no hard and fast guidelines about which machine to choose. It is important to establish the context in which the machine will be used, for example the selection may be different depending on whether the machine is to be used in hospital on an acute basis or in the long term at home. Each type of machine has differing features in terms of the mode of operation and ventilatory capacity, so it may not be possible to ventilate all types of patients using one type of ventilator.

When delivering a service the following resources are required:

- Experienced team with essential skills. Staff should be trained in the use and application of non-invasive ventilation and have recognized roles in the delivery of the service.
- A regular teaching programme which captures all new staff should be in place along with 24 hour cover by clinicians experienced in the delivery of non-invasive ventilation.
- Variety of machines and equipment, access to machines.
- Recognition of limitations.
- Access to ICU/HDU.
- Policies and procedures – there should also be written information in the form of procedures and policies in order to ensure that the service is carried out safely and effectively.

In delivering a service it may also be of use for the team to set criteria for treatment with non-invasive ventilation (Plant et al 1998). This allows the team to decide in advance which patients are appropriate for treatment with non-invasive ventilation and so avoids the difficult last minute decision making process. In addition the team could agree 'failure criteria', for example the point at which it would be considered that treatment with non-invasive ventilation had failed and that further interventions may be indicated, e.g. intubation. Plant et al (1998) chose the following failure criteria:

- pH 7.2–7.25 on 2 occasions 1 hour apart
- Glasgow coma score of < 8
- $PaCO_2 > 8$ kPa
- $PaO_2 < 6$ kPa despite maximal tolerated FiO_2
- cardiorespiratory arrest.

Cleaning of non-invasive ventilation equipment

Cleaning of reusable items should follow manufacturer's guidelines. All guidelines should also comply with local infection control policies.

Servicing

Servicing of equipment should take place on a regular basis and can either be performed on a contract basis by the manufacturer or in the hospital clinical equipment management department by a suitably qualified technician. All hospital equipment should be safety checked on a regular basis depending on the use of the machine. Inlet filters should be changed or washed according to the manufacturer's guidelines. Bacterial filters should be used where recommended by the manufacturer to protect the machine from contamination.

Domiciliary use

Machines for home use should be portable and compatible with the circumstances in which they are to be used at home. The patient must be confident and capable of using the machine successfully prior to discharge home with it.

Some patients using non-invasive ventilation at home may require the use of a portable machine with battery back up that can be attached to a wheelchair to enable them to maintain a degree of independence away from an electrical supply. The batteries need recharging by plugging into the mains and manufacturers will supply details of how long the batteries will last in constant use. Careful assessment should be made when choosing a machine with a battery back up to ensure that it meets the need of the patient. In some circumstances where the patient is ventilator dependent it may be necessary to supply a second machine at home in case of machine breakdown. It is also essential that the local electricity company is contacted to ensure that the patient's home will be reconnected as a matter of urgency in the event of a power failure.

Despite the added burden of being required to carry out so much treatment at home, Persson et al (1994) found that patients with restrictive ventilatory disorders using non-invasive ventilation did not describe themselves as having a poor quality of life, and indeed clinical experience tells us that despite needing to use non-invasive ventilation on a long term basis many patients still want to take holidays. For holidays taken in the UK this does not present too many difficulties apart from carrying the weight of the machine. It is important, however, that advice is given to patients travelling abroad, that correct information is given about voltages in the country of destination, and that the machine is carried as hand luggage on flights as airlines will not cover the cost of replacement of damaged equipment.

CONTINUOUS POSITIVE AIRWAY PRESSURE (CPAP)

CPAP can be delivered in two ways. Each method of delivery is applied in specific circumstances and they are not interchangeable. High flow CPAP delivers a mixture of oxygen and air and is used for the treatment of Type I respiratory failure. A CPAP machine for the treatment of obstructive sleep apnoea delivers compressed air to which oxygen can be entrained should it be required.

High flow continuous positive airway pressure (CPAP)

Definitions and indications for use

The use of high flow CPAP delivered from a flow generator has been developed to provide oxygen enriched continuous positive pressure (Fig. 8.13).

The flow generator delivers oxygen and entrained room air at between 50 and 80 L/min. The fraction of inspired oxygen delivered to the patient can be titrated using an oxygen analyser in the circuit. This system can deliver 35–90% oxygen, which can be delivered via a full face mask or sealing mouthpiece with the addition of humidification as indicated. It can also be delivered by an endotracheal or tracheostomy tube, but when delivered in this way should be humidified as high flow gas could cause drying of the airways and hence sputum retention.

Its primary use is in postoperative cases in the presence of Type I respiratory failure where the patient requires support for oxygenation and improvement in functional residual capacity. The use of CPAP as a ventilatory support is limited as

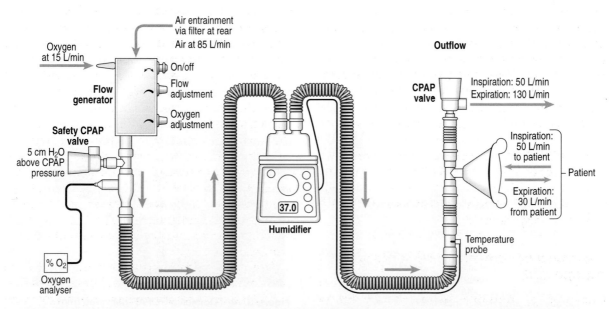

Figure 8.13   Diagram of set-up for delivering humidified high flow CPAP. Reproduced with permission from Medic-Aid Ltd.

Box 8.8 Use of high flow CPAP

The clinical indications for use are:
- atelectasis
- sputum retention
- reduced levels of arterial oxygen
- restrictive patterns of breathing

Contraindications for the use of high flow CPAP include:
- undrained pneumothorax
- epistaxis
- vomiting
- severe emphysematous bullae
- encephalopathy
- unstable facial fractures
- cardiovascular instability
- bronchial tumour in proximal airway
- Type II respiratory failure

---

it will not give the patient breaths and therefore will not eliminate carbon dioxide.

Outside of the ICU or HDU environment it is most likely that CPAP would be used for 10–15 minutes every hour as part of the physiotherapy treatment regime of patients with respiratory complications postoperatively. It is more accurate to describe this treatment as periodic continuous positive airway pressure (pCPAP) as it should be given on an intermittent or periodic basis. CPAP should only be used over longer periods of time with caution and with regular medical review.

CPAP for the treatment of obstructive sleep apnoea (OSA)

Definition and indications for use

The development of the use of nasal CPAP arose out of studies performed in Australia in the early

---

Box 8.9 Physiological effects of high flow CPAP

- Correction of hypoxaemia (Type I respiratory failure) (Andersen et al 1980)
- Increased functional residual capacity (FRC) (Gherini et al 1979, Lindner et al 1987, Stock et al 1985)
- Decreased work of breathing (Gherini et al 1979)
- Re-expansion of atelectatic areas
- Increased compliance (Hinds 1987)

1980s which postulated that CPAP could be successfully delivered via a nasal mask for the treatment of OSA (Sullivan et al 1981) (Fig. 8.14).

In this condition the upper airways are 'floppy' and collapse on expiration during sleep, causing them to vibrate and produce loud snoring as air is pushed through them. The symptoms of obstructive sleep apnoea are:

- loud snoring
- witnessed apnoeas
- choking
- disturbed sleep
- psychological disturbances/mood swings
- decreased libido/impotence
- inability to concentrate
- daytime somnolence.

The consequences of these symptoms are a reduction in the quality of life of the patient, resulting in the inability to work effectively, to drive and to lead a fulfilling life. Long term OSA has also been shown to increase the incidence of myocardial infarction and stroke (Stradling 1996). The use of a CPAP machine, powered by electricity and delivering a pre-set pressure to the patient via a nasal mask worn throughout the night, is largely confined to the treatment of OSA and has proved to be one of the most effective ways of treating this condition. It works by providing a positive pressure, usually between 5 and 15 cm H_2O, to keep the

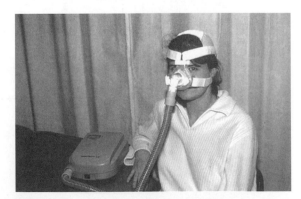

Figure 8.14 Domiciliary CPAP delivered from a compressor for the treatment of obstructive sleep apnoea.

upper airway open during expiration, allowing expired air to be breathed out effortlessly with the CPAP effectively forming a pneumatic splint for the airway.

Diagnosis and assessment of the severity of the condition can be made by overnight sleep study using polysomnography (Fig. 8.15a, 8.15b, Table 8.6).

Diagnosis is made when there are more than 15 apnoeas/hypopnoeas per hour during sleep and by psychological impact on sleep quality, oxygen saturation and cardiovascular function. Assessment of somnolence could be made by using a scale such as the Epworth sleepiness scale with daytime somnolence being the key to need for CPAP (Johns 1991) (Fig. 8.16).

Compliance in using the machine can be poor and for this reason it is important that the patient receives adequate education and advice about its use (Engelman et al 1994) (Table 8.7).

It may also be appropriate to refer the patient for dietetic advice as obesity predisposes patients to OSA.

Some patients with severe OSA dip into Type II respiratory failure, for example in cases where the patient has a combination of OSA and COPD, in the presence of morbid obesity or where the patient has respiratory muscle weakness. These patients may require a higher level of ventilatory support than a CPAP machine can provide and may need non-invasive ventilation in order to correct arterial blood gases in hospital before returning to the use of a CPAP machine once at home (Simonds 1996).

Table 8.6 Measurements taken during polysomnography	
Feature being measured	Mode of measurement
Arousals	Electroencephalogram (EEG)
Sleep stage	Electro-oculogram (EOG) Electromyogram (EMG)
SpO$_2$	Pulse oximetry
Apnoea/hypopnoea index	Airflow at nose and mouth Rib cage and abdominal movement
Posture in bed	Position monitor
Snoring	Microphone
Periodic leg movement	Leg movement

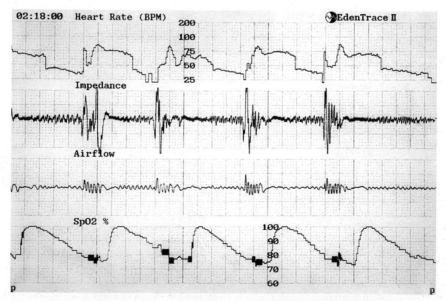

Figure 8.15a Sleep study trace showing uncorrected obstructive sleep apnoea.

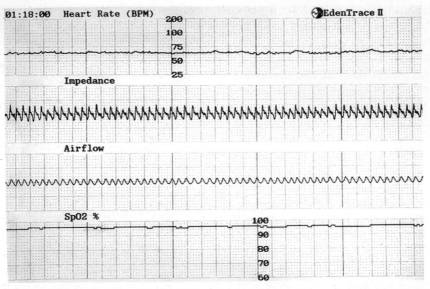

Figure 8.15b Sleep study showing corrected obstructive sleep apnoea using CPAP from a compressor.

THE EPWORTH SLEEPINESS SCALE

Name: ....

Today's date: .... Your age (years): ....

Your sex (male=M; female=F): ....

How likely are you to doze off or to fall asleep in the following situations, in contrast to feeling just tired? This refers to your usual way of life in recent times. Even if you have not done some of these things recently, try to work out how they would have affected you. Use the following scale to choose the *most appropriate number* for each situation:

     0 = would *never* doze
     1 = *slight* chance of dozing
     2 = *moderate* chance of dozing
     3 = *high* chance of dozing

Situation	Chance of dozing
Sitting and reading	....
Watching TV	....
Sitting, inactive in a public place (e.g., a theatre or a meeting)	....
As a passenger in a car for an hour without a break	....
Lying down to rest in the afternoon when circumstances permit	....
Sitting and talking to someone	....
Sitting quietly after a lunch without alcohol	....
In a car, while stopped for a few minutes in the traffic	....

Thank you for your cooperation

Figure 8.16 The Epworth sleepiness scale to identify the presence of obstructive sleep apnoea. Reproduced with permission from Johns 1991.

Table 8.7 Advice for patients using CPAP at home: questions and answers

Question	Answer
How does the machine work?	A motor generates compressed air which can be pre-set at different pressures
How will the machine help?	The pressure generated helps to keep the upper airway open during expiration to correct the symptoms of hypopnea/apnoea
When should the machine be used?	During sleep
How often should the machine be used?	Ideally every night; periods off the machine may be possible depending on the severity of the symptoms and with the guidance of the prescribing doctor
What if symptoms persist?	The prescribing doctor should be contacted for symptom review; pressure may need increasing
Who should be contacted in the event of machine failure?	A contact name and number should be supplied with written information about how to use the machine at home
How should the machine and circuit be cleaned?	Machine can be wiped clean with a damp cloth; circuit can be washed in warm soapy water. Make sure water does not get into the machine and circuit is dry before reuse
When will the machine need servicing?	Once a year for pressure check and electrical safety
Can the machine be taken abroad when travelling?	The voltage of the machine should be compatible with destination voltage or machine should have a universal transformer. Stow as hand luggage as airlines will not replace damaged machines. Include the item on the medical insurance. Take a letter from the prescribing doctor describing the purpose of the machine
Can driving be continued?	Driving Vehicle Licensing Agency (DVLA) should be informed under the guidance of the prescribing doctor
Will alcohol or sedatives affect my sleeping pattern?	It is advisable not to drink excessively 3–4 hours prior to retiring. Sedating agents should be avoided as these will further depress the respiratory system

CONCLUSIONS AND RECOMMENDATIONS

The use of any non-invasive respiratory support technique should only be considered following a multidisciplinary assessment. The benefits of the use of non-invasive ventilation are now well documented in patients with neuromuscular diseases, chest wall diseases, and in carefully selected COPD, cystic fibrosis and motor neurone disease cases. These techniques should be applied as part of a team approach to managing patients, with staff experienced in the techniques responsible for the management and monitoring of patients to ensure that patient care is both safe and effective. CPAP for OSA should not be confused with high flow CPAP, and it must be remembered that the application of high flow CPAP for the treatment of Type I respiratory failure is not interchangeable with non-invasive ventilation, which is used for the treatment of Type II respiratory failure. Criteria for use of the different types of respiratory support techniques need to be clearly defined and agreed by the multidisciplinary team.

REFERENCES

Ambrosino N, Foglio K, Rubini F et al 1995 Non-invasive mechanical ventilation in acute respiratory failure due to chronic obstructive pulmonary disease: correlates for success. Thorax 50(7): 755–757

American Thoracic Society 1986 Evaluation of impairment/disability secondary to respiratory disorders. American Review of Respiratory Disease 133: 1205–1209

Andersen J B, Olesen K P, Eikard B et al 1980 Periodic continuous positive airway pressure, CPAP, by mask in the treatment of atelectasis. European Journal of Respiratory Diseases 61: 20–25

Antonelli M, Conti G, Rocco M et al 1998 A comparison of non-invasive positive pressure ventilation and conventional mechanical ventilation in patients with acute respiratory failure. New England Journal of Medicine 339(7): 429–435

Bach J R, Alba A, Mosher R, Delaubier A 1987 Intermittent positive pressure ventilation via nasal access in the management of respiratory insufficiency. Chest 92(1): 169–170

Benhamou D, Muir J F, Raspaud C et al 1997 Long-term efficiency of home nasal mask ventilation in patients with diffuse bronchiectasis and severe respiratory failure: a case-control study. Chest 112(5): 1259–1266

Borasio G D, Voltz R 1998 Discontinuation of mechanical ventilation in patients with amyotrophic lateral sclerosis. Journal of Neurology 245(11): 717–722

Bott J, Carroll M P, Conway J H et al 1993 Randomized controlled trial of nasal ventilation in acute ventilatory failure due to chronic obstructive airways disease. Lancet 341: 1555–1557

Braun N M, Marino W D 1984 Effect of daily intermittent rest of respiratory muscles in patients with severe chronic airflow limitation (CAL). Chest 85 (suppl): 59s–60s

Brochard L, Rauss A, Benito S et al 1994 Comparison of three methods of gradual withdrawal from ventilatory support during weaning from mechanical ventilation. American Journal of Respiratory and Critical Care Medicine 150: 896–903

Brochard L, Mancebo J, Wysocki M et al 1995 Noninvasive ventilation for acute exacerbations of chronic obstructive pulmonary disease. New England Journal of Medicine 333: 817–822

Cazzolli P A, Oppenheimer E A 1996 Home mechanical ventilation for amyotrophic lateral sclerosis: nasal compared to tracheostomy intermittent positive pressure ventilation. Journal of Neurological Science 139: 123–128

Douglas N J, White D P, Pickett C K et al 1982 Respiration during sleep in normal man. Thorax 37: 840–844

Elliott M W 1999 Non-invasive ventilation – mechanisms of benefit. Medizinische Klinik 94 (1 Spec No): 2–6

Elliott M W, Simonds A K 1995 Nocturnal assisted ventilation using Bi-level positive pressure airway pressure: the effect of expiratory positive airway pressure. European Respiratory Journal 8: 436–440

Elliott M W, Mulvey D A, Moxham J et al 1991 Domiciliary nocturnal nasal intermittent positive pressure ventilation in COPD: mechanisms underlying changes in arterial blood gas tensions. European Respiratory Journal 4: 1044–1052

Elliott M W, Aquilina R, Green M et al 1994 A comparison of different modes of non-invasive respiratory support: effects on ventilation and inspiratory muscle effort. Anaesthesia 49: 279–283

Ellis E R, Bye P T P, Bruderer J W, Sullivan C E 1987 Treatment of respiratory failure in patients with neuromuscular disease. American Review of Respiratory Disease 135: 148–152

Ellis E R, Grunstein R R, Chan C S et al 1988 Treatment of nocturnal respiratory failure in kyphoscoliosis. Chest 94: 811–815

Engelman H M, Martin S E, Douglas N J 1994 Compliance with CPAP therapy in patients with sleep apnoea/hypopnea syndrome. Thorax 149: 263–266

Estes R J, Meduri G U 1995 The pathogenesis of ventilator-associated pneumonia via mechanisms of bacterial transcolonisation and airway inoculation. Intensive Care Medicine 21: 365–383

Gacouin A, Desrues B, Lena H et al 1996 Long-term nasal intermittent positive pressure ventilation (NIPPV) in sixteen consecutive patients with bronchiectasis: a retrospective study. European Respiratory Journal 9(6): 1246–1250

Gherini S, Peters R M, Virgilio R W 1979 Mechanical work on the lungs and work of breathing with positive end-expiratory pressure and continuous positive airway pressure. Chest 76: 251–256

Hill A T, Edenborough F P, Cayton R M, Stableforth D E 1998 Long term nasal intermittent positive pressure ventilation in patients with cystic fibrosis and hypercapnic respiratory failure (1991–1996). Respiratory Medicine 92(3): 523–526

Hinds C J 1987 Intensive care. Baillière Tindall, London

Hodson M E, Madden B P, Steven M H et al 1991 Non-invasive mechanical ventilation for cystic fibrosis patients – a potential bridge to transplantation. European Respiratory Journal 4: 524–527

Hotchkiss J R, Marini J J 1998 Non-invasive ventilation: an emerging supportive technique for the emergency department. Annals of Emergency Medicine 32: 470–479

Johns M W 1991 A new method for measuring daytime sleepiness: the Epworth sleepiness scale. Sleep 14: 540–545

Kerby G R, Mayer L S, Pingleton S K 1987 Nocturnal positive pressure ventilation via a nasal mask. American Journal of Respiratory Disease 135: 738–740

Kramer N, Meyer T J, Mehang J et al 1995 Randomized, prospective trial of noninvasive positive pressure ventilation in acute respiratory failure. American Journal of Respiratory and Critical Care Medicine 151: 1799–1806

Leger P, Jennequin J, Gerard M, Robert D 1989 Home positive pressure ventilation via nasal mask for patients with neuromuscular weakness or restrictive lung or chest-wall disease. Respiratory Care 34: 73–79

Leger P, Bedicam J M, Cornette A et al 1994 Nasal intermittent positive pressure ventilation. Chest 105: 100–105

Lindner K H, Lotz P, Ahnefeld F W 1987 Continuous positive airway pressure effect on functional residual capacity, vital capacity and its subdivisions. Chest 92: 66–70

Meecham-Jones D J, Wedzicha J A 1993 Comparison of pressure and volume pre-set nasal ventilator systems in stable chronic respiratory failure. European Respiratory Journal 6: 1060–1064

Meecham-Jones D J, Braid G, Wedzicha J A 1994 Nasal masks for domiciliary positive pressure ventilation: patient usage and complications. Thorax 49: 811–812

Meecham-Jones D J, Paul E A, Jones P W, Wedzicha J A 1995 Nasal pressure support ventilation plus oxygen compared with oxygen therapy alone in hypercapnic COPD. American Journal of Respiratory and Critical Care Medicine 152: 538–544

Persson K, Olofson J, Larsson S, Sullivan M 1994 Quality of life of patients treated by home mechanical ventilation due to restrictive ventilatory disorders. Respiratory Medicine 88: 21–26

Piper A J, Ellis E R 1998 Non-invasive ventilation. In: Webber B A, Pryor J A (eds) Physiotherapy for respiratory and cardiac problems, 2nd edn. Churchill Livingstone, Edinburgh

Piper A J, Parker S, Torzillo P J et al 1992 Nocturnal nasal IPPV stabilizes patients with cystic fibrosis and hypercapnic respiratory failure. Chest 102: 846–850

Plant P K, Owen J L, Elliott M W 1998 Non-invasive ventilation in acute exacerbations of COPD – The Yorkshire non-invasive ventilation trial. BTS Abstract, Winter meeting, December

Polkey M I, Lyall R A, Davidson A C et al 1999 Ethical and clinical issues in the use of home non-invasive mechanical ventilation for the palliation of breathlessness in motor neurone disease. Thorax 54(4): 367–371

Restrick L J, Scott A D, Ward A D et al 1993 Nasal intermittent positive-pressure ventilation in weaning intubated patients with chronic respiratory disease from assisted intermittent positive-pressure ventilation. Respiratory Medicine 87: 199–204

Simonds A K, 1996 Non-invasive respiratory support, 1st edn. Chapman & Hall, London

Simonds A K Elliott M W 1991 Use of BiPAP ventilator for non-invasive ventilation: advantages and

disadvantages. American Review of Respiratory Disease 143(S): A585

Simonds A K, Elliott M W 1995 Outcome of domiciliary nasal intermittent positive pressure ventilation in restrictive and obstructive disorders. Thorax 50: 604–609

Stock M C, Downs J B, Gauer P K et al 1985 Prevention of post-operative pulmonary complications with CPAP, incentive spirometry, and conservative therapy. Chest 87(2): 151–157

Stradling J R 1996 Longer term consequences of sleep apnoea. In: Simonds A K (ed) Non-invasive respiratory support, 1st edn. Chapman & Hall, London

Sullivan C E, Berthon-Jones M, Issa F G, Eves L 1981 Reversal of obstructive sleep apnoea by continuous positive airway pressure applied through the nose. Lancet 1: 862–865

Udwadia Z F, Santis G F, Steven M H, Simonds A K 1992 Nasal ventilation to facilitate weaning in patients with chronic respiratory insufficiency. Thorax 47(9): 715–718

Wedzicha J A 1996 Non-invasive ventilation for exacerbations of respiratory failure in chronic obstructive pulmonary disease. Thorax 51 (suppl 2): S35–S39

Younes M 1992 Proportional assist ventilation, a new approach to ventilatory support. American Review of Respiratory Disease 145: 114–120

USEFUL ADDRESSES

Convatec Ltd
Harrington House
Ickenham
Uxbridge UB10 8PU
(Supplies Granuflex)

Deva Medical Electronics
1 Chandlers Court
Picow Farm Road
Runcorn
Cheshire WA7 4UH
(Supplies Breas 401, 501, Monnal DCC)

Fisher and Paykel Healthcare Ltd
The Valley Centre
Gordon Road
Buckinghamshire
HP13 6EQ
(Supplies Fisher and Paykel heated humidifier systems)

Mallincrodt Nellcor Puritan Bennett
Nellcor Puritan Bennett UK Ltd
10 London Road
Bicester
Oxfordshire
OX6 0JX
(Supplies range of CPAP equipment and accessories and Adams CPAP circuit (nasal pillows))

Medic-Aid Ltd
Heath Place
Bognor Regis
West Sussex
PO22 9SL
(Medic-aid supplies Respironics equipment in UK: BiPAP S, BiPAP ST30, Respironics silicone and vinyl nasal masks, full face masks, Monarch mini-mask, Goldseal mask, Profile mask)

Resmed (UK) Ltd
67B Milton Park
Abingdon
Oxfordshire
OX14 4RX
(Supplies VPAP, VPAP II, Sullivan and
Mirage nasal and full face masks
and range of CPAP equipment and accessories)

Sunrise Medical Ltd
High Street
Wollaston
West Midlands
DY8 4PS
(Supplies range of CPAP equipment and accessories)

Spenco Medical (UK) Ltd
Burrell Road
Haywards Heath
West Sussex
RH16 1TW
(Supplies Spenco dermal pad)

PC Werth Ltd
Audiology House
45 Nightingale Lane
London
SW12 8SP
(Supplies Otoform K2 silicone impressioning
material for making prostheses to protect
vulnerable pressure areas)

9 Respiratory infections

Paul Hateley

Infections of the respiratory tract are potentially life threatening. They form a significant percentage of all hospital acquired and hospital treated infections and remain a significant cause of morbidity and mortality (National Audit Office 2000).

The normal host defence mechanisms will remove microbes that may transiently invade the bronchial tract or lung alveoli in a normal healthy person. These mechanisms keep the lower respiratory tract sterile and include:

- mechanical clearance of microbes by the upward movement of mucus produced by ciliated epithelial epithelium of the tracheobronchial tract
- phagocytosis, bipolymorphs and macrophages and a local production of licozyne, interferon and secretory IgI.

The bronchial tract may become colonized by organisms such as *Haemophilus influenzae* and *Streptococcus pneumoniae* when the host defence mechanisms are defective because of damage to the bronchial tract or the lungs, which can be due to advanced respiratory disease or trauma. Should this occur the patient is then at greater risk of developing recurrent or severe lower respiratory tract infections, which may be life threatening (British Thoracic Society and Public Health Laboratory Service 1987).

ACUTE BRONCHITIS

Many cases of acute tracheitis or bronchitis are caused by viral infections and amongst the commonest causes of acute infection of the trachea and bronchi are:

• rhinoviruses
• influenza
• parainfluenza.

Additionally bacterial infections, which are often secondary to a viral infection, may follow, often caused by *Streptococcus pneumoniae* or *Haemophilus influenzae. Staphylococcus aureus* is a possible, although not common secondary bacterial infection of the respiratory tract. With an increased incidence of methicillin resistance in *Staphylococcus aureus*, MRSA respiratory infections, although remaining uncommon, are increasing. Microbiological investigations of acute tracheitis or acute bronchitis are not usually indicated. Antimicrobial chemotherapy of secondary bacterial infections when needed is usually with a broad spectrum agent such as amoxicillin or erythromycin.

Infective exacerbation of chronic bronchitis

Viruses are often the main cause of exacerbations of chronic bronchitis, although secondary bacterial infections are not uncommon. Bacterial causes of infective exacerbations are particularly relevant when patients with chronic bronchitis produce mucopurulent (green or greenish yellow) sputum instead of the usual mucoid sputum. *Haemophilus influenzae* is probably the most common bacterial cause. This organism is often

isolated in small numbers and better results are obtained when cultured from an early morning sputum sample. In such circumstances positive isolation may indicate colonization. The evidence that is required to determine bacterial rather than viral infection as the cause of infective exacerbations includes:

• purulent sputum
• a decrease in the purulence of sputum with antimicrobial therapy
• clinical improvement.

As well as *Haemophilus influenzae, Streptococcus pneumoniae* and *Branhamella catarrhalis* may also cause infective exacerbations (British Thoracic Society 1997). Patients with severe disease have often had repeated courses of antimicrobial therapy with very little sensitivity testing and may therefore become infected by antibiotic resistant strains of bacteria, such as haemophilus strains, which will be resistant to first line therapy such as amoxicillin, ampicillin or co-trimoxazole (Austrian 1981, Everett et al 1977).

Microbiological investigations

Most patients who have infective causes of chronic respiratory tract infections do not require microbial investigations as the two main bacterial pathogens are *Haemophilus influenzae* and *Streptococcus pneumoniae* and their antibiotic susceptibility patterns remain, despite an increased resistance, reasonably predictable. Investigations may be effective and worthwhile in the minority of patients with advanced disease who develop severe infective exacerbations. These patients may be at risk of developing a life threatening respiratory tract infection which may be associated with a bacteraemia or septicaemia due to one of the less frequent and also antibiotic resistant pathogens. However, the majority of this type of patient will often be admitted to hospital, where it is more appropriate for the collection of sputum to be obtained, preferably before the start of antimicrobial therapy.

Treatment of infective exacerbation

Patients with chronic respiratory tract infections are best prescribed an antibiotic to keep at home and instructed to start a course as soon as the sputum becomes purulent. For most patients one of the following would be most appropriate:

- amoxicillin 500 mg 8-hourly before meals for 5–7 days
- ampicillin 500 mg 6-hourly for 5–7 days
- co-trimoxazole 2 tablets twice daily for 5–7 days
- oxytetracycline 250 mg 6-hourly for 7 days.

When there is a history of a possible allergic reaction to penicillin, tetracycline or co-trimoxa-zole can be given. New generation oral cephalo-sporins such as cefalexin and cefradine are not very active against many of the *Haemophilus influenzae* strains, although cefaclor remains reasonably sensitive. Erythromycin has limited activity against *Haemophilus influenzae* and therefore its true effect in the treatment of infective exacerbations can be questioned.

Patients with chronic bronchitis need careful assessment to determine whether treatment of their acute exacerbation takes place at home or in hospital. A simple tool (British Thoracic Society

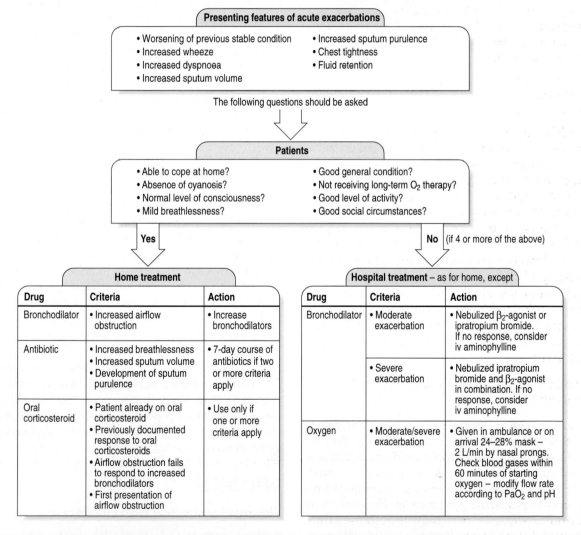

Figure 9.1 Tool for assessing home or hospital care for acute exacerbations of chronic obstructive pulmonary disease. Reproduced with permission from the British Medical Journal (British Thoracic Society 1997).

Case study 9.1

Eva Smith is a sprightly, 82-year-old, fiercely independent lady who loves bingo and smokes 11 cigarettes a day and has done so for 40 years. She says she has the occasional 'poorly chest'.

She has become more breathless so she makes an appointment to see her GP. On assessment and examination by her regular GP it was decided that this was bronchitis, which was an exacerbation of her underlying chronic obstructive pulmonary disease. This episode occurred following a flu-like illness, and had gradually worsened. Eva's symptoms were a 'hacking' cough, slight breathlessness and a temperature.

An assessment of Eva's physical and social conditions was carried out to determine if she should be treated at home or in hospital and the British Thoracic Society (BTS) COPD guidelines were used in the assessment process (British Thoracic Society 1997) (see Fig. 9.1).

Eva was able to cope at home as she had no signs of hypoxaemia and did not require oxygen, she was still quite active, had lots of family and friends who visited regularly and only had mild breathlessness.

The treatment Eva received was a 7 day course of an oral broad spectrum antibiotic, bronchodilators and a course of oral steroids.

She was successfully managed at home and returned to her pre-infection state and of course was able to attend bingo. During this treatment course a discussion regarding smoking cessation took place with Eva, who did not dismiss it altogether but did not feel she was quite ready. It was decided that this would be discussed further when Eva was next reviewed.

1997) has been developed to assist with this decision (Fig. 9.1).

Patients with severe chronic bronchitis with infective exacerbations should have sputum sent for microscopy, culture and sensitivity before blind antimicrobial therapy is started. In such situations amoxicillin is often the drug of choice. For patients who do not respond to initial chemotherapy because of antimicrobial resistance to the selected drug, a second line therapy will be commenced. Cefuroxime is another alternative which, unlike ampicillin and amoxicillin, remains active against many penicillinase reducing staphylococci strains with the exception of the methicillin resistant group. Cefuroxime and cefotaxime are parenteral cephalosporins highly active against *Haemophilus influenzae* strains and remain sensitive to the increasing ampicillin resistant

strains. The dosage will be recommended by a clinical microbiologist, but essentially for an adult is around 750 mg 8-hourly, preferably intravenously but also available as intramuscular injection. Oral cefuroxime is also available and can be useful in selected cases.

As well as treating the infection that has triggered the acute exacerbation, optimization of other treatments needs to be addressed otherwise there will be further deterioration in the patient's condition.

Prevention

Patients who have chronic respiratory disease should be advised as a health promotion strategy:

- not to smoke
- to have influenza immunization at the start of the seasonal variation peak
- to avoid going out in the cold foggy weather.

Chemoprophylaxis in such patients can be questioned, although it is still prescribed for patients with severe respiratory disease. If chemoprophylaxis is going to be given, amoxicillin or ampicillin are not recommended because of the association with gastrointestinal complications that may result in *Clostridium difficile* diarrhoea. In such cases, oxytetracycline would be a drug of choice as prophylaxis. However, in areas where the incidence of *Streptococcus pneumoniae* or *Haemophilus influenzae* resistance is high, trimethoprim may be an appropriate alternative. However, prophylaxis is questionable. The best course of action for most patients with severe chronic bronchitis is to start an appropriate 5 day antimicrobial therapy course within 24 hours of developing purulent sputum. Continuous prophylaxis should probably only be considered for a minority of patients when the latter approach has proved unsuccessful.

INFLUENZA

The causative organisms of influenza are:

- myxoviruses
- influenza Types A, B and C.

Influenza remains essentially an unconquered infectious disease. The epidemiological characteristics remain difficult to predict accurately (Webster 1997). There are seasonal variations and documented pandemic outbreaks.

Influenza A

Pandemics due to 'new' Influenza A viral strains that show an antigenic move have appeared over the last 15 years. Influenza A viruses mainly affect man but may also cause infection in a range of animals, mammals and birds. New strains emerging throughout the last decade between mammals and birds and in densely populated areas in both China and Asia are documented. When this antigenic shift occurs, a pandemic lasts for up to 4 months and thereafter continues with smaller numbers of cases during subsequent months and even years. Influenza A virus caused a pandemic between 1977 and 1979 after an absence of about 20 years (Tillett et al 1983). Interestingly those affected were mainly young people under the age of 26 years of age who had no immunity to Influenza Type A. This pandemic, it is believed, started in 1977 in China before crossing to Russia and affecting eastern and then western Europe between 1978 and 1979, and was thus termed Russian Influenza. Two years later, between 1980 and 1981, there were still documented cases of influenza due to the same strain being identified in both Europe and the Americas.

Influenza B

Influenza B viruses usually cause much smaller epidemics, milder illnesses and tend to be seasonal and every 2–3 years, often affecting institutions, children and the elderly. There is little change between the surface antigens of Influenza B viruses and this is often referred to as a minor drift and rarely a shift.

Influenza C

Influenza C, again an important pathogen, usually only causes mild and sporadic infection, is usually self-limiting and has rarely caused the type of outbreaks associated with Influenza A and, to a lesser extent, with Influenza B.

Transmission of influenza

All the influenza viruses are transmitted by respiratory droplets during:

- coughing
- sneezing
- close contact.

As with all respiratory viruses, they are often spread by the hands or by fomites in the environment contaminated by respiratory secretions from the carrier. Amongst susceptible individuals, other patients, carers, family, friends and healthcare workers, spread may be rapid.

Influenza incubation period

The incubation period is between 1 and 3 days. The virus multiplies in the epithelium of the upper and lower respiratory tract, damaging the ciliated mucosa of the trachea and the bronchi. Multiplication of organisms stimulates the production of interferon and local IgA with systemic serum antibodies that remain active against the haemagglutin and other surface antigens of the virus. The latter defence mechanisms gradually help the patient to overcome the infection. In a minority of patients the virus may directly infect the alveoli, which may result in an intense and rapidly fatal alveolitis.

Clinical signs and symptoms of influenza

Classically influenza has a rapid onset associated with:

- headache
- fever
- malaise
- cough
- general body muscle aching
- loss of appetite
- sore throat.

Initial symptoms may subside within a week but tiredness, often depression and associated secondary problems may persist for days if not weeks. The great majority of all influenza illnesses are due to Influenza Type A viruses.

Secondary complications of influenza

Secondary bacterial infections frequently complicate influenza, particularly in the elderly and those with underlying respiratory disease such as chronic obstructive pulmonary disease, cystic fibrosis and bronchiectasis, but they can also occur in young healthy people. The main bacterial pathogens are:

- *Staphylococcus aureus*
- *Streptococcus pneumoniae*
- *Streptococcus pyogenes*
- *Haemophilus influenzae*.

Pneumonia due to *Staphylococcus aureus* or, less frequently, *Streptococcus pyogenes* may be rapidly progressive, resulting in the death of a patient within a few days despite antimicrobial therapy.

Primary influenza virus pneumonia is far less frequent a complication than secondary bacterial infection but when it does occur the morbidity rates are higher. The patient's general condition will rapidly worsen, which is associated with severe respiratory distress and hypoxaemia. Death may occur within a few hours of onset. Essentially the lungs are characteristically congested and oedematous with a tracheobronchial ciliated epithelium. Pneumonitis is usually viral without significant bacterial infection. Other complications, although much rarer, include:

- myocarditis
- encephalitis
- polyneuropathy
- pericarditis.

Patients with severe influenzal illness requiring hospitalization or patients involved in an institutional outbreak of influenza must have samples obtained for virological and bacteriological investigations. Simple Gram staining of sputa will give a rapid indication of secondary bacterial infection, for example a potential *Staphylococcus aureus*.

Virus isolation and rapid diagnosis

A throat swab or nasopharyngeal washing should be obtained as early as possible and transported in viral transport medium. Virus isolation can then be undertaken in the appropriate virological laboratory. Rapid diagnosis is possible using direct immunofluorescent techniques on respiratory secretions from the patients.

An acute serum and a convalescent serum collected up to 2 weeks later are both tested by an Influenza A complement fixation test to detect a > 4-fold antibody titre rise. An Influenza B complement fixation test is usually carried out at the same time.

Alternatively, influenza haemagglutin inhibition tests can also be performed. However, this is group specific, either Group A or Group B, and therefore is really only applicable during an epidemic due to a known strain of influenza.

Treatment

General measures such as bed rest and an antipyretic such as paracetamol are usually sufficient. Bacterial complications often arise and therefore prompt treatment with a combination of antimicrobial drugs effective against *Staphylococcus aureus*, *Streptococcus pneumoniae* and *Haemophilus influenzae* should be given. Patients with underlying respiratory disease who develop severe bacterial complications usually require urgent hospital admission and require the following investigations and treatment:

- sputum microscopy, culture and sensitivity
- blood cultures
- chest X-ray
- prompt parenteral antimicrobial therapy
- physiotherapy
- humidified oxygen
- hydration.

When a patient is admitted with suspected influenza, isolation with respiratory precautions must be undertaken to prevent the spread of infection to other patients and to limit the spread to healthcare workers.

Prevention of influenza

Immunization against influenza is recommended in patients with known respiratory or heart disease and in the elderly (Salisbury & Begg 1996). The influenza virus strains included in the killed vaccine will include currently prevalent strains. The vaccine is given by subcutaneous or intramuscular injection and seasonal variations would advise that this be given during September or early October to give adequate protection during winter months. Various studies have shown varying degrees of protection but it is generally thought that protection is afforded to between 60% and 80% of those who receive immunization.

Even when new Influenza A strains are detected a new modified recombinant vaccine containing the appropriate protective haemagglutin antigens is developed even before the new strain reaches Europe. Rarely, serious complications of influenza vaccine may occur, such as Guillain-Barré syndrome which followed the use of the swine influenza vaccine in the USA during the late 1970s.

Antiviral drug therapy is expensive; amantadine is one such drug which is effective against Influenza A viruses. If given to contacts of a patient with Influenza A, successful prophylaxis against infection may be achieved.

Parainfluenza

Parainfluenza viruses Types I–IV often cause upper respiratory tract infections and tracheitis in adults, but the illness is usually of a less severe nature than influenza viruses. These viruses may cause severe lower respiratory tract infections in infants, with parainfluenza virus Type III being one of the commonest causes of croup in the young. Investigations for parainfluenza are similar to those for influenza, with serological tests also being available to complement fixation antigens of parainfluenza Types I, III and IV.

PNEUMONIA

Pneumonia is a leading cause of illness and death with approximately 5 million deaths occurring worldwide (Farr 1997). Classic symptoms of pneumonia include:

> **Box 9.1   Types of pneumonia**
>
> - Pneumococcal pneumonia
> - Streptococcus pneumoniae
> - Aspiration pneumonia
> - Anaerobic bacterial pneumonia
> - Influenza
> - Atypical pneumonias
> - Legionnaires' disease
> - Pneumocystis carinii pneumonia (PCP)

- cough
- pleuritic chest pain
- pyrexia.

In the early phases, the cough is often non-productive with bacterial pneumonia, but subsequently there is increased production of mucopurulent yellowy/green sputum. Patients with atypical pneumonias characteristically have a non-productive dry cough. Physical signs include diminished movement of the infective side of the lung, with associated crepitations. This may be associated with a pleural effusion. The chest X-ray usually shows signs of consolidation (Fig. 9.2), and there may be abnormal physical signs with radiological changes in the early stages.

Pneumonias due to bacteria are more acute and are of greater severity than atypical pneumonias caused by a mycoplasma or other organism; however it must be highlighted that these are often indistinguishable clinically.

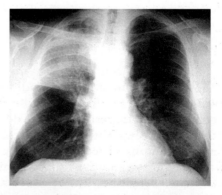

Figure 9.2   Chest X-ray showing a lobar pneumonia. Reproduced with permission from Webber & Pryor 1993.

Pulmonary tuberculosis, for example, may also occasionally present clinically as an acute pneumonia. *Streptococcus pneumoniae* is the commonest cause of pneumonia in both patients in the community and hospitalized patients. There are over eighty pneumococcal serotypes. *Streptococcus pneumoniae* Type III is one of the most virulent organisms and is frequently associated with a severe pneumonia and associated bacteraemia and often septicaemia. *Streptococcus pneumoniae* is probably the most common cause of pneumonia in over two-thirds of patients seen by GPs. Pneumococcal pneumonia is often seen as a secondary cause, where the factors present for predisposing to pneumonia are usually:

- impaired respiratory defences
- old age
- underlying respiratory disease
- secondary influenza
- aspiration of vomit or associated with chronic diseases such as alcoholism, hepatic and renal disease.

Pneumococcal disease, however, can also cause primary pneumonias in previously healthy people. Historically, classical pneumococcal lobar pneumonia was common, and this was followed by what was referred to as either crisis or lysis. Recovery after a pneumococcal lobal pneumonia was followed by immunity to the infecting capsular serotype, but a fatal pneumococcal pneumonia could subsequently occur due to a different serotype. This classic type of lobal pneumonia remains uncommon today, compared with other types of pneumonia. Complications of pneumococcal pneumonia include both meningitis and empyema. Death occurs most often in the elderly and those with debilitating chronic conditions.

Staphylococcus aureus is more likely to cause a pneumonia in hospitalized patients. However, when there is also an influenza epidemic within a community, staphylococcal respiratory infections and pneumonias are not uncommon. *Staphylococcus aureus* is also an important secondary cause of pneumonia in infants with rare congenital disorders and in intravenous drug users, particularly heroin addicts. Complications include:

- multiple lung abscess
- empyema
- bacteraemias
- septicaemias
- death, especially in patients who have had a recent influenza.

Haemophilus influenzae strains, often mixed with *Streptococcus pneumoniae*, are occasionally causes of secondary pneumonia in patients with chronic bronchitis. However, the documented evidence regarding the national incidence is not available as it is not a notifiable disease. Estimates remain between 20% and 35% (Macfarlane et al 1982).

Coliforms rarely cause pneumonia in patients within the community; however they are occasionally seen in patients with a history of alcohol abuse, who have aspirated on vomit. In hospitalized patients, coliforms and particularly *Pseudomonas* species are an important pathogen for pneumonia, particularly amongst patients in intensive care units, whereby intubation has allowed easy access into the respiratory tract. In particular both *Pseudomonas* and *Klebsiella* are important primary causes of pneumonia in patients in intensive care units.

Anaerobic bacteria usually mixed with other organisms, either from the upper respiratory tract or the bowel, can also contribute to severe aspiration pneumonia and to a pneumonia in patients who have got an obstructive disease of the respiratory tract, such as a foreign body that has been inhaled.

Atypical pneumonias

Various other important causes of pneumonia include:

- *Mycoplasma*
- *Chlamydia*
- *Coxiella burnetii*

Classically the characteristics of an atypical pneumonia include an unproductive dry cough and a remittent fever. There are rarely marked physical signs in the chest. A full bood count (FBC) may show no leukocytes, whereas in many cases of bacterial pneumonia, leukocytosis is evident. Chest X-ray will inevitably show patchy consolidation. Of note among the atypical pneumonias is Legionnaires' disease, which is occasionally diagnosed clinically as an atypical pneumonia and will be discussed in more detail later in the chapter.

Variances of age

Streptococcus pneumoniae is an important cause of pneumonia at all ages. However, the overwhelming prevalence is in the elderly. The mortality rate for pneumococcal pneumonia is greatest in patients in excess of 70 years. *Staphylococcus aureus* is also an important but uncommon cause in infants. *Legionella pneumophila* is most often a cause of serious pneumonia in patients over 45 years of age. *Haemophilus influenzae* Type B rarely causes pneumonia, but when it does it mainly occurs in infants. Viruses such as respiratory syncitial virus (RSV), parainfluenza viruses and adenoviruses are frequent causes of pneumonitis in infants. *Chlamydia trachomatis*, which may be acquired by the infant from an infected mother during delivery, has mainly been reported in the Americas as causing pneumonia during the neonatal period, but is seen as a more important cause of pneumonia in immunocompromised patients in western Europe.

Zoonosis

A history of recent close contact with birds, including ducks, parrots, budgerigars and turkeys, should raise the possibility of zoonosis with patients who are presenting with an atypical pneumonia, either ornithosis or psitticosis. However, a history of recent contact with birds is only obtained in about one-third of affected patients.

Contact with either cattle or sheep and the drinking of unpasteurized milk should also raise the possibility of infectious pathogens, such as Q fever. If the patient presenting with a pneumonia has an occupation that involves handling raw meat animal products, Q fever must be considered. Additionally laboratory staff who have contact with samples, such as microbiology workers (MLSOs), who develop pneumonia may have acquired a psitticosis or a tuberculosis whilst handling sputum specimens.

Seasonal variations

Patients who develop flu-like illness leading to pneumonia during or soon after a visit abroad, particularly during the British summer season, must have Legionnaires' disease excluded. Legionnaires' disease is endemic in Britain but characteristically is most frequently acquired in the summer months whereas pneumococcal pneumonia most often occurs during the winter season.

Unresolving pneumonias

Patients who have already been given antimicrobial therapy and who have an unresolving pneumonia may have received inappropriate antibiotic treatment. For example, an antimicrobial agent may have been prescribed blindly prior to antimicrobial sensitivities being available and therefore the organism may be resistant to the antimicrobial agent prescribed, thus the pneumonia will be unresolving. Other causes for unresolving pneumonias include a primary atypical pneumonia treated with a broad spectrum antibiotic when in fact causes of atypicals include *Mycoplasma pneumoniae*, psitticosis and *Mycobacterium* spp. Additionally, Legionnaires' disease will not respond to initial treatment with beta-lactam antimicrobial therapy or aminoglycosides but should respond effectively to erythromycin or tetracycline. Secondary bacterial infection associated with an obstruction of the respiratory tract may be associated with a foreign body or carcinoma of the respiratory tract. Therefore, a secondary infection would be more difficult to treat and may not respond to first line therapies. Tuberculosis is often misdiagnosed, treated as a chest infection and only when no improvement is made are further investigations undertaken and tuberculosis considered.

Opportunistic conditions

Opportunistic infections in patients with HIV and AIDS, neoplastic disease and other causes of immunosuppression may well have an unresolving pneumonia as a first presenting factor, such as pneumocystis, fungal or various viral infections. Protozoal infections, especially *Pneumocystis carinii* pneumonias, frequently cause an acute pneumonia in patients who are immunocompromised, especially those with HIV and AIDS. Many factors predispose to opportunistic pneumonias, including:

- frequent severe previous lower respiratory tract infections
- general debilitation
- intensive care unit (ICU) management with intubation
- prolonged broad spectrum antimicrobial therapy
- steroids
- cytotoxic therapy
- instrumentation
- immunodeficiency diseases.

Microbiological investigations of pneumonia

Investigations are indicated in all patients with a pneumonia to:

- identify the cause
- deliver appropriate treatment
- rule out other causes of disease.

Microbiological investigations of pneumonia include:

- sputum microscopy, culture and sensitivity
- blood cultures
- white cell count
- pleural fluid microscopy, culture and sensitivity
- pneumococcal antigen tests
- serological tests.

Sputum microscopy, culture and sensitivity

Sputum for microscopy, culture and antibiotic sensitivities is important. Sputum is rarely collected well. Saliva samples are unsuitable for the above tests yet continue to be sent. What is required is mucopurulent or purulent sputum collected before antimicrobial therapy is commenced. If this is difficult, although with a true respiratory infection it probably will not be, a physiotherapist can help in obtaining specimens. Sputum should never be left for long periods before being transferred to a laboratory otherwise an overgrowth with Gram negative organisms may occur, then the laboratory will identify the predisposing organism as a Gram negative organism which may mask pathogens causing the pneumonia.

Specimens obtained through tracheal suctioning are particularly useful for diagnosis of both anaerobic and fungal infections as there is less contamination from oral flora, although this is rarely performed in the United Kingdom because of the rare complications associated with the procedure. Certainly it should be considered more often for investigation of serious unrelenting pneumonia. For bronchoscopies undertaken, any purulent secretion should be obtained for microscopy, culture and sensitivity. More invasive techniques may be justified if the investigation of opportunistic respiratory disease is to be carried forward.

Sputa are cultured after homogenization to reduce the risk of sampling errors. A dilution method of sputum culture is preferred to give a semi-quantitative idea of the number of organisms present. The diluted homogenized sputum specimen is routinely cultured on blood agar and chocolate agar for up to 48 hours in an aerobic atmosphere.

Blood cultures

Blood cultures should be collected from all patients with a pneumonia prior to antimicrobial therapy being commenced. Should a bacteraemia or septicaemia occur with the same organisms as are causing the primary pneumonia, therapy can be altered accordingly.

White cell count

White blood cell count and differential film are often useful in distinguishing bacterial pneumonias from non-bacterial pneumonias and Legionnaires' disease. Bacterial pneumonias usually have raised total white count and a neutrophilia often > 12 000 mm³. However, non-bacterials and Legionnaires' disease do not.

Pleural fluid

If a patient presents with a pleural effusion the fluid should be collected in a sterile container for microscopy and in another sterile container for culture and sensitivities.

Pneumococcal antigens

These tests are for pneumococcal antigens and can be carried out by immunoelectrophoresis. They are particularly useful when antimicrobial therapy has already been commenced.

Specific serological tests

Antibody rising titres 4-fold or greater are the criteria used to diagnose the cause of a primary atypical pneumonia indicative of active infection due to respective organisms. They are:

- complement fixation tests, antigens against *Mycoplasma pneumoniae*, psitticosis, *Coxiella burnetii* and Influenza A and B
- fluorescent antibody tests carried out against *Legionella pneumophila* (the cause of Legionnaires' disease) using a specific legionella antigen, titres > 1 in 128 suggest diagnosis, although preferably a rising antibody titre should also be demonstrated.

Treatment of pneumonia

Most adults who need antimicrobial therapy for the treatment of pneumonia will require drugs that are active against *Pneumococci* and if the patient also has chronic respiratory disease the antimicrobial therapy should also be active against *Haemophilus influenzae*. For both of these organisms, oral amoxicillin or ampicillin is suitable. *Staphylococcus aureus* need only be considered as a cause of pneumonia during an epidemic or outbreak of influenza. During this time if *Staphylococcus aureus* is considered a potential, or proven through microbial culture, then flucloxacillin would be the drug of choice, or a combination of amoxicillin and flucloxacillin (Shanson et al 1984). For patients who are proven to have an allergic reaction to the pencillins, erythromycin is an alternative.

Patients who are admitted to hospital with pneumonia usually have sputum taken at the earliest opportunity for microbial examination, including microscopy, culture and sensitivity. Investigations can give a rapid and valuable assistance in guiding the management of the patient's respiratory tract infection. Gram staining will indicate the Gram positive or Gram negative nature of the organism, although culture will take a minimum of 24 hours, and longer with some organisms, particularly mycobacteria which are very slow growing and can take between 4 and 12 weeks.

In the majority of situations, bacteriological data are not available for patients who are admitted to hospital with respiratory tract infections, prior to the commencement of treatment. Therefore broad spectrum antimicrobial therapy will be commenced but this must be reviewed in line with microbiological data and full sensitivities and antibiogram of the drug used for treatment of the organism.

Prevention of pneumonia

Prevention is better than cure. Prevention of penumonia throughout the population depends on many factors (Woodhead et al 1987), of which most are non-specific but include:

- poverty
- housing
- nutrition
- environment including exposure to pollutants
- smoking both active and passive
- alcohol consumption.

Additionally it is well documented that more specific factors include immunization of children against childhood infectious diseases including both measles and pertussis (whooping cough). A

Case study 9.2

Gary is a 22-year-old philosophy student with a part time job in a bar who visited his GP with a lingering cough which he put down to pre-exam nerves.

Following an examination the GP prescribed a course of erythromycin 500 mg qds orally. He felt that Gary had a lower respiratory infection as he was producing light green sputum.

A few days later Gary's cough became worse and he noticed his sputum was dark green with flecks of blood. Gary felt hot and cold at times and experienced episodes of breathlessness, especially when climbing the stairs in his halls of residence. A friend called an ambulance when Gary was unable to get out of bed and he was admitted to hospital.

A chest X-ray was performed, a sputum specimen obtained for microscopy, culture and sensitivity and full blood count, urea, electrolytes, liver function tests and blood cultures were taken. Gary was diagnosed as having a lobar pneumonia.

Gary's saturations were between 90% and 92% so he was administered humidified 28% oxygen and intravenous fluids and was commenced on intravenous amoxicillin and flucloxacillin. He had physiotherapy twice a day.

Gary began to feel better within 48 hours, his appetite improved, he was able to mobilize unaided and was discharged home to his parents after a week in hospital.

pneumococcal vaccine is available (Salisbury & Begg 1996) which, although still in terms of vaccines is a fairly new vaccination, may well in time prove extremely useful in preventing pneumococcal respiratory infections especially in those patients known to have predisposing factors.

LEGIONNAIRES' DISEASE

Legionnaires' disease was identified in the latter quarter of the last century as an atypical pneumonia due to a Gram negative bacillus, *Legionella haemophila*. The disease became recognized following a large explosive outbreak of a pneumonia-type illness with many fatalities amongst war veterans (Legionnaires) attending a convention in America during the summer of 1976 (van Arsdal et al 1983). The Communicable Disease Center (CDC) in Atlanta isolated the causative organism from the lungs of those who had died. It is believed that the organism had not previously been recognized and it did not appear clearly as a Gram stainable organism. However, ultimately, when cultured, Gram stains of colonies showed that it was a Gram negative bacillus.

Epidemiological data from this original outbreak in Philadelphia identified that the route of spread was airborne with an incubation period of less than 7 days and no evidence of person-to-person spread (Fraser et al 1997). Pneumonitis inevitably followed inhalation of the air contaminated by the water containing legionella bacilli. Following on from this outbreak there have been many documented outbreaks throughout the world, mainly during the summer or warmer seasons. It is considered that up to 3% of undiagnosed pneumonias may be caused by *Legionella pneumophila*. Essentially, fit healthy people usually under 45 years of age who smoke cigarettes or with a history of previous respiratory disease are identified as those most at risk of developing Legionnaires' pneumonia. The mortality rate is around 15%. Men are twice as likely as women to become infected (Murray & Tuazon 1980).

Clinical features of Legionnaires' disease

Clinical features of Legionnaires' disease are similar to a flu-like illness with a dry cough and in the latter stages mental confusion, often mistaken for acute psychiatric illness or the neurological features indicative of neurological trauma or neoplasm (Sanford 1979). Often by the time the patient is admitted to hospital there is gross consolidation of the lungs identifying a lobal pneumonia. Many patients who are admitted to hospital have been treated in the community by their GPs with antimicrobial therapies in the preceding days or weeks.

Microbiological diagnosis of Legionnaires' disease

Specific microbiological diagnosis is usually made by looking at the titre level of serum immunofluorescent antibody to legionella. There are six serotypes of legionella but serotype 1 accounts for the majority of cases. Rapid diagnosis may sometimes be achieved by the use of an enzyme linked immunosorbent assay (ELISA) test to detect legionella antigen excreted through urine.

Antibiotic treatment

Erythromycin, tetracycline and ciprofloxacin have greater activity against legionella than many other antimicrobial drugs. However, the drug of choice is usually erythromycin. If Legionnaires' disease is indicated, usually high dose erythromycin should be given intravenously. If patients do not appear to respond to this treatment and Legionnaires' is still strongly suspected or confirmed, rifampicin would be a drug of choice.

ASPERGILLUS BRONCHOPULMONARY DISEASES

Spores of the *Aspergillus* species may be inhaled to reach most parts of the lower respiratory tract including the alveoli. *Aspergillus* can cause:

- asthma in patients who have an allergic reaction to *Aspergillus*
- an allergic bronchopulmonary aspergillosis (ABPA) where spores other than the *Aspergilli* reach the lungs and lower respiratory tract and stimulate an allergic bronchoalveolitis
- aspergilloma when *Aspergillus fumigatus* or *flavus* or other species cause a chronic infection in a particularly damaged area of the lung
- disseminated aspergillosis where invasive lung infection by *Aspergillus* occurs.

Microbiological investigations

Mucus plugs in the sputum stained by silver stains may show the *Aspergillus* in patients with allergic bronchopulmonary aspergillosis. Culture of the *Aspergillus* species can be carried out but the colonies may sometimes be difficult to identify due to contamination of transient colonization with other organisms of the respiratory tract. Negative fungal cultures especially from sputa are often obtained in patients who have got an overwhelming fungal infection.

Treatment

Treatment of the allergic response with oral steroids without having to give antifungal therapy is often sufficient in patients who have asthma or an allergic bronchopulmonary aspergillosis. Treatment with long term steroids (oral and/or inhaled) may be necessary. Antifungal therapy such as amphotericin is often not indicated in the treatment of aspergilloma unless there is evidence of coexistent dissemination of the *Aspergillus*.

CYSTIC FIBROSIS

Cystic fibrosis is the most common recessive genetic disorder affecting one in every 2500 births. The main cause of morbidity and mortality in cystic fibrosis (CF) is bacterial lung infection. A background of chronic lung sepsis, in which *Staphylococcus aureus*, *Haemophilus influenzae*, *Pseudomonas aeruginosa* and *Burkholderia cepacia* are the bacteria most frequently involved, is punctuated at increasingly frequent intervals by acute infective exacerbations. In response to persistent inflammation, pulmonary fibrosis and bronchiectasis progress, culminating in respiratory failure and death.

An acute exacerbation is characterized by some or all of the following symptoms:

- increasing breathlessness
- change in sputum volume, colour and viscosity (may have reduced sputum volume as unable to perform physiotherapy/expectorate as effectively)
- tiredness
- loss of appetite/weight loss.

Treatment

Treatment depends on the severity of both the exacerbation and the underlying lung disease. The aim of treatment is to maintain lung function which can be achieved by:

- regular physiotherapy
- early and effective antibiotic treatment of acute exacerbations
- optimal bronchodilation
- attention to optimal nutrition.

Physiotherapy

The aim of physiotherapy is to clear bronchial secretions and to delay progression of lung damage. Patients with cystic fibrosis are taught to self-manage but may need additional assistance during acute exacerbations. Physiotherapy treatment will depend on each patient's assessment and may include:

- active cycle of breathing (Fig. 9.3)
- postural drainage (Fig. 9.4)
- PEP mask +/– postural drainage
- exercise.

Antibiotic therapy

The choice of antibiotic will vary and depends on the most recent sputum culture result, the previous clinical response to agents already used and allergies. The quinolones (e.g. ciprofloxacin), being the only available class of oral anti-pseudomonal agents, may be the best first line oral therapy, although the response is unlikely to be of benefit if

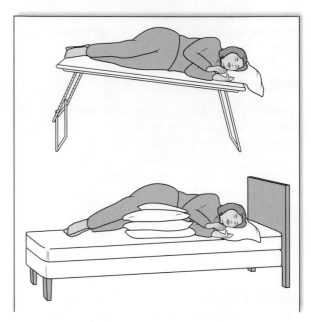

Figure 9.4   Postural drainage for physiotherapy.

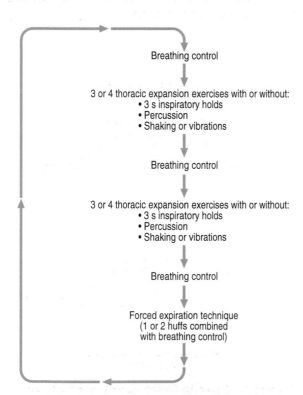

Breathing control

⬇

3 or 4 thoracic expansion exercises with or without:
- 3 s inspiratory holds
- Percussion
- Shaking or vibrations

⬇

Breathing control

⬇

3 or 4 thoracic expansion exercises with or without:
- 3 s inspiratory holds
- Percussion
- Shaking or vibrations

⬇

Breathing control

⬇

Forced expiration technique
(1 or 2 huffs combined
with breathing control)

Figure 9.3   Active cycle of breathing technique.

the patient has recently received ciprofloxacin. Some other broad spectrum oral agents (oxytetracycline or erythromycin) should be considered as these may improve lung function (probably by treating other pathogens and reducing exoenzyme production by *Pseudomonas aeruginosa*).

The UK Cystic Fibrosis Trust's Antibiotic Group (2000) have produced guidance for use of antibiotics in cystic fibrosis patients. The microbiology of cystic fibrosis sputum requires specific expertise with the use of selective media and multiple antibiotic sensitivity tests. Sputum should be sent for microbiology before such treatment is given. For intravenous anti-pseudomonal therapy, the most common first line approach is a combination of a beta-lactam or penicillin derivative and an aminoglycoside (Fig. 9.5).

If the patient is known to harbour *Staphylococcus aureus*, flucloxacillin should also be used. Anti-staphylococcal agents are sometimes given indefinitely following the isolation of *Staphylococcus aureus* (i.e. flucloxacillin).

Anti-pseudomonal agents may be given via the nebulized route so that the antibiotics can reach the most distal airways. The most frequently

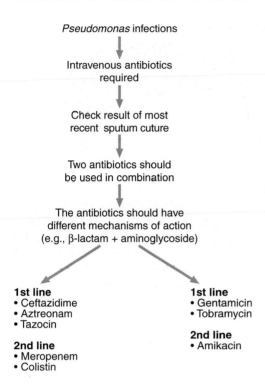

Pseudomonas infections

↓

Intravenous antibiotics required

↓

Check result of most recent sputum culture

↓

Two antibiotics should be used in combination

↓

The antibiotics should have different mechanisms of action (e.g., β-lactam + aminoglycoside)

1st line
- Ceftazidime
- Aztreonam
- Tazocin

2nd line
- Meropenem
- Colistin

1st line
- Gentamicin
- Tobramycin

2nd line
- Amikacin

Figure 9.5   Choosing intravenous antibiotics for patients with cystic fibrosis who have pseudomonal infection.

used antibiotics for nebulization are colistin, tobramycin/TOBI and gentamicin. The use of bronchodilators and pre-nebulized antibiotics can prevent bronchospasm related to nebulized antibiotics. In general, patients are asked to take bronchodilators (usually nebulized) before physiotherapy, which is itself performed before nebulized antibiotics.

Burkholderia cepacia has been identified as a significant respiratory pathogen in cystic fibrosis. The acquisition of *Burkholderia cepacia* may pose a particular threat to the cystic fibrosis patient because the organism is often multi-resistant to antipseudomonal agents. Patients can have transient *Burkholderia cepacia* or can become colonized with the organism. Clinical outcome following colonization can affect patients in different ways. They may remain clinically stable, they may deteriorate gradually, or in some cases they may deteriorate rapidly. The poor prognosis in patients with *Burkholderia cepacia* may be due to severe lung dis-

ease at the time of onset and the poor response to antibiotics. Cross-infection between cystic fibrosis patients in the hospital and outside the hospital setting during social contact has been described.

Home versus hospital antibiotics treatment

Patients can self-administer intravenous antibiotics at home (Wolter et al 1997) provided there is adequate education and support (Fig. 9.6). Selection of patients' suitability should be done on an individual basis with motivation, home stability and family support all being assessed. The aim of home intravenous antibiotic therapy is to allow patients to have minimal disruption to their lifestyle whilst maintaining equal efficacy to hospital care. If this can not be achieved then the patient should not be considered for home intravenous antibiotic therapy.

BRONCHIECTASIS

Bronchiectasis is defined as a chronic dilation of the bronchi which is caused by:

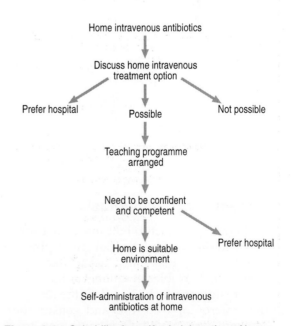

Home intravenous antibiotics

↓

Discuss home intravenous treatment option

Prefer hospital   Possible   Not possible

↓

Teaching programme arranged

↓

Need to be confident and competent   Prefer hospital

↓

Home is suitable environment

↓

Self-administration of intravenous antibiotics at home

Figure 9.6   Suitability for self-administration of home intravenous antibiotics.

- childhood infections (i.e. pertussis, bronchiolitis)
- immunodeficiency syndromes (i.e. hypogammaglobulinaemia)
- allergic bronchopulmonary aspergillosis
- pneumonia
- cystic fibrosis
- tuberculosis
- alpha-1 antitrypsin.

Collections of necrotic material and bronchial secretions in the dilated bronchi may result in inflammation which causes secondary bacterial infection and fibrosis in the lung. This will result in recurrent and persistent lower respiratory tract infections. Clinical features include:

- production of large amounts of purulent sputum
- bronchoconstriction
- cough
- haemoptysis.

Microbiological investigations

Sputum microscopy and culture during an acute respiratory tract infection should be obtained with a sputum specimen being collected before the commencement of antimicrobial therapy. For severe infections, blood cultures should also be obtained. During this time, the most frequent pathogens isolated are *Haemophilus influenzae*, *Streptococcus pneumoniae*, *Staphylococcus aureus*, a variety of anaerobes and coliforms and *Aspergillus* species. In advanced disease the patient will become colonized with *Pseudomonas aeruginosa*.

Treatment of bronchiectasis

Physiotherapy and postural drainage are usually necessary in the treatment of severe respiratory tract infections that are associated with bronchiectasis. Sensible yet rational antimicrobial therapy treatment may be based on the results of sputum microscopy culture and sensitivities. Unless there is an overwhelming infection, treatment should not be started until these data are available. The principles of treatment are the same as for cystic fibrosis.

LUNG ABSCESS

Lung abscess may develop in any patient who has had a localized lung infection, but is more common in those who have had infections with organisms such as *Staphylococcus aureus* and *Klebsiella* species. Intravenous drug users and patients who develop Influenza A infections are most at risk of developing staphylococcal lung abscess leading to multiple lung abscesses. Clinically the patient will be physically unwell with a swinging pyrexia and respiratory symptoms. However, diagnosis is usually identified from a chest X-ray that will identify the cavitated lesions.

Microbiological investigations

Sputum and blood cultures are collected to identify causative organisms.

Treatment

Postural drainage and antimicrobial therapy are usually successful if there is not an associated obstruction present that may require a surgical intervention. In a small minority of patients who do not respond to antimicrobial therapy and postural drainage, surgery can be undertaken where open surgical drainage of any abscess may become necessary. The choice of antimicrobial therapy should always be based on results from sensitivities of the organism to antimicrobials so the patient is not treated blindly, the specific organism is targeted and hopefully this will reduce the incidence of the development of resistance to antimicrobial therapies.

EMPYEMA

Empyema, or pus in a pleural cavity, is resultant from a previous episode of pneumonia. A range of organisms have been isolated from empyema pus, including *Staphylococci*, *Streptococci*, various anaerobes, a variety of Gram negative bacilli and mycobacteria. Microbiological diagnosis is usually easy as the pus is examined by Gram stain, acid fast and auramine stains for a presumptive diagnosis of tuberculosis, and cultured both anaerobically and aerobically. Antimicrobial therapy depends on the results of antimicrobial sensitivity tests but must be given in conjunction with the draining of the pus.

MYCOBACTERIAL INFECTIONS

Mycobacteria are seen as long red acid alcohol-fast bacilli in a Ziehl–Neelsen test. *Mycobacterium tuberculosis*, the commonest mycobacterium seen, has an abundance of wax and lipids in the cell wall allowing it to multiply intracellularly in macrophages as well as extracellularly. Infection with a mycobacterium leads to a delayed hypersensitivity type of immune response.

Tuberculosis

Tuberculosis is still a common notifiable infectious disease which kills more than 3 million people worldwide each year. In 1993 the World Health Organization declared tuberculosis a global emergency. Tuberculosis has two infection phases, firstly the initial primary infection with tubercle bacilli and then the development

of active smear positive tuberculosis. Soon after the primary infection enters the lung, the inflammatory response occurs and a calcified lesion is left. The primary infection remains dormant but may be reactivated (post primary infection) and if the immune system is weakened active open tuberculosis can be a result (Fig. 9.7). At the time of the primary infection tubercle bacilli are carried to lymph nodes by macrophages, allowing them to enter the blood stream (Taylor 1996), hence tuberculosis can be found in other parts of the body such as the spine and kidneys.

Predisposing factors for development of pulmonary tuberculosis include:

- immunodeficiency (i.e. HIV and AIDS)
- malnutrition
- old age
- history of alcohol abuse
- immunosuppression (i.e. steroids, chemotherapy)
- chronic respiratory disease.

Clinical features include:

- chronic cough
- haemoptysis
- weight loss
- pyrexia

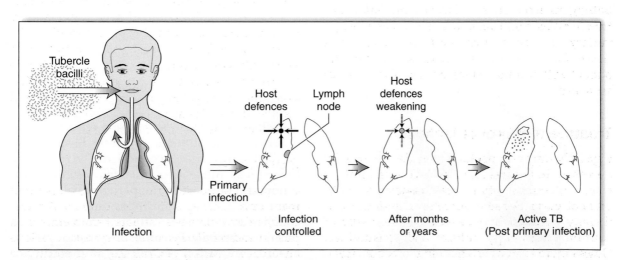

Figure 9.7 Primary and post primary tuberculosis infection.

- night sweats
- general malaise.

Chest X-ray changes are often seen which indicate pulmonary tuberculosis (Fig. 9.8). Open pulmonary tuberculosis should be considered in patients who have any of the predisposing factors and in any patient who has an unresolving pneumonia. Cavitating lesions of the lungs are due to a human type tubercle bacilli in more than 98% of cases and opportunistic mycobacteria account for around 2% of cases.

About 75% of patients with pulmonary tuberculosis in the UK present with an acute respiratory infection with a history indicative of tuberculosis. Most commonly, sites of infection with post primary tuberculosis are in the apical region of the lower lobes or in the upper lobes of the lungs. Cavitation is most characteristic in post primary tuberculosis. Tubercle bacilli are expectorated in the sputum and respiratory droplet nuclei expelled during coughing and sneezing. Open tuberculosis and contacts may be infected by inhaling this tubercle bacilli containing the droplet nuclei.

Treatment of pulmonary tuberculosis

The British Thoracic Society (1998) produced guidelines on chemotherapy and management of tuberculosis in the UK. Currently for fully sensitive tuberculosis, a six month treatment regimen is recommended consisting of rifampicin, izoniazid, pyrazinamide and ethambutol or streptomycin for 2 months and then rifampicin and

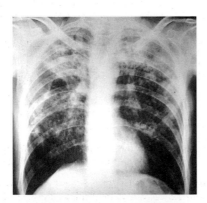

Figure 9.8 Chest X-ray showing tuberculosis.

Case study 9.3

Patrick is a 69-year-old retired sailor with a long history of alcohol abuse, and has been living in various hostels in London for the last few years. He was found collapsed and admitted to hospital via A&E.

Patrick was a poor health historian, feeling angry at being kept in hospital. A chest X-ray was abnormal and sputum was obtained for acid fast bacillus as pulmonary tuberculosis was suspected. Patrick was nursed in isolation and the diagnosis was confirmed.

Patrick was commenced on the treatment regimen of rifampicin and isoniazid for 6 months with the addition of pyrazinamide and ethambutol for the first 2 months (BTS 1998).

The main challenge with Patrick was his homelessness and his reluctance to take his medication. Once accommodation was found the community TB nurse visited Patrick on a regular basis. Although directly observed therapy (DOT) was considered it was found unnecessary as Patrick agreed to take his medication. He successfully completed his 6 month course of treatment, put on weight and had more energy.

isoniazid for a futher 4 months. The fourth drug, ethambutol or streptomycin, can be omitted when patients have a low risk of developing resistance to isoniazid (Table 9.1).

Pulmonary tuberculosis is a treatable condition but with inadequate initial therapy or non-completion of the course of treatment multi-drug resistant tuberculosis (MDR TB) will develop. The reasons for this occurring are:

- inadequate treatment (monotherapy or low dose)
- failure to complete course of antibiotics
- asymptomatic after 2–4 weeks of treatment
- lack of knowledge and understanding
- inability to access healthcare.

With an increased resistance in reported cases of tuberculosis, strategies must be developed to ensure the incidence is controlled. The role of the tuberculosis nurse is essential in providing education and support to the patient during treatment and thereby improving adherence and completion of therapy. Patients must be assessed on an individual basis and stategies adopted to ensure completion of courses of therapy, for example the use of directly observed therapy

Table 9.1 Tuberculosis treatment for active open tuberculosis

Drug	Duration	Side effects	Advantages
Rifampicin	6 months	• Gastrointestinal disturbance • Urine may turn red / orange • Hepatocellular viral infections	• Well absorbed in mouth • Allows reduced treatment time
Isoniazid	6 months	• Nausea and vomiting • Rashes • Hepatocellular damage	• Effectively kills replicating mycobacteria
Pyrazinamide	2 months	• Rashes • Hepatoxicity • Triggers acute gout	• Well absorbed, especially in cerebrospinal fluid
Ethambutol	2 months	• Optic neuritis • Visual impairment • Reduced ability to distinguish red/green	

(DOT), where patients are observed taking their therapy by a healthcare professional.

CONCLUSION

Respiratory infections can affect everyone in society and most people will experience the symptoms of influenza during their lives. However, for those with underlying respiratory disease and the young and elderly, respiratory infections can be life threatening. As well as treating infections, it is essential to take infection control seriously particularly in light of the increasing number of resistant organisms. Awareness of the different types of respiratory infections, microbiological investigations and treatment regimens will ensure early detection and intervention.

REFERENCES

Austrian R 1981 Some observations on the pneumococcus and on the current status of pneumococcal disease and its prevention. Review of Infectious Diseases 3 (suppl): S1–S17

British Thoracic Society 1997 Guidelines for the management of chronic obstructive pulmonary disease. Thorax 52 (suppl 5): S1–S28

British Thoracic Society 1998 Chemotherapy and management of tuberculosis in the United Kingdom: recommendations. Thorax 53: 536–548

British Thoracic Society and Public Health Laboratory Service 1987 Community-acquired pneumonia in adults and British hospitals in 1982–1983. A survey of aetiology, mortality, prognostic factors and outcome. Journal of Medicine 239: 195–200

Everett E D, Rahm A E J, Adantya M R 1977 *Haemophilus influenzae* pneumonia in adults. Journal of the American Medical Association 283: 319–321

Farr B 1997 Prognosis and decisions in pneumonia. New England Journal of Medicine 336(4): 228–289

Fraser D W, Tsai T R, Orenstein W et al 1997 Legionnaires' disease: description of an epidemic of pneumonia. New England Journal of Medicine 297: 1189–1203

Macfarlane J T, Finch R G, Ward M J, Macrae A D 1982 Hospital study of adult community acquired pneumonia. Lancet ii: 255–258

Murray H W, Tuazon C U 1980 Atypical pneumonias. Medical Clinics of North America 64: 507

National Audit Office 2000 The management and control of hospital acquired infection in acute NHS trusts in England. The Stationery Office, London

Salisbury D, Begg N 1996 Immunisation against infectious disease. HMSO, London

Sanford J P 1979 Legionnaires disease – the first thousand days. New England Journal of Medicine 300: 654–656

Shanson C C, McNabb W R, Williams T D M, Lant A F 1984 Erythromycin compared with a combination of ampicillin plus flucloxacillin for the treatment of community acquired pneumonia in adults. Journal of Antimicrobial Chemotherapy 14: 75–79

Taylor D 1996 Tuberculosis: knowledge and practice. Nursing Times 92(42): 1–4

Tillett H E, Smith J W, Gooch C D 1983 Excess deaths attributable to influenza in England and Wales: age at death and certified cause. International Journal of Epidemiology 12: 344–350

UK Cystic Fibrosis Trust's Antibiotic Group 2000 Report of the UK CF Trust's Antibiotic Group. Cystic Fibrosis Trust, Bromley

van Arsdal J A, Wunderlich J C, Meto D 1983 The manifestations of Legionnaires' disease. Journal of Infection 7: 51–62

Webber B A, Pryor J A 1993 Physiotherapy for respiratory and cardiac problems. Churchill Livingstone, Edinburgh

Webster R G 1997 Predictions for future human influenza pandemics. Journal of Infectious Diseases 176 (suppl 1): 514–519

Wolter J M, Bowler S D, Nolan P J, McCormack J G 1997 Home intravenous therapy in cystic fibrosis: a prospective randomized trial examining clinical, quality of life and cost aspects. European Respiratory Journal 10(4): 896–900

Woodhead M A, Macfarlane J T, McCracken J S, Rose D H, Finch R G 1987 Prospective study of the aetiology and outcome of pneumonia in the community. Lancet i: 671–674

Nutrition

Tracy Parker

Balanced nutrition in the respiratory patient is one aspect of respiratory therapy that can help prevent further progression of the disease as well as optimizing physical fitness and function of other organs. Traditionally, the interest has focused on the effects on lung function of being underweight rather than overweight. However, descriptions of the pink puffer (Body Mass Index (BMI) < 20) and blue bloater (BMI > 27) highlight the range of nutritional dilemmas that respiratory patients pose for practitioners involved in their care (Fig. 10.1).

The association between chronic respiratory disease and weight loss contributes towards a decline in lung function and hence the clinical condition is well recognized (Wilson et al 1985, 1989). On the one hand malnutrition increases with the severity of respiratory disease and on the other, malnutrition results in reduced respiratory muscle mass and muscle strength, reduced ventilatory drive and immune competence and hence a decline in lung function (Driver et al 1982, Gray-Donald et al 1996). Malnutrition also

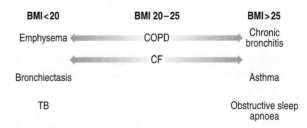

Figure 10.1 Body Mass Index (BMI) range and nutritional needs of respiratory patients.

Box 10.1 Clinical effects of malnutrition

- Respiratory system
  - reduced diaphragmatic function
  - reduced respiratory rate
  - reduced depth of ventilation
  - reduced ventilatory response to hypoxaemia and hypercapnia
- Immune system
  - impaired antibody response
  - depressed process of phagocytosis
  - reduced epithelial integrity – poor wound healing
- Gastrointestinal system
  - atrophy of villi – malabsorption
  - reduced activity of enzymes at the brush border
  - increased incidence of bacterial translocation
- Cardiac system
  - reduced cardiac output
  - increased liability to heart failure and renal dysfunction

has adverse effects on other organ systems (Box 10.1) and it is known that mortality is higher in the malnourished patient, independently of the severity of airway disease.

Being overweight also places extra metabolic stress on the cardiorespiratory system, causing hypercapnia. Eating and breathing at the same time can become a problem, especially during periods of acute exacerbations, and these patients are also at risk of being malnourished. Weight loss is frequently masked by oedema, so patients may have increased or static weight, but be nutritionally depleted. Malnutrition has been shown to be present in 50% of the population with chronic obstructive pulmonary disease (COPD) regardless of Body Mass Index (BMI) (Sahebjami et al 1994) (Table 10.1).

There is potential for reversibility, and nutritional supplementation has led to weight gain and improvements in respiratory muscle strength and endurance (Efthimiou et al 1988, Scott Whittaker et

Table 10.1 Instance of malnutrition in COPD patients

BMI (kcal/m²)	Percentage (%)
< 20	20%
20–27	53%
> 27	24%

al 1990). However, despite the awareness of the importance of good nutrition, the assessment of nutritional status remains infrequently performed. Malnutrition is a major negative prognostic factor; therefore, of equal clinical importance to the provision of optimal nutrition, is the identification and the evaluation of nutritional status and assessment of body composition. Early identification can have a favourable impact on the management of these patients.

MECHANISM OF WEIGHT LOSS

Weight loss is an independent prognostic indication of mortality and is associated with increased morbidity and decreased health related quality of life (Congleton 1999). Unfavourable energy balance seems to be the cause of weight loss in the respiratory patient, rather than an inherent component of the disease (Muers & Green 1993). Energy balance is determined by three factors:

- energy expenditure
- energy losses
- energy intake.

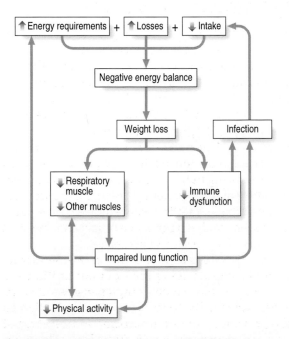

Figure 10.2 Negative feedback cycle between nutrition and lung function.

Negative energy balance occurs when energy expenditure and energy losses exceed energy intake (Fig. 10.2). Therefore, weight loss will occur as a result of inadequate energy intake in relation to energy needs.

Patients may lose weight acutely, during periods of exacerbation of the disease when oral intake is low and nutritional requirements are raised due to the increased work of breathing and infection, but they usually regain it upon recovery. However, in the majority of patients, as respiratory disease worsens, there appears to be a gradual stepwise decline in weight. There seems to be an interaction between declining nutritional status and declining lung function, but the causal relationship between nutrition and lung function remains unclear – does poor nutrition lead to worsening lung disease or does lung disease lead to poor nutrition, or both? By providing adequate nutritional support the negative feedback cycle between poor nutritional status and decline in lung function could be interrupted (Fig. 10.2). An integral part of this process is the identification and assessment of those patients at risk of malnutrition.

NUTRITIONAL SCREENING

50% of COPD patients in outpatients have been shown to have lost 10% or more of their ideal body weight with associated abnormalities in anthropometric, biochemical and immunological indices of poor nutritional status (Hunter et al 1981). However, most nutritional problems are only identified in hospitalized patients with advanced respiratory disease when it is often too late to correct nutritional deficits. In view of the likelihood of pre-existing nutritional deficits, improved identification of these patients is necessary, especially in the outpatient setting where they are most regularly seen, so that aggressive nutritional support can be initiated early in the disease.

Nutritional screening is a process of identifying patients who are at high risk of malnutrition and who may require a more comprehensive nutritional assessment. The King's Fund report highlighted the prevalence of undernutrition in hospitalized patients, identifying that 35–50% of patients admitted to medical and surgical wards are malnour-

ished (Lennard-Jones 1992). As part of the report it was recommended that a simple assessment of nutritional status should form part of the standard routine admissions procedure and should also be part of screening strategies in the community. The approach to nutritional support should be multidisciplinary so screening tools need to be simple, easy to use and acceptable to patients. A number of nutritional screening tools have been developed and although they vary in design and content they all include core questions relating to known risk factors for malnutrition, such as body weight changes, appetite, feeding difficulties and medical diagnosis. These are scored to give an overall indication of relative risk of malnutrition. Figure 10.3 is an example of a screening tool developed by the Department of Nutrition and Dietetics at Barts and The London NHS Trust which is based on the Birmingham Heartland's validated nutritional screening tool (Reilly et al 1995).

A simpler approach could be to ask questions related to the risks of malnutrition:

- Has there been any unexpected weight change?
- What is your usual weight and height?
- Are meals being missed or is less being eaten at meal times?
- Are there long periods without food or drink?
- Have you any physical problems with eating (i.e. problems with swallowing)?

ESTIMATION OF NUTRITIONAL STATUS

Nutritional assessment is a more complex process that involves the use of certain measurements to determine nutritional status. Nutritional assessments are used to:

- identify patients who are likely to benefit from nutritional support (i.e. those at risk of developing protein/calorie malnutrition or those, at the other end of the nutritional spectrum, who are overweight)
- help determine methods and goals of nutritional therapy
- act as a baseline to monitor the adequacy of nutritional therapy.

NUTRITIONAL ASSESSMENT SCORE

Assessment	Date	Weight	BMI	Score	Action taken	Name
Initial (IA)						
Week 2						
Week 3						
Week 4						
Week 5						

Usual weight ....

Height ....

MAC ....

| | SCORE | | | | IA | W2 | W3 | W4 | W5 |
	0	1	2	3					
WEIGHT Unintentional loss in last 3 months	No weight loss	0–3 kg weight loss	3–6 kg weight loss	6 kg or more					
BMI (Body Mass Index)	20 or more	18 or 19	15–17	Less than 15					
APPETITE/INTAKE	Good appetite, manages most of 3 meals/day		Poor appetite or poor intake – leaving > half of meals provided	Unable/unwilling to eat, NBM (for > 3 days)					
ABILITY TO EAT	No difficulties eating. No vomiting	Physical difficulty with feeding, e.g. arthritis, poor coordination, mild nausea, regurgitation	Difficulty chewing or swallowing, affecting food intake. Partial dysphagia requiring modified consistency. Slow to feed. Nausea + vomiting. Needs nursing help to feed	Unable to take food orally. Severe vomiting					
STRESS FACTOR	No stress factor. Apyrexial	Minor infection. Temperature 37–38°C	Infections, temperature 38–39°C. Major surgery. Single fracture. Pressure sores. Chemotherapy. Radiotherapy	Multiple injuries. Multiple fractures/burns. Severe sepsis. Temperature > 39°C					
			TOTAL SCORE						

Unable to swallow: refer immediately to Speech and Language Therapist <u>and</u> Dietitian

0–3 Minimal risk
4–5 Moderate risk
6–15 High risk

Action for patients at minimal risk (Score = 0–3)

1 Weigh on admission and then once a week
2 Review weekly. If it becomes appropriate take action as detailed above

Action for patients at moderate risk (Score = 4–5)

1 Weigh on admission, then twice weekly
2 Help with feeding if necessary
3 Keep food record chart
4 Give patient HP menu (yellow)
5 Offer one Build-up per day (use Ensure Plus for RENAL patients)
6 Replace uneaten meals with Build-up soup or Build-up drink (use Ensure Plus for RENAL patients)
7 Review weekly and if no improvement inform medical staff and ask them to refer to Dietitian
8 Document as part of the nursing process
9 On discharge: liaise with Dietitian regarding follow-up

Action for patients at high risk (Score = 6–15)

1 Inform medical staff and ask them to refer to Dietitian for advice
2 Weigh on admission, and then twice weekly
3 Help with feeding if necessary
4 Keep food record chart
5 Ensure Dietitian's recommendations are followed
6 Review weekly and liaise with Dietitian
7 Document as part of nursing process

Figure 10.3 Nutritional assessment tool. Reproduced with permission from Barts and The London NHS Trust.

As there is no single generally accepted non-invasive measure of nutritional status, it is necessary to use a combination of methods to avoid the shortcomings of a single approach. The measurements should be cheap, easy to perform without discomfort to the patient and should be regularly repeated to provide serial measurements to assess change in body mass and composition. A combination of measurements is required to give an accurate picture of a patient's nutritional status and these include:

- dietary history
- clinical examination
- anthropometric measurements
- laboratory measurements.

The summary of the findings can then be used to identify the specific nutritional problems and develop a comprehensive and individual care plan, the outcome of which can then be evaluated.

Anthropometric measurements

Anthropometry uses common quantitative measurements to identify changes in body composition by recording body weight, height, skin fold thickness and mid arm circumference.

Body weight and Body Mass Index

Carefully measured weight and height remain the most easily performed and useful determinants of nutritional status and predictors of mortality of the general population. Ideal or desirable weights have been associated with the lowest mortality and the Body Mass Index (BMI) is now the de facto criterion for defining desirable weight. It is calculated by:

$$\frac{\text{weight (kg)}}{\text{height (m}^2)}$$

It is an index of weight in proportion to height and indicates the relative fatness of individuals. Table 10.2 summarizes the interpretation of the BMI calculation (Garrow 1981).

A BMI either above or below the ideal range is associated with worsened health and increased mortality (Kushner 1993). From this percentage ideal body weight (IBW) can be calculated by:

Table 10.2   Interpretation of BMI (kcal/m²)

BMI (kcal/m²)	Description
< 19	Underweight
20–25	Ideal/healthy weight
26–30	Overweight
31–40	Obese
> 40	Severely obese

$$\frac{\text{current weight (kg)}}{\text{ideal weight (kg)}} \times 100$$

Malnutrition is defined as body weight below 80% IBW. Although BMI is easy to calculate there are limitations to its interpretation:

- It does not take into account the effect of change in body water because of dehydration, oedema and ascites. Weight can fluctuate between 1 kg with minimal peripheral oedema and 10 kg with severe oedema (Madden & Morgan 1994). Therefore, it is important to document not only actual weight at the time of assessment, but usual steady weight.
- It provides only limited information about body composition and changes that occur in response to fitness, illness and ageing. For example a high BMI in athletes does not mean they are obese as they have an increased weight of lean body mass (LBM) relative to height, and in older people LBM declines with ageing, but BMI remains the same as there is an increase in fat mass.

A high BMI does not preclude malnutrition in existing obesity where lean tissue may have been lost. Sustained weight loss and other measurements of fat and muscle stores therefore need to be considered to provide a more complete assessment of nutritional status.

Percentage weight loss

By documenting usual body weight, percentage body weight loss can also be calculated. This provides information on recent weight loss and therefore weight change can be considered on an individual basis. Percentage weight loss is calculated by:

$$\frac{\text{Usual weight (kg)} - \text{actual weight (kg)}}{\text{Usual weight (kg)}} \times 100$$

Percentage weight loss over time is a better indicator of the risk of malnutrition. These percentage weight losses are considered high risks of malnutrition:

- 1–2% weight loss in a week
- 5% weight loss in one month
- > 10% weight loss during the preceding three months.

However, it can be difficult to determine true weight loss because of:

- errors in recall
- presence of oedema, organomegaly, tumour growth.

Table 10.3 gives examples of action to be taken in relation to percentage weight loss.

Body composition measures

The primary goal of nutritional intervention is repletion or preservation of lean body mass (LBM), so methods that determine body composition are useful parameters to monitor changes in nutritional status. Although these measures are not as useful in detecting short term changes, they can be monitored serially to determine body composition and are accessible, non-invasive and inexpensive.

Mid arm circumference

Mid arm circumference (MAC) is a useful measure of muscle protein stores. The non-dominant arm should be measured while hanging relaxed and vertical at the side. The point of measurement is the midpoint of the upper arm, halfway between the tip of the shoulder and the tip of the elbow. The circumference of the upper arm should be measured at this midpoint. A non-stretch tape measure, which does not compress underlying tissue, should be used. The average of three measurements is recorded.

Triceps skin fold thickness

Triceps skin fold thickness (TSF) provides an estimate of body fat reserves. It measures the thickness of fat fold at the midpoint of the non-dominant arm (mm) using high-resolution callipers with scale reading accurate to $+/- 0.1$ mm and standard pressure of $10\,g/mm^2$. The average of three measurements is recorded. Based on TSF and MAC, mid arm muscle circumference (MAMC) can be calculated:

$$MAC\ (cm) - (0.3142 \times TSF\ (mm)).$$

This reflects the amount of muscle or lean tissue in the body. Actual measured TSF, MAC and

Table 10.3	Examples of use of % weight loss as a marker of nutritional status
Assessment	**Action**
Height 1.7 m Usual weight 58 kg; BMI 20 Actual weight 53 kg; BMI 18 % weight loss = 10.3%	BMI < 20 – nutritional intervention regardless of time over which weight is lost
Height 1.7 m Usual weight 72 kg; BMI 25 Actual weight 63 kg; BMI 23 % weight loss = 8% over 6 weeks	Monitor regarding healthy versus unhealthy weight loss
Height 1.7 m Usual weight 65 kg; BMI 22 Oedematous weight 60 kg; BMI 21 Flesh weight (mild oedema) 55 kg; BMI 19 % weight loss = 15%	Nutritional intervention regardless of time
Height 1.7 m Usual weight 78 kg; BMI 27 Actual weight 64 kg; BMI 22 % weight loss = 18% over 2 years	Encouragement to maintain weight

MAMC values can be compared to standard values for age and sex (Bishop et al 1981). As with BMI the influence of age, hydration and physical activity can introduce potential interpretation error, but markedly abnormal values (below the 5th percentile) are associated with poor clinical outcome. For the respiratory patient regular screening of body weight is indicated and the use of anthropometry to measure body composition and depletion of LBM (McWhirter et al 1994) (Table 10.4).

Bioelectrical impedance

This is a relatively new technique for assessing body composition. The principle of bioelectrical impedance (BI) is based upon the conductance through body fluids of an electrical current. Conductivity is higher in fat free mass (FFM), which contains all body fluids and electrolytes, than in fat. Electrodes are placed at a unilateral hand and foot and resistance is measured with the body supine. Theoretically FFM is linearly related to:

$$\frac{body\ height^2}{body\ resistance}\ or$$

$$\frac{body\ height^2}{body\ impedance}$$

BI is well validated in normal populations, but lacks substantiation in ill, obese or malnourished individuals. In the respiratory patient oedema, malnutrition or the use of steroids may influence fluid status and hence affect BI measurements. However, Schols et al (1991a) have found that BI is a useful measure of body composition in patients with stable severe COPD. It is also more preferable than TSF for use in the elderly with COPD as TSF has been shown to overestimate LBM and hence patients at risk of malnutrition can be missed.

Biochemical parameters

Biochemical assessment of various body fluids has also been advocated as a marker of nutritional status.

Serum protein concentrations

Proteins, which circulate in the plasma and include the hepatic secretory proteins, are influenced by dietary intake and are therefore often used to assess the adequacy of protein and calorie intake. They include:

- albumin
- prealbumin
- transferrin.

Albumin and transferrin are used as indices of visceral protein stores. However, hypoalbumineamia in adults is a marker of associated disease such as cardiac, intestinal, renal and liver disease, cancer, inflammation, wounds, burns and peritonitis, rather than a feature of protein/energy malnutrition. Albumin levels are not usually affected by nutritional intake and will not increase in stressed patients until the stress remits (Blunt et al 1998). Also, the

Table 10.4 Interpretation of anthropometric measurements

Interpretation	Measurements
Mildly undernourished	BMI 20 TSF/MAC 15th percentile
Moderate undernutrition	BMI < 18 TSF/MAC 5th percentile
Severe undernutrition	BMI < 16 TSF/MAC < 5th percentile
Unintentional weight loss before illness of more than 10% in the previous 3 months indicates undernutrition	

circulating half-life of albumin is 18 days so the benefits of any nutritional intervention will not be reflected until several weeks later. During periods of starvation and decreased energy supply, the body appears to maintain serum albumin concentrations at the expense of other protein sources, predominantly muscle. Malnourished COPD patients present with depleted body weight and anthropometric indices often have normal serum albumin or transferrin levels (Donahoe & Roger 1990, Efthimiou et al 1988). The influence of other disease, infection and steroid therapy also complicates the use of these indices and therefore they are unreliable indicators of malnutrition when used alone in assessing nutritional status (Jeejeebhoy 1994, Margarson & Soni 1998).

Total lymphocyte count

Achieving optimum immune response is another goal of nutritional therapy. Total lymphocyte count to below $1200/mm^3$ is reported in malnutrition and correlates with cellular immune status. Low lymphocyte counts have been reported in respiratory failure patients (Driver et al 1982), but stable malnourished respiratory patients often reveal normal counts (Knowles et al 1988, Otte et al 1984). Many conditions in addition to malnutrition affect the immune response, for example anaesthesia and surgery, infections, and steroids. Therefore, used alone its utility as a nutritional parameter needs careful interpretation.

Nitrogen balance

Nitrogen balance is not performed for the assessment of tissue stores but to indicate how current dietary intake is meeting the body's protein needs and to assess whether an anabolic state has been reached in response to nutritional therapy. It is a particularly useful measurement during periods of tube enteral feeding to ensure adequate calories and proteins are being given. Calculations of nitrogen balance are based on a 24 h urine collection for urea content

(Todorovic & Micklewright 1997). It is also useful to measure sodium and potassium at the same time:

$$\text{nitrogen output} = \text{urinary urea}/\text{mmol}/24\,\text{h} \times 0.033$$

A constant of 3 g is added to account for obligatory losses, for example through hair, skin, faeces and any extra renal losses such as pyrexia, GI fistulae and inflammatory bowel disease (IBD). Nitrogen intake is determined from dietary intake of protein over the same period:

$$\text{nitrogen balance} = \text{nitrogen intake} - \text{nitrogen output}$$

Positive values put the patient in positive nitrogen balance and anabolism and negative ones indicate catabolism.

Muscle function testing

Muscle function tests are the newest approach for evaluating nutritional status. Handgrip strength has been shown to be better than weight loss and other anthropometric measurements as a predictor of postoperative complications (Hunt et al 1985). Changes in muscle function can be induced by nutritional therapy and improvement in handgrip strength with weight gain after oral nutritional support in COPD patients has been reported (Efthimiou et al 1988). It provides an inexpensive and simple means of assessing muscle function and is easily obtained in both an outpatient and inpatient setting. Serial measurements can be used to monitor nutritional progress.

Micronutrients, especially potassium, calcium, magnesium and phosphate, are important contributors to respiratory muscle strength and therefore play a role in muscle function and the nutritional status of patients with respiratory disease. The combination of many factors, including poor dietary intake, steroids and diuretics, can cause marked depletion of these electrolytes, so monitoring of electrolytes should also form part of a nutritional assessment. Box 10.3 summarizes the methods to assess changes in body composition.

Box 10.3 Summary of methods to assess changes in body composition

- Protein status
  - MAC
  - MAMC
  - serum protein (albumin)
  - hand grip strength
  - nitrogen balance

- Fat stores
  - TSF
  - BMI

- Body water
  - BI
  - biochemistry
  - fluid balance
  - rapid weight change
  - girth/pitting ankles

Dietary assessment

A diet history should form an assessment of nutritional, medical and socio-economic factors that affect adequate nutrient intake. It should include:

- eating habits in health and in sickness
- type and quantity of food eaten
- ethnic and cultural background, e.g. restrictions of usual home diet
- socio-economic background such as facilities for preparing and storing food
- physical disability and degree of reliance on home help, family and friends
- factors affecting intake such as dysphagia, dyspnoea, impaired taste or smell, nausea, diarrhoea, constipation
- psychosocial factors regarding preparation of meals and eating arrangements
- use of food, nutritional or vitamin supplements
- drugs that could affect nutritional status or intake
- history of weight loss or gain and note of any oedema.

Dietary assessment is thought to be a simple technique, but it still remains difficult to obtain accurate and valid dietary assessments. There are various methods to assess dietary food intake and the method chosen will depend on the needs of the patient.

Weighed food record

This is thought to be the gold standard of dietary assessment methods. The patient is taught how to weigh and record the food immediately before eating and to weigh any left overs. Due to its probable greater accuracy it is usually the preferred method in research. The main problems are that a weighed food record can not be used for some disabled or illiterate people and it requires a high degree of cooperation from patients. There also may be inaccuracy from the scales, and habitual food intake maybe altered when individuals know the diets are to be analysed.

Recorded intakes using household measures

This involves keeping a diary of all food consumed using household measures such as spoonfuls, cupfuls, and bowls as well as labels from packaged foods to provide information about portion size and ingredients. This method may be less demanding on the patient, but still requires the patient to be trained how to record and estimate portion sizes. If it is known that a patient is attending an outpatient appointment with a nutritional/weight problem, it is useful to get the patient to fill out a food intake diary before attending. This means that nutritional action can be initiated after the first consultation.

24 hour recall method

This retrospective method is one of the most widely used techniques for dietary assessment. It can be based on pre-designed forms or questions relating to specific meal times, snacks and special eating occasions and a check list can be used to ensure that as many as possible of the foods eaten are remembered. It is quick and simple to perform, places minimal burden on the patient and is applicable to most groups

Case study 10.1

Andrew is a 30-year-old with cystic fibrosis, not requiring pancreatic enzymes. He is normally a well person with a full time job and is a fitness instructor in his spare time. He was admitted to hospital with considerable abdominal pain and a 2 week history of 5 kg weight loss; his bowels were not open for 7 days, followed by diarrhoea. Pre-admission nutritional assessment (stable for the last few years) was:

- weight 75 kg
- height 1.7 m
- BMI 25 kg/m²
- MAC 32.3 cm (75th percentile)
- estimated average requirements (EAR) 2700–3500 kcal (120–150% EAR)
- actual intake 2700 kcal (120% EAR) with 40% of energy from fat.

The diagnosis was distal intestinal obstruction syndrome (DIOS) (bowel blockage) thought to be as a result of not taking pancreatic enzymes. This was treated with lactulose and acetylcysteine. Admission assessment was:

- weight 68 kg
- BMI 23 kg/m²
- MAC 31 cm
- % weight loss 7% in 2 weeks
- intake remained 120% EAR.

Creon was started, as he presented with classic symptoms. Six months later his assessment was:

- weight 76 kg
- BMI 26 kg/m²
- MAC 32 cm
- pancreatic enzymes Creon 10 000 – 10/day
- intake 120% EAR.

Andrew's dietary intake remained the same throughout, emphasizing the effect of malabsorption on weight. This was corrected by pancreatic supplementation. There were no further problems and he maintained the weight he had regained.

regardless of their background. However, it does rely heavily on memory and is the least accurate of all methods. This tends to be the method used in the inpatient setting to get an overview of current and normal dietary intakes.

Asking simple questions relating to how often certain foods are consumed can help identify specific nutrient deficiencies, for example red meat, chicken, fish and eggs for iron, and dairy products for calcium.

NUTRITIONAL INTERVENTION

The aim of nutritional support is to:

- preserve physiologically important lean tissue thereby improving respiratory muscle and lung function
- maintain or gain weight
- improve mobility and exercise tolerance
- reduce mortality.

Calorie requirements

As already discussed, the respiratory patient is at risk of undernutrition as a result of inadequate dietary intake for energy expenditure.

Energy expenditure

Patients with compromised lung function have rates of energy expenditure 10–20% higher than predicted. This has primarily been attributed to the increased work of breathing, especially in patients with advanced respiratory disease with decreased ventilatory muscle efficiency (Donahoe & Roger 1990, Schols et al 1991b, Sridhar et al 1994). Exacerbations of respiratory disease further increase energy expenditure associated with infection and inflammatory activity.

Adults with cystic fibrosis have on average a 20–50% higher resting energy expenditure than healthy age matched patients (Murphy et al 1995). At a cellular level it is thought that the abnormal

---

Box 10.4 Factors affecting the nutritional health of the hospitalized patient

- Failure to record the height and weight of a patient on admission
- Rotation of the hospital staff and diffusion of responsibility for the patient's nutritional care
- Withholding meals for diagnostic tests
- Physiotherapy, IV antibiotic treatments before meal times
- Delay of nutritional support until the patient is in an advanced state of nutritional depletion
- Poor nutritional screening when the patient enters hospital
- Lack of appreciation of the role of adequate nutrition in the treatment and prevention of respiratory disease

functions of the cystic fibrosis transfer regulator (CFTR) gene are energy requiring. Progressive respiratory disease during the second and third decades also increases energy demands, and over inflation of the lungs increases energy demands by 10%. In addition, these patients also have faecal nutrient losses from malabsorption. For example:

- 18 year old male needs 2700 kcal/day
- 18 year old male with cystic fibrosis needs 3300–4100 kcal/day.

Other factors which could stimulate metabolism have also been considered to contribute towards weight loss, such as the production of cytokines at the time of infection. Monocytes and macrophages produce tumour necrosis factor (TNF) which mediates an increase in energy expenditure, hypermetabolism, as well as mobilization of amino acids and muscle catabolism, hence can result in weight loss. Cytokines are increased in periods of respiratory infection, so could be associated with the weight loss and hypermetabolism seen in respiratory patients.

Energy losses

There are energy losses in sputum and sweat. Cystic fibrosis patients are particularly prone to energy losses as a result of malabsorption. 85% of cystic fibrosis patients have pancreatic insufficiency that is characterized by steatorrhoea, gastrointestinal symptoms such as pain, abdominal distension and weight loss. Pancreatic enzyme therapy should correct the malabsorption symptoms; however, despite apparent adequate pancreatic enzyme supplementation cystic fibrosis patients still lose about 15% of energy taken orally (normal amount of energy lost is 5%). Therefore, these patients have to ensure that they follow a high calorie diet whilst optimizing enzyme supplementation. The number of or need for pancreatic enzymes increases with age.

Energy intake

Providing adequate nutritional intake is an important part of the care of the respiratory patient, but unfortunately food is always the first thing to be missed out at the expense of other treatments or investigations (Box 10.4). The respiratory patient also suffers from a number of physical and practical problems that limit food intake. Often simple, practical advice is all that is needed to facilitate the patient's ability to maintain an adequate nutritional intake. Communication between dietitians, physiotherapists, nursing staff and physicians is vital to ensure that chest physiotherapy, intravenous (IV) antibiotic therapy and meal times do not all happen at once.

Factors affecting intake

Breathlessness

The effort of breathing for these patients is often so great that they have little energy left to eat and drink. The most common complaint from respiratory patients is that they can not chew, swallow and breathe at the same time (Smith et al 1989). Large meals can cause bloating and increased breathlessness and therefore lead to early satiety.

Advice:

- Eat little and often.
- Concentrate on energy dense foods, e.g. cheese sandwich, two chocolate biscuits and a glass of milk rather than a plate of vegetables, potatoes and two lamb chops.
- Drinking calories is often easier so the use of high calorie drinks is encouraged. Prescribed nutritional supplements available in the community are useful.
- Avoid drinking before meals to avoid bloating and a lower calorie intake.
- Have readily prepared meals to reduce fatigue before eating.

Dry mouth and throat

This is often due to general breathlessness and oxygen therapy and dry hard food becomes more difficult to swallow.

Advice:

- Have moist food rather than extra fluid with meals to wash food down with.

- Encourage extra gravy and sauces with meals.
- Suck boiled sweets or chew on dental gum to produce extra saliva.

Dysphagia

Regardless of the cause of dysphagia assessment by a speech and language therapist is recommended to ensure the patient is not at risk of aspiration. Altered food textures or placement of a nasogastric tube may be indicated.

Taste changes/nausea

This is a common problem in cancer patients receiving chemotherapy. Many patients on antibiotic therapy are prone to oral candida, so early identification and treatment can prevent poor food intake. Drug therapy, nebulized or oral, can leave a lingering unpleasant taste in the mouth; sputum does not taste good either.
  Advice:

- Go for sharp tasting food and drinks, e.g. lemon sorbet, jellies made with fruit juice, fruit juices on their own or diluted with fizzy water.
- Suck on boiled sweets or chew dental gum.

Constipation

Dehydration and immobility combined with a poor food intake, especially fibre, can cause constipation. This in turn can lead to increased abdominal distension and discomfort, breathlessness, nausea and increased patient anxiety that ultimately affects appetite and intake.
  Advice:

- Ensure adequate fluid intake: 8–10 cups per day.
- Encourage increased fibre: wholegrain cereals or bread and increased fruit are a good start.
- Incorporate exercise as tolerated.
- Laxatives should be prescribed where necessary.

Diarrhoea

More often than not this is a side effect of antibiotic treatment, but it is a major reason for patients to stop eating. Patients receiving nasogastric or gastrostomy feeding often have their feeds discontinued as a result of diarrhoea. Feeds should not be stopped or altered until it has been confirmed that infection is not the cause of the diarrhoea.
  Advice:

- Ensure adequate fluid intake to prevent dehydration.
- Avoid high fibre foods.
- Try foods that are light and easily digested, e.g. white fish, chicken, mashed potato and milk puddings.

Position and posture

Many patients try to eat lying supine in bed, hunched over their tray, or perched on the end of the bed. These all cause problems of feeling uncomfortable, difficulties in swallowing and bloatedness, which result in half eaten or missed meals. Small frequent meals and the use of liquid supplements can be beneficial.

Oxygen therapy

An oxygen mask can present a physical barrier to eating. Patients are often reluctant to remove the mask at meal times as it compounds the problem of breathlessness. Providing patients with nasal cannulae, if appropriate, for use during meal times can help to ensure an adequate intake is maintained.

Nasal ventilation

This is often required in Type II respiratory failure and eating and drinking is not encouraged to avoid aspiration of food and fluid. It is therefore important to ensure that time off the ventilator coincides with meal times to ensure adequate intake and that the patient is allowed time to adapt to being off the ventilator before attempting to eat. Those patients requiring continuous nasal ventilation can have a fine bore nasogastric tube placed. Using a fine bore nasogastric tube allows the seal of the face mask to be maintained and ensures nutrition is maintained.

Composition of requirements

Calories

There has been much discussion and research into the composition of nutritional intervention for patients with respiratory disease, in particular that of carbohydrate versus fat calories (Dark et al 1985, Koretz 1985). The metabolism of food produces carbon dioxide and utilizes oxygen. Carbon dioxide production is higher when carbohydrates are the main energy source and lower when fat is mainly oxidized. Therefore, carbohydrate loads could induce or worsen hypercapnia in patients with ventilatory limitation because of their reduced capacity to excrete the resulting carbon dioxide load. Respiratory failure precipitated by a high carbohydrate load has been reported in ventilated patients receiving total parenteral nutrition (TPN) (Dark et al 1985). However, it is not contraindicated in respiratory patients who have non-functioning gastrointestinal tracts as the fat to carbohydrate composition of the TPN is always closely monitored and can be altered as appropriate. To try and prevent an associated increase in carbon dioxide when feeding respiratory compromised patients there has been an interest in specialized products for respiratory patients. The formulations have a high fat and low carbohydrate content which is suitable for enteral tube feeding or oral nutritional supplementation. However, it appears that preventing gross overfeeding, rather than choice of energy source of a feed, is more important in avoiding nutritionally related increases in carbon dioxide production in mechanically ventilated patients (Talpers et al 1992). Accurate calculation of nutritional requirements is, therefore, an essential part of a patient's nutritional assessment.

Nutritional requirement calculations should be based on ideal or desired body weight rather than actual body weight. This will prevent over feeding in the obese patients and ensure adequate nutrition in the underweight ones. It is also reported that stable ambulatory COPD patients seem to tolerate high carbohydrate loads without difficulty (Schols et al 1991b). Therefore, there seems little reason to favour a 50% fat to 30% carbohydrate formulation over a standard formulation of 30% fat to 50% carbohydrate formulation. The advantage of encouraging a higher intake of carbohydrate is that carbohydrate spares protein breakdown more than fat. It is far more important to achieve an adequate energy intake from foods which the patients find palatable than to limit carbohydrate in patients who are prone to weight loss as a result of inadequate dietary intake for energy expenditure. The high cost to benefit factor of these specialist feeds, compared to standard feeding formulas, also needs to be considered before deciding to use them.

Cystic fibrosis patients have specific nutrient requirements related to nutritional composition and this can be demonstrated when comparing cystic fibrosis recommendations (Ramsey et al 1992) and healthy eating guidelines (Department of Health 1991) (Table 10.5). Although cystic fibrosis is characterized by malabsorption, the traditional low fat diets are now contraindicated for these patients (Corey et al 1988, Nir et al 1996). A high energy, high protein diet without the restriction of dietary fat is required because of their need for a calorie dense diet (Littlewood & MacDonald 1987). The enteric coated microsphere pancreatic preparations have been a major factor in permitting the introduction of more liberal amounts of fat.

It is generally recommended that 50% of these patients' calories come from fat. The use of unsaturated fats is now recommended in the light of patients living much longer and being at risk of

Table 10.5 Cystic fibrosis recommendations compared to healthy eating guidelines

	Cystic fibrosis	Healthy eating
Energy	120–150% EAR	100% EAR
Fat	40% total energy (TE)	30–35% TE
Type	Unsaturated	Unsaturated
Carbohydrate	40% TE	50–55% TE
Sugar	Allowed freely	25 g/day
Protein	20% TE	10–15% TE
Salt	Increase	Decrease

heart disease. Protein requirements are increased by the need for nutritional repletion and by nitrogen losses in the sputum. 20% of calorie requirements need to come from protein. This is not normally a problem to achieve as the general population has a higher intake of protein than recommended intake anyway. The loss of nutrients in sweat, particularly salt, in warm weather, requires that salt consumption remains unrestricted and salty foods and table salt are consumed. Salt tablets are often advised when travelling abroad.

Vitamins and minerals

As with all dietary manipulation, vitamin and mineral requirements also have to be considered. Respiratory defence mechanisms depend on the integrity of respiratory epithelium and the immune system. Malnutrition is associated with a loss of humoral and cell mediated immunity and therefore in malnourished respiratory patients this could increase premorbid susceptibility to infection. Infection compromises lung function which in turn can compromise nutritional status (Hunter et al 1981).

Nutritional depletion also has an effect on the lungs' antioxidant system. Tissue damage in lung disease is an inflammatory phenomenon resulting from unopposed oxidant activity, including the oxidants in tobacco smoke, polluted air, products of phagocytic cells, and the action of other free radicals (Heffner & Repine 1989). Certain vitamins known as antioxidants, vitamins A, C and E and selenium, and in particular B-carotene, are thought to protect against free radicals and oxidative damage. Groups particularly at risk of micronutrient deficiencies are:

- malnourished individuals who will have both macro- and micronutrient deficiencies
- smokers who require higher vitamin C intakes
- high intake alcohol users are generally malnourished and particularly require vitamin C and the B vitamins (thiamine and folic acid).

As advocated in patients with cardiovascular disease and cancer, a diet high in fresh fruit and fish oils, with their high antioxidant and anti-inflammatory activity, offers protection against such damage (Alpha-tocopherol beta carotene cancer prevention study group 1994). So perhaps effective advice for the respiratory patient, apart from 'stop smoking', should be 'and eat plenty of fruit and vegetables' (Sridhar 1995). Multi-vitamin preparations may be of benefit in those patients who are not meeting nutritional requirements.

For patients whose drug therapy includes the use of long term oral steroids, for example

Table 10.6 Fat soluble vitamins

Vitamin	Role	Recommended amount	Food source
Vitamin A	Is an antioxidant, and has a role in lung function and immunity	8000 iu (2 multivitamins)	Dairy products, liver, oily fish, carrots and green vegetables
Vitamin D	Is needed for the absorption of dietary calcium and phosphate to maintain healthy bones	Deficiency is rare as most vitamin D comes from exposure to sunlight. Monitoring of high risk patients is required	Cod liver oil, oily fish, eggs, dairy products
Vitamin E	Is an antioxidant, has a protective role during the inflammatory response to infection. Prolonged deficiency can result in irreversible neurological damage	200 mg in addition to 2 multivitamins	Vegetable oils, eggs, wheatgerm, green vegetables
Vitamin K	Is needed to ensure normal blood clotting	Is not routinely supplemented as it is mostly synthesized by intestinal flora	Green vegetables, cereals, dairy products

COPD, asthma and cystic fibrosis patients (Donovan et al 1988), there is an increased risk of developing osteoporosis particularly if they are smokers, and the condition will be accelerated in malnourished patients. Fractured ribs secondary to osteoporosis can result in pain, a decrease in respiratory depth, reluctance to cough and expectorate and a consequent increase in the risk of infection. Good intakes of calcium are therefore encouraged with a need for adjunct vitamin D supplementation, especially if mobility and exposure to sunlight are limited. The prevalence of vitamin D deficiency in the cystic fibrosis population is 38% (Haworth 1999) due to malabsorption or defects in metabolism due to liver disease.

Cystic fibrosis patients have particular increased micronutrient needs primarily as a result of malabsorption. They have a higher need for the fat soluble vitamins A, D, E and K (Table 10.6). It is generally agreed that there are no deficiency problems with water soluble vitamins. Patients most at risk appear to be those with poorly controlled malabsorption, poor compliance, liver disease, bowel resection or following late diagnosis. Poor patient compliance is probably the most common cause of vitamin deficiency. Patients tend to focus on the short term benefits of treatment and the ending of unpleasant symptoms, for example they tend to take insulin and pancreatic supplements but give a low priority to vitamins as they do not see any physical benefits.

Regular individual nutritional assessment and monitoring is essential, as many patients may not understand the importance of vitamin supplementation. Also much more research is required on the mechanisms of vitamin transport in cystic fibrosis and the potential risk of liver toxicity related to long term vitamin supplements, the use of vitamin fortified supplement drinks and enteral feeds and the increased life expectancy.

Nutritional support

The thermogenic effect of a large meal creates a significant metabolic and ventilatory load, which often increases symptoms of breathlessness, bloating and early satiety, and consequently a decreased nutritional intake. The aim, therefore, is to increase calorie intake without increasing the amount eaten, especially at one sitting. This can be achieved by:

- normal diet plus between meal snacks
- normal diet fortified with fat, milk powder, glucose polymers, e.g. Maxijul, Hycal
- supplementary feeding.

Palatable enteral feeding preparations can be administered orally to those patients who are eating insufficient quantities of normal food. There are two categories of enteral feeding preparations:

- High protein supplements such as Ensure Plus, Fortisip, Entera, Fresubin and Build up all provide complete nutrition which includes protein, calories, vitamins and minerals. Scandishake is a good source of energy, but does not have a complete vitamin and mineral profile, therefore can not be a sole source of nutrition. All are suitable for diabetics and are prescribable for disease related malnutrition.

- High calorie supplements such as Maxijul and Polycal are also prescribable. They provide only energy therefore are not suitable for diabetics.

If adequate nutrition can not be maintained by oral intake, supplementary enteral tube feeding has to be considered in the form of:

- nasogastric feeding
- gastrostomy feeding.

Choice depends on the length of time feeding will be required. For the majority of respiratory patients, standard isotonic 1 kcal/ml (i.e. Osmolite) or slightly hypertonic 1.5 kcal/ml (i.e. Ensure Plus enteral feeds) are used.

Supplementary overnight gastrostomy feeding in cystic fibrosis patients is frequently used (particularly for those patients who fall below 85% ideal body weight for height), but only after dietary intervention, enzyme therapy and diabetes control are optimized. It is not a substitute for eating. It is thought of as adjunct therapy,

Case study 10.2

Carlos is a 38-year-old gentleman diagnosed with tuberculosis. He is South American, single, lives alone in a hostel, is a smoker and an alcoholic. He has a history of sweating, cough, poor appetite, especially when pyrexial, and weight loss of 10 kg in 3 months.

Assessment

- Normal weight 68 kg, height 1.7 m, BMI 23 kg/m^2.
- Current weight 58 kg, height 1.7 m, BMI 20 kg/m^2.
- % weight loss: 10% over 18 months.
- Requirements: 2500 kcal/day.

Diet history:

- Breakfast: cereal and milk (no specific type of either), no sugar.
- Lunch: 'liquid' lunch at the pub 5–7 pints (approx 1500 kcal).
- Evening meal: take-aways from friends' restaurants.
- Current intake: approx 2300 kcal (65% of energy from alcohol).

Other factors that would need to be considered as part of the assessment:

- cooking/storage facilities in the hostel
- any meals provided by the hostel
- nutritional deficiencies – smoker/alcoholic.

The hostel provided a cooked breakfast, he was not up in time; he had access to limited cooking facilities which included a kettle, toaster and 2 ring cooker but no fridge or storage room.

Recommendations

- Make use of the breakfast, especially if meals missed during the day.
- Use full fat milk with meals or to drink – aim one pint/day (380 kcal).
- Have available tinned foods (cheap, have a long shelf life, easy to use at any time, e.g. baked beans and soup).
- Ready made nutritional supplements were encouraged for a period of one month and to be reassessed after this time –1/day (300 kcal).
- Commenced on a multivitamin.

6 weeks later

- Weight 60 kg, BMI 21 kg/m^2.

Diet history:

- Breakfast: cooked breakfast 4 out of 7 days + pint of milk.
- Lunch: 2–3 pints +/– pub sandwich.
- Evening meal: continued take-aways.
- Occasional use of hostel's limited cooking facilities for pot noodle and beans on toast.
- Taking a multivitamin, poor compliance with nutritional supplements – has supplements from clinic and never renewed prescription.
- Intake: 2600 kcal (22% energy from alcohol).

Weight gain was achieved with Carlos. This was probably due to clinical improvement of symptoms as well as a slightly improved dietary intake. Points to remember:

- take into account individuals' lifestyles
- simple and practical dietary changes can and do make a difference especially when compliance is a problem.

providing up to 50–75% of the estimated average requirements (EAR) (Moore et al 1986), and should be considered as an early intervention rather than one of last resort (Walker & Gozal 1988).

Obesity

Consideration of the other end of the nutritional support spectrum is also important in respiratory disease. Many patients requiring oxygen therapy may be obese. This is often as a result of a combination of medical, physical and dietary factors, but inevitably follows chronic energy consumption in excess of energy expenditure. Long term steroid therapy can lead to gradual weight gain which, along with a reduction in physical activity due to compromised lung function, can become the start of a vicious circle.

Obesity is defined as body weight 20% greater than ideal body weight; however, anatomic localization of body fat seems to determine health risk more than does overall body fat, i.e. apple versus pear fat distribution. Upper body, centrally located fat is associated with increased risk of heart disease, hypertension, diabetes and certain cancers. Lower body fat is relatively insignificant with respect to health risks. The implications of obesity in respiratory patients are related to limitations of function. Metabolically inactive fat mass when centrally localized can impede lung function to a greater degree than in other areas because of its impairment of ventilatory apparatus (Chen et al 1993). It increases the load of an already compromised respiratory system, particularly during weight bearing exercise. The latter is often already limited due to joint pain, which has an implication in the role of exercise in encouraging weight loss.

Obesity is notoriously resistant to treatment, but that should not be a reason to ignore the problem. However, it does depend on the patient's recognition and willingness to address the fact of a weight problem. Intervention needs to include not only modest calorie restriction, but behavioural modification techniques (Prochaska & DiClemente 1982), exercise and an emphasis on slow weight loss (0.5–1 lb/week). Weight cycling should be discouraged as it contributes to loss of lean body mass and increased body fat and weight and makes long term weight maintenance more difficult. The availability of skilled clinicians who can implement and monitor change and provide support for relapse prevention is vital and helps to keep patients motivated.

During acute respiratory distress or infective exacerbation there should be no dietary restrictions. Dietary intake is likely to be poor and the primary objective should be to ensure nutritional requirements are met with any foods the patient is able to eat. Weight reduction at this time may exacerbate an existing risk for weight loss associated with disease and lead to further decline in lung function. The importance of nutritional screening and assessment is highlighted once again. The weight reducing diet can be resumed when the patient's appetite has improved.

Case study 10.3

Tom is a known COPD patient with increasing breathlessness, particularly on exertion, is obese and is not very mobile. He has recently been told to give up smoking and referred for weight reducing advice.

Assessment
Weight 124 kg, height 1.7 m, BMI 43 kg/m^2

A 24 hour diet history revealed that his diet was high in fat and sugar (butter, fried foods, non-diet squashes, evaporated milk, and a daily Mars bar). He often missed lunch, which meant that he snacked in the afternoon on sweets and had very large portions for the evening meal. He enjoyed fruit and complex carbohydrates (i.e. bread, potatoes, pasta, rice) but thought the latter were fattening. He lived on his own, was happy cooking for himself and had a microwave oven.

Calories from a small can of evaporated milk, Mars bar and sweets: 600 kcal.

Advice

This was based on simple, realistic changes:
- cooking methods – avoid frying
- have low fat alternatives – semi-skimmed milk, low fat spread
- choose diet or sugar free drinks
- ensure he had something at lunchtime based on complex carbohydrate – explained that these foods were filling and not fattening
- reduce the Mars bars to 3 a week, watch sweets and have more fruit instead
- decrease his protein portions (e.g. 4 lamb chops to 2) and have more vegetables instead.

Target weight 110 kg, BMI 38 kg/m^2 over 4 months

Follow-up assessment 4 weeks later
Weight 120 kg, BMI 41 kg/m^2

Good weight loss, approximately 1 kg/week. He had made most of the recommended changes. He had tried to follow a one week diet based on 'healthy' soup, but found that he was hungry all the time so did not continue with it. It was explained that the 'diet' had inadequate carbohydrate sources, which was why he was feeling hungry and therefore likely to snack on high fat and sugar snacks, and that it was not teaching him lifetime healthy changes.

His clothes were looser and he felt his breathing was better. Continued 4–6 week follow-up was recommended.

Diabetes

People with respiratory disease often develop diabetes as a result of steroid therapy, referred to as steroid induced diabetes. High dose steroids, commonly > 30 mg, can cause raised blood sugars which may or may not resolve when the steroid dose decreases. Blood sugar levels can be controlled with diet alone but oral hypoglycaemics or insulin may be needed. Dietary advice for this group of patients follows the recommendations of the British Diabetic Association (British Dietetic Association 1982):

- a diet high in fibre-rich carbohydrate
- low in fat
- controlled in energy content
- avoidance of rapidly absorbed carbohydrate consumed in isolated form.

In cystic fibrosis the prevalence of diabetes increases with age. It is not the classical Type I or Type II diabetes but is referred to as CF related diabetes (CFRD). Insulin is generally considered the medical therapy of choice especially if the patient is underweight. The choice of insulin regimen needs to be individualized with regard to lifestyles, inconsistent food intakes and sickness; however, multiple injection therapy seems to offer the best control for those reasons. Cystic fibrosis patients with diabetes tend to have accelerated weight loss and deterioration of lung function, so the nutritional goal is still to secure optimal nutritional status. The advice is not to follow the traditional low fat, low sugar diabetic diet. Restricting sugar and fat will decrease daily energy intake and result in further weight loss. Fat continues to be encouraged with no significant decrease in simple sugars. Refined carbohydrates are recommended to be evenly distributed throughout the day or eaten as part of a meal. If patients are taking supplements with a high sugar content or are on nocturnal supplementary feeds the insulin should be adjusted accordingly.

Summary

- All healthcare professionals need to take part in nutritional screening and assessment.
- A multidisciplinary approach to nutritional support can optimize treatment.
- Simple assessment tools, such as questions about dietary intake and documentation of initial weight and weight trends, should be used so that nutritional support can be implemented at the earliest moment.
- Monitoring progress allows for appropriate adjustment of any intervention where necessary.

CONCLUSION

Malnutrition is no longer considered an inevitable consequence of respiratory disease. Whether nutritional therapy can improve morbidity and reduce mortality still remains unanswered. However, careful nutritional support and the correction of a poor energy intake is crucial in enhancing physical wellbeing and function and reducing the risk of acute respiratory failure.

REFERENCES

Alpha-tocopherol beta carotene cancer prevention study group 1994 The effect of vitamin E and beta carotene on the incidence of lung cancer and other cancers in male smokers. New England Journal of Medicine 330: 1029–1035

Bishop C W, Bowen P E, Ritchey S J 1981 Norms for nutritional assessment of American adults by upper arm anthropometry. American Journal of Clinical Nutrition 34: 2530–2539

Blunt M C, Nicholson J P, Park G R 1998 Serum albumin and colloid osmotic pressure in survivors and non-survivors of prolonged critical illness. Anaesthesia 53: 755–761

British Dietetic Association 1982 Dietary recommendations for diabetics of the 1980s. Human Nutrition Applied Nutrition 36A: 378–394

Chen Y, Horne S L, Dosman J A 1993 Body weight and weight gain related to pulmonary function decline in adults: a 6 year follow-up study. Thorax 48: 375–380

Congleton J 1999 Pulmonary cachexia syndrome: aspects of energy balance. Proceedings of the Nutrition Society 58(2): 321–328

Corey M, McLauglin F J, Williams M, Levinson H 1988 A comparison of survival, growth and pulmonary function in patients with cystic fibrosis in Boston and Toronto. Journal of Epidemiology 41: 583–591

Dark D S, Pingleton S K, Dorley G R 1985 Hypercapnia during weaning. A complication of nutritional support. Chest 88: 141–143

Department of Health 1991 Dietary reference values for food energy and nutrients for the United Kingdom: report of the panel on dietary reference values. Committee on Medical Aspects of Food Policy, HMSO, London

Donahoe M, Roger A M 1990 Nutritional assessment and support in chronic obstructive pulmonary disease. Clinics in Chest Medicine 11: 487–504

Donovan D S, Papdopoulos A, Staron K B et al 1988 Bone mass and vitamin D deficiency in adults with advanced cystic fibrosis lung disease. American Journal of Critical Care Medicine 157: 1892–1899

Driver A G, McAlevy M T, Smith J L 1982 Nutritional assessment of patients with chronic obstructive pulmonary disease and acute respiratory failure. Chest 5: 568–571

Efthimiou J, Flemming J, Gomes C, Spiro S G 1988 The effect of supplementary oral nutrition in poorly nourished patients with chronic obstructive pulmonary disease. American Review of Respiratory Disease 137: 1075–1082

Garrow J S 1981 Treat obesity seriously. Churchill Livingstone, Edinburgh

Gray-Donald C, Gibbons L, Shapiro S H et al 1996 Nutritional status and mortality in chronic obstructive pulmonary disease. American Journal of Critical Care Medicine 139: 1435–1438

Haworth C S 1999 Low bone mineral density in adults with CF. Thorax 54(11): 961–967

Heffner J E, Repine J E 1989 State of the art: pulmonary strategies of antioxidant defence. American Review of Respiratory Disease 140(2): 531–554

Hunt D R, Rowlands B J, Johnston D 1985 Hand grip strength: a simple prognostic indicator in surgical patients. Journal of Parenteral and Enteral Nutrition 36: 680–690

Hunter A M B, Carey M A, Larsh H W 1981 The nutritional status of patients with chronic obstructive pulmonary disease. American Review of Respiratory Diseases 124: 376–381

Jeejeebhoy K N 1994 Nutrition and albumin levels (editorial). Nutrition 10: 353

Knowles J B, Fairbarn M S, Wiggs B J et al 1988 Dietary supplementation in respiratory muscle performance in patients with COPD. Chest 93: 977–983

Koretz R L 1985 Nutritional support: whether or not some is good, more is not better. Chest 88(1): 2–3

Kushner R F 1993 Body weight and mortality. Nutrition Reviews 51(5): 127–136

Lennard-Jones J E 1992 A positive approach to nutrition as treatment. King's Fund, London

Littlewood J M, MacDonald A 1987 Rationale of modern dietary recommendations in cystic fibrosis. Journal of the Royal Society of Medicine 80(15): 16–24

McWhirter J P, Pennington C R, Christopher R 1994 Incidence and recognition of malnutrition in hospital. British Medical Journal 308: 945–948

Madden A M, Morgan M Y 1994 A comparison of skinfold anthropometry and bioelectrical impedence analysis for measuring percentage body fat in patients with cirrhosis. Journal of Hepatology 21(55): 878–883

Margarson M P, Soni N 1998 Serum albumin: touchstone or totem? Anaesthesia 53: 789–803

Moore M C, Greene H L, Donald W D, Dunn G D 1986 Enteral-tube feeding as adjunct therapy in malnourished patients with cystic fibrosis: a clinical study and literature review. American Journal of Clinical Nutrition 44: 33–41

Muers M F, Green J H 1993 Weight loss in chronic obstructive pulmonary disease. European Respiratory Journal 6: 729–734

Murphy M A, Ireton-Jones C S, Hilman B C et al 1995 Resting energy expenditures measured by indirect colorimetry are higher in preadolescent children with cystic fibrosis than expenditures calculated from prediction equations. Journal of the American Dietetic Association 95(1): 30–33

Nir M, Lanng S, Johansen H K, Koch C 1996 Long term survival and nutritional data in patients with cystic fibrosis treated in a Danish centre. Thorax 51: 1023–1027

Otte K E, Ahlburg P, D'Amore F 1984 Nutritional repletion in malnourished patients with emphysema. Journal of Parenteral and Enteral Nutrition 143: 152–156

Prochaska J D, DiClemente C C 1982 Transtheoretical therapy: toward a more integrative model of change. Psychotherapy Theory and Practice 129: 276–288

Ramsey B W, Farrell P M, Pencharz P, Consensus Committee 1992 Nutritional assessment and management in cystic fibrosis: a consensus report. American Journal of Clinical Nutrition 55: 108–116

Reilly H M, Martineau J K, Moran A, Kennedy H 1995 Nutritional screening – evaluation and implementation of a simple nutritional risk score. Clinical Nutrition 14: 269–273

Sahebjami H, Doers J T, Render M L, Bond T L 1994 Anthropometric and pulmonary function test profiles of outpatients with stable chronic obstructive pulmonary disease. American Journal of Medicine 94: 469–474

Schols A M W J, Wouters E F M, Soeters P B, Westerterp K R 1991a Body composition by bioelectrical-impedence analysis compared with deuterium dilution and skinfold anthropometry in patients with chronic obstructive pulmonary disease. American Society for Clinical Nutrition 53: 421–424

Schols A M, Mostert R, Cobben N, Soeters P, Wouters E 1991b Transcutaneous oxygen saturation and CO_2 tension during meals in patients with chronic obstructive pulmonary disease. Chest 100: 1287–1292

Scott Whittaker J, Ryan F, Buckley P A, Road J D 1990 The effects of refeeding on peripheral and respiratory muscle function in malnourished chronic obstructive pulmonary disease patients. American Review of Respiratory Disease 142: 283–288

Smith J, Wolkove N, Colacone A, Kreisman H 1989 Co-ordination of eating, drinking and breathing in adults. Chest 96: 578–582

Sridhar M K 1995 Nutrition and lung health: should people at risk of chronic obstructive lung disease eat more fruit and vegetables? British Medical Journal 310: 75–76

Sridhar M K, Carter R, Lean M E J, Banham S W 1994 Resting energy expenditure and nutritional state of patients with increased oxygen cost of breathing due to emphysema, scoliosis and thoracoplasty. Thorax 49: 781–785

Talpers S S, Romberger D J, Bunce S B, Pingleton S K 1992 Nutritionally associated increased carbon dioxide production. Excess total calories vs. high proportion of carbohydrate calories. Chest 102: 551–555

Todorovic V E, Micklewright A 1997 A pocket guide to clinical nutrition, 2nd edn. Parenteral and Enteral

Nutrition Group of the British Dietetic Association. British Dietetic Association, Birmingham

Walker S A, Gozal D 1988 Pulmonary function correlates in the prediction of long term weight gain in cystic fibrosis patients with gastrostomy feeding. Journal of Paediatric Gastroenterology and Nutrition 27: 53–56

Wilson D O, Rogers R M, Hoffman R M 1985 Nutrition and lung disease. American Review of Respiratory Disease 132(6): 1347–1365

Wilson D O, Rogers R M, Wright E C, Anthonisen N R 1989 Body weight in chronic obstructive pulmonary disease. American Review of Respiratory Disease 139: 1435–1438

11

Pulmonary rehabilitation

Sharon Rudkin

CHAPTER CONTENTS

Breathlessness has a major impact on the lives of patients with chronic respiratory disease and their families, although the presence of symptoms can be extremely variable and often not related to the severity of the disease. Drug therapies have some effect in controlling patients' symptoms, but medical management often has little to offer in terms of symptom control and slowing disease progression. Pulmonary rehabilitation can help patients whose lives are adversely affected by chronic breathlessness. Pulmonary rehabilitation begins with the premise that medical management cannot further improve the underlying condition. This form of multidisciplinary care is aimed at helping patients to achieve their highest possible level of functioning and quality of life.

ORIGINS OF PULMONARY REHABILITATION

Pulmonary rehabilitation is not a new concept; as early as 1895 patients with tuberculosis were advised to exercise to improve their wellbeing. Formal rehabilitation programmes were available in the USA in the 1960s, although it was 1981 before the American Thoracic Society (ATS) endorsed respiratory rehabilitation as an integral part of patient care and 1993 before they were joined by the European Respiratory Society (ERS). Unfortunately it took the British Thoracic Society (BTS) somewhat longer and it was 1997 before the BTS guidelines recommended pulmonary rehabilitation as an additional treatment in moderate to severe chronic obstructive pulmonary disease (COPD) (BTS 1997).

Fortunately the growth in rehabilitation programmes began before this time and rehabilitation is already becoming widely available. There is, however, a wide variation in the type and content of regional programmes and there is no uniform approach to rehabilitation in the United Kingdom. When considering setting up a pulmonary rehabilitation programme it is necessary to consider:

- aims of pulmonary rehabilitation
- components and organization of a programme
- evaluation of a programme.

DEFINITION OF PULMONARY REHABILITATION

There is a wide variety of definitions available of what rehabilitation should and should not be. However, although they all vary, the recurring themes remain the same. One often quoted definition is from the National Institutes of Health (NHI) workshop on rehabilitation held in 1994, which states: 'Pulmonary rehabilitation is a multidimensional continuum of services directed to persons with pulmonary disease and their families usually by an interdisciplinary team of specialists, with the goal of achieving, and maintaining the individual's maximum level of independence and functioning in the community.' (National Institutes of Health (NIH) 1994).

This defines the aim of rehabilitation as reducing the impact of the disability and incorporates the following key concepts:

- patient and family care
- multidisciplinary team work
- community care.

Pulmonary rehabilitation has a focus that is different from rehabilitation offered to patients with other conditions. It is understood that there is no cure and the patient does not have the potential to return to pre-disease state as does, for example, a patient following a myocardial infarction. It is all about the patients achieving their own maximal potential within the limits of their own disease and being able to live with a respiratory disability.

Research has largely focused on the medical nature of the condition leaving the social impact on the patient and their family a relatively neglected area. This neglect may reflect a wider public attitude surrounding smoking related chronic illness and its treatment. Chronic lung diseases tend to strike in later life and are often incurable and thus are relatively low profile illnesses. They can be perceived as self-inflicted and hold a certain stigma because of this. As with many other chronic conditions the daily reality of living with breathlessness goes on in the home and is the life experience of both the patient and their family.

Chronic illness has often been viewed using the World Health Organization's *International classification of impairments, disabilities and handicaps* (World Health Organization 1980):

- Impairment is defined as 'any loss or abnormality of psychological, physiological or anatomical structure or function'.
- Disability is defined as 'any restriction or lack (resulting from an impairment) of ability to perform an activity in the manner or within the range considered normal for a human being'.
- Handicap is defined as 'a disadvantage for a given individual resulting from an impairment or a disability that limits or prevents the fulfilment of a role that is normal for that individual'.

These classifications are useful to apply to help understand the effects of chronic lung disease. An important principle to recognize in the management of this condition is that much of the resulting disability stems from the secondary effects of the respiratory disease rather than from damage to the lung itself.

Impairment

This is characterized mainly by ventilatory impairment and is the area that has been most widely studied. Of interest is the repeated finding that airflow obstruction is poorly related to the degree of breathlessness, or quality of life (Jones 1995). Baseline measures of FEV_1 have been used in an attempt to classify patients and predict those who will benefit from pulmonary rehabilitation, but it has been shown that there can be as much as 86% variance in both dyspnoea and physical disability after taking lung function into account (Sweer & Zwillich 1990), suggesting that the relationship between physiological impairment and symptoms is poor (Ries et al 1995). There appears to be a greater relationship between ventilatory effort during exercise and physiological impairment and the sensation of dyspnoea increases when ventilation reaches a substantial proportion of maximum ventilatory capacity. Leblane et al (1986) found that breathlessness was closely related to ventilatory effort and that the ability to predict breathlessness at any point during cycle ergometry was excellent.

Disability

This describes the main effects of impairment due to chronic respiratory disease. Healthcare professionals and carers of patients with chronic respiratory disease commonly experience the frustration of trying to help a patient with breathlessness. The degree of dyspnoea may often be disproportional to the degree of impairment in lung function. Standard pharmacological treatment and medical management are often unable to relieve this symptom.

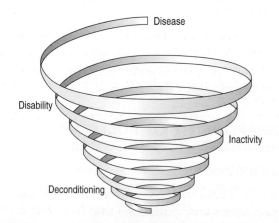

Figure 11.1 Dyspnoea spiral of deconditioning. Reproduced with permission from Casaburi & Petty 1996.

Dyspnoea or breathlessness is a perceived symptom rather than a measurable physical variable. The dyspnoea spiral of deconditioning is a schematic representation of the effects of chronic dyspnoea in COPD (Casaburi & Petty 1996) (Fig. 11.1). Respiratory impairment causes dyspnoea with activity and activity is then restricted to avoid dyspnoea. This reduction in activity results in physical deconditioning which increases dyspnoea with mild exercise and thus causes further reluctance to be active. Thus the progressive spiral has increasingly greater impact on the patient's lifestyle. A major goal of pulmonary rehabilitation is to interrupt this downward spiral by increasing fitness levels and enabling patients to achieve a higher level of activity.

Handicap

The impact of chronic respiratory disease is a neglected medical and social problem. Handicap is the social and/or physical impact of the disability on the patient's life, such as lack of employment, and is generally assessed by subjective measures of quality of life. A quality of life questionnaire can be a useful tool but must be chosen carefully as not all are specific to the area of handicap. The chronic respiratory disease questionnaire (Guyatt et al 1987) explores all three areas of impairment, disability and handicap. It offers a useful reflection of the patient's quality of life if used during the assessment for rehabilitation.

SETTING UP A PULMONARY REHABILITATION PROGRAMME

The object of setting up a rehabilitation programme is to complement rather than replace existing healthcare resources. The previously discussed definition of rehabilitation provides the rationale for this type of service, but accessing the required funding may be a more difficult task. The composition of the team will depend on time and funding issues. A programme may start with a skeleton team that grows and diversifies as the programme grows and funding allows.

Box 11.1 Members of a comprehensive rehabilitation team

- Chest physician
- Programme coordinator
- Physiotherapist
- Respiratory nurse specialist
- Occupational therapist
- Clinical psychologist
- Dietitian

Facilities are required for the baseline assessments of medical management and for lung function and exercise testing. Where these take place may be determined by the setting of the programme. There are three settings where pulmonary rehabilitation can take place:

- Inpatient: the patient is required to stay overnight in the hospital, often for a period of days or weeks.
- Outpatient: the patient visits the hospital several times a week for a specified time period, e.g. 2–4 hours
- Home based: the patient undertakes exercise and receives education in their own home.

Some programmes may involve a combination of settings, for example initiating the programme as an outpatient and, once the patient has confidence, continuing the programme at home. The setting and associated facilities will also determine the mode of exercise training that will be used. However, potential programme coordinators should not be put off by simplicity. Simple programmes can be as effective as more comprehensive programmes in improving quality of life. A useful comparison is between a programme that was set up and run in a district general hospital on an outpatient basis which used existing resources and simple and minimal equipment (White et al 1997), and an inpatient programme that was intensive with patients spending 8 weeks in hospital followed by 16 weeks supervised outpatient care (Goldstein et al 1994). Both were able to show improvements in quality of life and exercise capacity following the rehabilitation programme. Less sophisticated rehabilitation programmes may be as effective as the more comprehensive ones in improving health related

Case study 11.1

Norman is a 67-year-old, who has smoked for many years and finds it impossible to give up. He first noticed breathlessness with physical activity about 10 years ago and although it has become progressively worse he has avoided going to the doctor believing that it was self-inflicted by his smoking habits.

Last winter he had a severe chest infection and since that time he has become less active and reluctant to leave the house because of his breathlessness. He was encouraged to visit the GP by his wife, and from there he was referred for assessment to the medical team. Following medical assessment and optimal pharmacological management he remained breathless on minimal activity such as walking up stairs at home and gardening.

He was a reluctant rehabilitation member as he felt that his condition was due to his smoking and therefore self-inflicted. He was enrolled in a 6 week group outpatient based programme. By the end of his first week he told the coordinator that he didn't realize that there were people as breathless as him. He met other group members with similar smoking histories and realized he was not alone!

The physiotherapist adapted the exercise routine to make it manageable for Norman. He soon became comfortable with the fact that breathlessness was not harmful to him and increased the repetition of his exercise as his physical condition and confidence improved. He enjoyed the educational component of the programme and valued the experience of others who also suffered from breathlessness.

By the end of the 6 week programme he was able to plan some new daily activities and resume walking to the local paper shop. The programme physiotherapist adapted the outpatient based programme to one which could be completed in Norman's own home. He became a member of the rehabilitation support group and maintains contact with the other members of his rehabilitation group.

quality of life provided that the health professionals are motivated and that the programme is well thought through.

COMPONENTS OF PULMONARY REHABILITATION PROGRAMMES

Comprehensive rehabilitation programmes have the following components:

- assessment and patient selection
- exercise training
- education

- psychosocial intervention
- outcome assessment.

These components should be delivered by a multidisciplinary team.

Patient selection

Any patient who is limited by respiratory dyspnoea is eligible for pulmonary rehabilitation but first should have:

- optimal medical management
- a reduced exercise tolerance
- experienced a reduction in daily activities.

It is symptoms, disability and handicap, not the disease severity, that dictate the need for rehabilitation. Indeed the evidence to date suggests that benefit from rehabilitation is independent of the starting level of lung function (Lacasse et al 1997). It may be that in relative terms those with a lower FEV_1 gain more. Patients are generally unsuitable for rehabilitation if they have significant co-morbidities which will interfere with the process, or cardiac problems which make exercise unsafe. This may include conditions such as arthritis which make it difficult for the patient to mobilize, although programmes can very often be adapted to make the most of any patient's limitations.

Motivation is difficult to assess, but patients who actively want to take part and improve their lifestyle appear to be more successful, although patients who are poorly motivated may change when attending rehabilitation, particularly with the influence of a group setting. It is important not to exclude patients who are depressed as Wijkstra et al (1999) found that patients who were more depressed initially showed the greatest improvements in quality of life after receiving home pulmonary rehabilitation.

Assessment for rehabilitation

A medical history and physical assessment should be performed to determine that the patient is being treated optimally and has no signs of other co-morbidity. Lung function test-

---

Box 11.2   Summary of assessments

- Medical history
- Physical assessment
- Lung function testing
- Quality of life assessment
- Exercise capacity
- Psychological assessment

---

ing determines the level of severity and stability of the patient's disease. Outcomes committees of the American Association of Cardiovascular and Pulmonary Rehabilitation recommended that programmes evaluate dyspnoea and quality of life as these domains have the potential for improvement (Ries 1997). General and disease specific questionnaires allow an assessment of quality of life and psychological assessment evaluates the effects of anxiety and depression on the patient's disease. Rehabilitation programmes aim to result in improvements in exercise endurance and therefore the assessment should also include a test of exercise capacity. This is also useful information on which to base the patient's initial exercise prescription.

CONTENT OF A REHABILITATION PROGRAMME

The content of programmes varies from one hospital to the next, and the discussion as to the essential components continues. The common components of everyday pulmonary rehabilitation programmes include:

- exercise
- education
- psychosocial intervention.

Although most clinicians now agree that exercise is an essential component of rehabilitation, there remains much discussion as to the intensity and specificity of exercise required.

Exercise

Deterioration in skeletal muscle function contributes to disability in chronic respiratory disease. This, coupled with other causes such as hypoxaemia and malnutrition, leads to the deconditioning seen in many pre-rehabilitation patients (Sweer & Zwillich 1990). In healthy subjects this can be corrected through a process of physical training, and patients with chronic respiratory disease can achieve benefits in the same way. In healthy people, aerobic training is usually targeted at 60–90% of the predicted maximal heart rate or 50–80% of the maximal oxygen uptake (ATS 1999). This level is sustained for 20–45 minutes and repeated 3–4 times a week.

Until recently it has been suggested that patients with severe COPD have ventilatory limitation which prevents them from achieving the aerobic training levels needed for physiologic adaptation. However, Ries (1997) demonstrated that improvement with exercise training has occurred in patients with COPD even though patients have been trained below the effective threshold.

Casaburi et al (1991) addressed the physiological basis for exercise training in COPD by comparing high and low intensity exercise training and found that COPD patients can achieve physiologic training by establishing a training intensity. It has also been shown that both treadmill training and simple homestyle exercises in a hospital outpatient setting can improve both exercise capacity and quality of life (White et al 1997). The main issues to consider are:

- mode of exercise
- intensity of exercise
- frequency and duration of exercise.

Mode

In chronic respiratory disease, particularly COPD, much discussion is focused on upper versus lower extremity exercise training. Upper limb training is frequently used as it is suggested that most activities of daily living involve the upper extremities and thus this form of exercise should have a greater impact on patients' quality of life (ERS 1991).

Ries et al (1988) evaluated two upper extremity exercise programmes and found that those who underwent upper limb training improved their tests of arm function. Instruments to evaluate the effect of upper limb training are not well described and upper extremity training only improves arm specific mechanisms of exercise capacity. This relates to improvements in daily activities such as hanging out the washing.

Examples of upper extremity arm exercise (Fig. 11.2) include:

- lifting weights
- pulleys
- theraband exercise
- broomstick exercise.

Lower extremity training is easier to evaluate and has been shown to produce improvements in functional performance in virtually every programme that has been studied (Lacasse et al 1997). Lower limb training can also be achieved without the need for any equipment and specific rehabilitation setting. Many simple rehabilitation programmes that consist of exercise training alone may be as effective in improving exercise capacity and quality of life as the more comprehensive ones (Lacasse et al 1997). Improvements

Case study 11.2

Edna presented for assessment to enter the pulmonary rehabilitation programme. She was a well groomed 72-year-old lady accompanied by her husband. Her assessment suggested that her main problems were breathlessness with upper arm movements, particularly when doing her hair. Edna and her husband used to enjoy dancing but they recently stopped going as she found she became too breathless.

The rehabilitation team designed a programme for her that involved simple arm raising, wall chest press and walking exercise. Initially the arm raising was unrestricted and she was instructed to raise her arms above her head and then drop them to her sides again. After 2 weeks she was able to complete this exercise holding a simple rubber coil. She was also asked to walk around a simple corridor in the rehabilitation unit. She was advised to stop when she became too breathless to continue, but after regaining her breath she was asked to continue walking again for a 5 minute period. She performed these exercise both during the programme and at home on a twice daily basis.

Edna gained confidence in her ability to do more and the upper arm strength to do her hair without the assistance of her husband. Edna and her husband had the long term goal of being able to dance again.

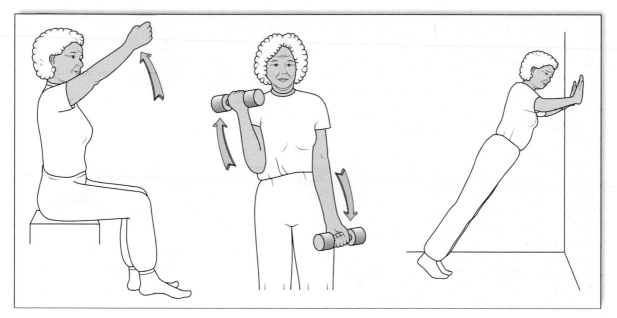

Figure 11.2   Upper arm exercises.

in lower limb training can be related to more functional activities of daily living such as walking around the home and upstairs (Fig. 11.3).

Examples of lower extremity exercise include:

- walking
- treadmill walking
- bicycle
- sit to stand
- stairs training.

Intensity and frequency

Most rehabilitation programmes focus on two types of exercise programmes (ATS 1999):

- Endurance training uses periods of sustained exercise for about 20–30 minutes 2–5 times a week. Training in this way is possible for some but not all patients.
- Interval training consists of 2–3 minutes of high intensity training alternating with equal periods of rest (Ries 1997). In healthy subjects interval training has been shown to produce training effects similar to those of endurance training.

Target level of training intensity should be 60% of the maximal oxygen consumption and a target

heart rate is often used to estimate this. Heart rate monitoring in patients with chronic respiratory disease is an added encumbrance to an exercise schedule and recent studies have examined the use of target dyspnoea rating as an alternative method of exercise prescription. Mejia et al (1999) compared the accuracy and reliability of patients' ability to produce exercise intensity using target dyspnoea rate and target heart rate. They found that patients could use both methods to accurately produce an expected exercise intensity for 10 minutes of sub-maximal exertion. If patients are able to modify their exercise levels using dyspnoea ratings, yet still maintain their own target heart rates, with correct instruction they should be able to achieve a training effect.

The majority of rehabilitation programmes now use interval training programmes. This type of training allows patients to exercise safely and learn how to control their dyspnoea whilst exercising.

Duration

Rehabilitation programmes vary in their duration and intensity. Obviously the setting also plays a part in defining the optimal duration,

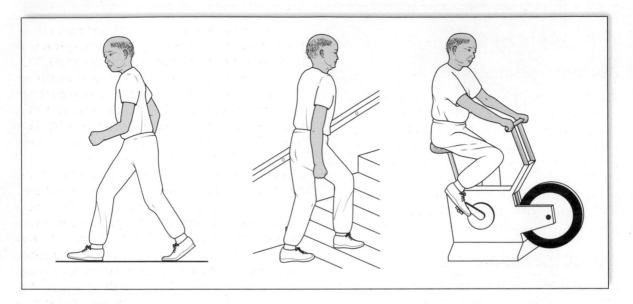

Figure 11.3   Lower limb exercises.

and home programmes are generally longer in duration than inpatient and outpatient based programmes. Lacasse et al (1996) identify that a programme of twice a week for 6–8 weeks is the

Case study 11.3

Stan is a 68-year-old man who used to be a bus driver. He has a very outgoing jovial personality and presented with a 4 year history of increasing breathlessness. He gave up work at age 62.

At his assessment for the pulmonary rehabilitation programme he said he would like to go and watch his grandson play football. He had not been doing this because he was worried about becoming breathless on walking between the car and the football field, especially when the weather was cold.

His programme involved a treadmill walking exercise as well as a range of other activities. He was taught strategies to increase his confidence and ability to cope with breathlessness attacks. In discussion with the rehabilitation team he set his personal goal to attend a football match by the end of the programme. The team discussed which match this should be and the distance from the car to the field was assessed.

Towards the end of the programme he was able to meet his goal and fulfill his role as a grandfather within the confines of his breathlessness.

minimum programme duration to see clinically significant improvements.

Education

Education is now an integral component of all comprehensive rehabilitation programmes and because of this it is difficult to determine its effect in isolation. Through the educational process the patient becomes more adherent and skilled at self-management (Lacasse et al 1997). The educational component should be tailored to the patients' needs and their disease process.

The topics of education sessions generally cover self-management issues, use of medications, dietary advice and aids to activities of daily living. Examples of education topics used in pulmonary rehabilitation programmes include:

- How our lungs work
- Stress, breathlessness and relaxation
- Breathing and breathing control
- Chronic bronchitis and emphysema
- Chest infections
- Steroids
- Living with breathlessness
- Diet and the lungs

- When to call your general practitioner
- Lung function tests
- Using inhalers and nebulizers.

Psychosocial interventions

The psychological component of rehabilitation programmes is very variable and often dependent on the members of the rehabilitation team. Psychosocial interventions are often a supplemental part of an exercise training regime (Blake et al 1990) and use a combination of relaxation and interactive behaviour. It has been demonstrated that psychological interventions can reduce dyspnoea and anxiety (Emery et al 1991, 1998).

OUTCOME MEASURES

If the aim of pulmonary rehabilitation is to help patients achieve their highest possible level of functioning and quality of life then any intervention should be evaluated. The outcome measures that can be used include:

- measures of exercise capacity
- quality of life questionnaires
- psychological evaluations
- measures of functional ability.

Measures of exercise capacity

Objective measures of disability are important for the assessment of patients who are limited by dyspnoea. This is a particularly important assessment for rehabilitation where the rationale and emphasis is on improving exercise capacity. Tests of maximal exercise capacity have limited use in respiratory disease. They are also not widely available and accessible and often the patient can be intimidated by the test before it even starts. Clinically based tests are most commonly used to evaluate pulmonary rehabilitation programmes as they can be administered easily in the rehabilitation setting and do not require specialized equipment. The most commonly used clinically based tests are:

- the self-paced 6 minute walking test
- the incremental standardized shuttle walking test.

Six minute walking test

This was first developed as a timed run, where the distance covered during a 12 minute run was measured and correlations were shown with VO_2 max in healthy people. A 12 minute walk rather than a run was then developed to demonstrate correlation between distance covered and VO_2 max in COPD patients (McGavin et al 1977). This type of self-paced walking test has since been adapted to the six minute walking test.

Self-paced tests can be susceptible to patient motivation and three separate walks are required before the results are reproducible. When performing this self-paced test the patient is instructed to walk as far as possible in 6 minutes. The test should be conducted in a flat marked corridor where the patient will not be impeded or distracted. The assessor should record the patient's distance walked but not actively encourage them in any way. The assessor may inform the patient at 1 minute intervals of the time left to walk. The patient decides when to stop because of breathlessness and also decides when to continue walking. The patient is asked to walk as though late for an appointment but ultimately patients will select a pace which is comfortable for them, rather than stressing themselves, and in this way patients fall far short of achieving their VO_2 max or VO_2 peak. This theory is supported by the work of McGavin et al (1977) who found only a moderate relationship between the walk and VO_2 max. Thus the simplicity of this test limits the information that can be assessed about the physiological and symptomatic changes that occur during exercise. The 6 minute walk reflects the patient's normal walking pattern in COPD and can be used as a tool to teach patients about pacing and managing breathlessness.

Shuttle walking distance

The shuttle walking test is an incremental and progressive test stressing the patient to a symptom-limited maximal performance. The test requires the patient to walk between two cones set 10 metres apart at a speed directed by an audio signal. Standard instructions are played to patients on a cassette tape. For the first shuttle (or

10 metre circuit) patients are accompanied by the assessor, a method which has been advocated by Singh et al (1992), to adapt the patient to the initial slow walking speed. The speed of walking remains the same for each minute and the patient is reminded that at the sound of the triple bleep the tape will get faster and thus the walking speed will increase. The test is terminated when patients can not maintain the required speed or feel they are too breathless to continue. This is determined by the patient or by the assessor if the patient does not reach within 0.5 metres of the cone on two consecutive occasions. Studies have shown that this test is reproducible after one practice walk.

During its development the shuttle walk was compared to the self-paced 6 minute walk. Singh et al (1992) found that there was a significant relationship between the distance walked in 6 minutes and the shuttle distance, but that the shuttle walk showed a graded cardiovascular response that the 6 minute walk did not. The shuttle walk is externally paced and it removes the possibility of influence by encouragement or assessor bias. There is a correlation between the shuttle distance walked and the determined VO_2 max on the treadmill. The shuttle walk can be used to predict the patient's VO_2 max and thus shuttle performance can be used as a basis for planning a patient's training schedule in chronic respiratory disease (Singh et al 1994).

Quality of life measurement in pulmonary rehabilitation programmes

There is increasing interest in the development of instruments to measure quality of life. Health related quality of life measures demonstrate the impact of an individual's health on his or her ability to enjoy the activities of daily life. Questionnaires vary and include:

- disease specific questionnaires aimed at a specific disease process or symptom
- generic global assessments.

Quality of life measures need to be practical to use as well as validated within the population they are aimed at. They also need to match

their purpose depending on whether they are being used to discriminate changes in individual patients at a single time point, to predict prognosis or to evaluate change within a given individual over time as is apparent following rehabilitation. A variety of measures have been used to evaluate rehabilitation programmes; these generally include a combination of disease specific and generic questionnaires. Commonly used quality of life questionnaires to evaluate pulmonary rehabilitation programmes are:

- Disease specific:
  - chronic respiratory disease questionnaire (CRDQ)
  - St George's respiratory questionnaire
- Generic:
  - sickness impact profile (SIP)
  - short form 36

Chronic respiratory disease questionnaire

The chronic respiratory disease questionnaire (CRDQ) was the first disease specific questionnaire designed to examine the effect of treatment on quality of life in chronic respiratory disease. Patients with chronic airflow limitation and an FEV_1 of less than 70% of predicted value were questioned during its design. They were asked about how they felt their life was affected by respiratory disease. Its authors suggest this is a questionnaire that allows a direct measurement of the impact of respiratory disease on the patients' lives. During the development phase Guyatt et al (1987) found that patients were affected in four broad areas:

- shortness of breath
- fatigue
- emotional function
- mastery.

The items associated with dyspnoea varied greatly according to the patients' sex, level of activity and disability. To overcome this problem the authors built in an individualized component to the dyspnoea dimension. The disadvantage of this is that between-patient comparison is lost, but

Box 11.3 The chronic respiratory disease questionnaire (CRDQ)

To administer the CRDQ the interviewer asks the patient to: 'Think of the activities that you have done during the last 2 weeks that have made you feel short of breath. These should be activities which you do frequently and which are important in your day-to-day life.'

Guyatt's examples of activities that induce breathlessness are:

1. Being ANGRY or upset
2. Having a BATH or shower
3. BENDING
4. CARRYING, such as carrying groceries
5. DRESSING
6. EATING
7. GOING for a walk
8. Doing your HOUSEWORK
9. HURRYING
10. MAKING a bed
11. MOPPING or scrubbing the floor
12. MOVING furniture
13. PLAYING with children or grandchildren
14. PLAYING sports
15. REACHING over your head
16. RUNNING such as for a bus
17. SHOPPING
18. While trying to SLEEP
19. TALKING
20. VACUUMING
21. WALKING around your own home
22. WALKING uphill
23. WALKING upstairs
24. WALKING with others on level ground
25. PREPARING meals

it has the advantage that each patient's individual response to dyspnoea is relevant and this in turn may improve the questionnaire's sensitivity to change. It also goes some way to answering critics' arguments regarding the individualized nature of quality of life. However, Wijkstra et al (1994 a, b) found that the consistency of the dyspnoea component was not as high as the other three components and therefore suggested that this dimension should be analysed in isolation. The questionnaire has 20 items and provides one overall score and four sub-scale scores in the areas previously identified by Guyatt et al (1987). There appears to be little emphasis on social dimensions, thus it may well be complemented by simultaneous use of a generic questionnaire (Morgan 1991).

The CRDQ is interviewer administered and the patient is asked to respond from a 7 point likert scale. With repeated administration of the questionnaire patients are 'informed' of their previous response. This results in a decrease in the variance or random error in the measurement of dyspnoea, fatigue and emotional function (Guyatt et al 1989).

The CRDQ has been used to evaluate many studies on pulmonary rehabilitation. Goldstein et al (1994) found improvements in all four components following rehabilitation and Vale et al (1993) found similar improvements although they could find no correlation between improvements in walking distance and the CRDQ.

The St George's respiratory questionnaire

This questionnaire was designed specifically to examine health gains obtained from differing types of therapy in both the asthma and the COPD population. It was designed to be used in long term studies and has been fully standarized. The questionnaire has three components:

- symptoms – distress due to respiratory symptoms
- activity – disturbance of physical activity
- impacts – overall impact on daily life and wellbeing.

A total score is also calculated and Jones et al (1992) suggest that this questionnaire can track changes in health over one year. This questionnaire was not designed to be used to assess short term changes. It has been successfully used to show changes in a pulmonary rehabilitation programme over a period of one year (Griffiths et al 2000).

Box 11.4 Examples of questions from the St George's respiratory questionnaire

True or false answers:

- My cough or breathing is embarrassing in public
- My chest trouble is a bother to my family, friends or neighbours
- I get afraid or panic when I cannot get my breath
- I feel that I am not in control of my chest problem
- I do not expect my chest to get any better
- I have become frail or an invalid because of my chest
- Exercise is not safe for me
- Everything seems too much of an effort

Sickness impact profile (SIP)

One of the earliest measures of quality of life was the sickness impact profile (SIP) first published in 1976 (Bergner et al 1976). The SIP was developed as a measure of perceived health status designed to be used with a wide range of diseases and problems. The SIP focuses on behaviours rather than actual disease.

During development, items were generated from a pool of over 1000 questionnaires and the original 312 items were piloted with 246 subjects from both inpatient and outpatient settings as well as healthy subjects. The current version of SIP consists of 136 statements forming 3 general categories from 12 sub-scales. This questionnaire may be self or interviewer administered and it takes about 20–30 minutes to complete. Patients are given 136 scenarios, which cover 12 different sub-scales. They are asked to respond yes or no to their ability to perform each of these activities. All the statements are weighted for scoring and the final scores are expressed as a percentage of impairment. Scores range from 0% to 100% with 10% or less considered normal. McSweeny et al (1982) suggest that any change in the SIP from one administration to another should in itself be a valuable indicator of clinically significant change in health. They further state that some SIP scales are more sensitive than others, which may help to identify specific problem areas for patients with COPD.

There are two major criticisms of the SIP. Firstly, it focuses only on negative functioning, thus when using this questionnaire in milder disease there may be a high degree of non-response. Secondly, the patient is required to respond only to the positive answers, therefore when there is no response there is no way of knowing if the item has been omitted deliberately or in error.

Short form 36

The short form 36 questionnaire (SF36) is a well known generic measure, developed by the medical outcomes study (Ware & Sherbourne 1992). The aim of development was to test the feasibility of self-administered patient questionnaires in subjects with chronic conditions and particularly the elderly. Ware & Sherbourne (1992) suggest the SF36 is universally valued and not age, disease or treatment specific.

Over 22 000 adult patients took part in a 2 year observational study during the initial development stage. The modified 36 item version became available in 1992. It has since been widely used to evaluate many different health care interventions including pulmonary rehabilitation programmes.

The SF36 has the advantage of being fairly short and practical because it can be self-administered. It looks at physical and mental health from a functional, disability and patients' evaluation point of view. The domains are:

- Limitations in physical activities because of health problems
- Role limitations because of health problems
- Limitations in social activities due to health problems
- Vitality (or energy and fatigue)
- Bodily pain
- General mental health
- Limitations in role activities because of emotional problems
- General health perceptions.

Scoring is done by adding the scores for each item within a dimension, averaging these scores according to the number of questions in the dimension, and transforming the value to a 0–100 scale, with 100 reflecting a positive state of health.

The SF36 is based heavily on the likert type response (i.e. it uses categories of responses such as 'a little', 'slight', 'moderate', etc.). It has been suggested that likert type responses allow for greater precision and sensitivity to different states of health, although there is little convincing evidence that the SF36 has any greater sensitivity in COPD because of this. Mahler & Mackowiak (1995) evaluated the use of the SF36 in relation to quality of life in COPD. Their study examined the validity of the SF36 by assessing its relationship with dyspnoea ratings and lung function.

Psychological evaluations

There are several other instruments available that have been designed to measure distinct psychological traits and properties. Many have been widely used in psychological research. They have often been mistaken for quality of life questionnaires in their own right although they are focused on a particular problem. Most studies of psychological factors in patients with chronic respiratory disease indicate that symptoms of anxiety and depression are common, although these symptoms may not necessarily be caused by the respiratory disease (Emery et al 1991). Scales which detect these symptoms are now in common use when evaluating these patients and include the hospital anxiety and depression scale.

Hospital anxiety and depression scale

The hospital anxiety and depression (HAD) scale has become increasingly popular. This questionnaire was first developed in 1983 by Zigmond and Snaith (Zigmond & Snaith 1983). They set out to develop a questionnaire to enable GPs to assess the emotional components of their patients' illnesses. Their original work examines internal consistency and reliability and stresses that care has been taken to avoid questions relating to somatic rather than emotional symptoms.

Box 11.5 Examples of statements used to examine the patient's psychological state

- I feel tense or wound up
- I still enjoy the things I used to enjoy
- I get a frightened sort of feeling as if something awful is about to happen
- I can laugh and see the funny side of things
- Worrying thoughts go through my mind
- I feel cheerful
- I can sit at ease and feel relaxed
- I feel as if I am slowed down in my thinking
- I get a frightened sort of feeling like 'butterflies' in the stomach
- I have lost interest in my appearance
- I feel restless as if I have to be on the move
- I look forward with enjoyment to things
- I get sudden feelings of panic
- I can enjoy a good book or TV programme

Each dimension is scored out of a range of 0–21. Scores of 10 or more are indicative of clinically significant anxiety or depression.

Other questionnaires are available for examining these symptoms and they have been used to evaluate rehabilitation. Emery et al (1991) examined the effects of an outpatient rehabilitation programme on psychological symptoms by using the psychological wellbeing index which is an American questionnaire with 22 items, including subjective assessment of patients' wellbeing. This work showed that patients experienced reductions in anxiety and depression following rehabilitation and supports the inclusion of a psychological assessment.

Measures of functional ability

Functional assessment is an integral part of patient evaluation. Goals of rehabilitation address overall functioning rather than merely a clinically based exercise test. Again functional disability scales can be grouped into generic and disease specific questionnaires.

Examples of functional ability scales include:

- Nottingham extended activities of daily living scale
- London chest activity of daily living scale.

Nottingham extended activities of daily living scale

Patients self-complete the Nottingham extended activities of daily living (NEADL) questionnaire. This is a short scale with 22 items, originally designed for use in stroke patients (Nouri & Lincoln 1987). It is divided into four sections, mobility, domestic tasks, leisure activities and kitchen tasks, and there is an overall score of disability. When completing the questions, patients are asked to score activities as they currently perform them, not as they think they could perform them. Lower scores suggest high degrees of disability. Although this questionnaire is not specific to COPD it has been used in studies and shown to correlate well with the severity of disease (Garrod et al 2000). However, its ability to determine sensitivity to change following rehabilitation has yet to be defined.

London chest activity of daily living scale

The London chest activity of daily living scale is a 15-item questionnaire designed specifically to measure dyspnoea during routine activities of daily living in patients with chronic lung disease. It consists of 4 components (self-care, domestic, physical and leisure). Patients score from 0 ('I wouldn't do it anyway') to 5 ('Someone else does this for me (or helps)'), with higher scores representing maximal disability (Garrod et al 2000).

CONTINUING PATIENT MOTIVATION

Dramatic improvements can occur in a respiratory patient during the few short weeks that they undergo intensive pulmonary rehabilitation. Maintaining these improvements in the months and years that follow is a challenge for everyone concerned. Maintaining a regular exercise programme is often difficult even for physically fit individuals. Patients with respiratory diseases have to continue to cope with their symptoms. Without the support and encouragement of the pulmonary rehabilitation team this can be difficult to maintain.

Some programmes offer maintenance classes, with the same staff usually at the same location as the original programme. Maintenance classes require less supervision but fulfil a useful role in maintaining and reinforcing exercise regimes. It is becoming increasingly popular for local sports centres to set up follow on programmes, which allow the patient to exercise with other post-rehabilitation participants. Also 'Healthy Living Centres' based in primary care are beginning to emerge which could allow continuation of pulmonary rehabilitation on a more long term basis. Other programmes have such limited resources that they must discharge patients who have completed a pulmonary rehabilitation programme to enable them to devote their scarce resources to new patients. Programmes need to focus on patient independence, encouraging the patient to build exercise into the normal daily routine as a lifetime treatment.

Summary

- It is important to identify and select patients who are optimally medically managed
- Programmes and goals should be individualized to the patient's needs and disease process
- Education is an integral part of pulmonary rehabilitation and needs to be relevant
- Appropriate outcome measures to assess effectiveness of intervention should be used
- Programmes and facilities should be made accessible to more patients
- There needs to be a motivated multidisciplinary team who believe in the concept of rehabilitation

CONCLUSION

All patients whose lifestyle is being adversely affected by chronic breathlessness can be helped by pulmonary rehabilitation. Programmes can be adapted to meet the needs of individuals patients and encompass differing diagnoses. Although the programmes' exercise and educational content may differ the philosophy of treatment and the aims of the programmes remain the same, the main principle being that the elements of pulmonary rehabilitation are delivered by individual prescription through a multidisciplinary team.

Chronic breathlessness is the major symptom of most respiratory disorders and thus there is a huge patient population who can potentially benefit from pulmonary rehabilitation. At present it seems that only a small number are seen and offered access to these resources because of a lack of facilities. Where facilities are available many patients experience difficulty in attending due to transport problems. The current literature would suggest that programmes at home may be equally effective in improving quality of life for these patients. It seems that it is not the setting but the treatment that is effective and it is likely that patients with all degrees of ventilatory impairment could achieve improved exercise capacity if given clear advice regarding home exercise and some form of continued support.

Numerous clinical studies have shown that pulmonary rehabilitation does improve quality of life and exercise capacity. There are now many well validated and recognized tools for measuring these improvements following rehabilitation programmes. These tools are easy to administer and can be incorporated into everyday clinical practice.

For the individual patient, the benefits of pulmonary rehabilitation will be the reduction in symptoms, improved functional capacity and independence in daily life.

REFERENCES

American Thoracic Society 1999 Pulmonary rehabilitation. American Journal of Respiratory and Critical Care Medicine 159: 1666–1682

Bergner M, Bobbitt R A, Pollard W E et al 1976 The sickness impact profile: validation of a health status measure. Medical Care 14: 57–67

Blake R B, Vandiver T A, Braun S et al 1990 A randomised controlled evaluation of psychosocial intervention in adults with chronic lung disease. Family Medicine 2: 365–370

British Thoracic Society 1997 Guidelines for the management of chronic obstructive pulmonary disease. Thorax 52 (suppl 5): S1–S28

Casaburi R, Petty T L 1996 Principles and practice of pulmonary rehabilitation. W B Saunders, Philadelphia

Casaburi R, Patessio A, Loli F et al 1991 Reductions in exercise lactic acidosis and ventilation as a result of exercise training in patients with obstructive lung disease. American Review of Respiratory Disease 143: 9–18

Emery C F, Leutherman N E, Burker E J, McIntyre N R 1991 Psychological outcomes of a pulmonary rehabilitation programme. Chest 103: 613–617

Emery C F, Sceir R L, Hanck E R, MacIntyre N R 1998 Psychological and cognitive outcomes of a randomised trial of exercise among patients with chronic obstructive pulmonary disease. Health Psychology 17(3): 232–240

European Respiratory Society Rehabilitation and Chronic Care Scientific Group 1991 Pulmonary rehabilitation in COPD, with recommendations for its use. European Respiratory Journal 1: 463–569

Garrod R, Bestall J L, Jones P W 2000 Development and validation of a standardised measure of activities of daily living in patients with COPD. The London chest activities of daily living scale (LCADL). Respiratory medicine. (In press)

Goldstein R S, Gort E H, Stubbing D, Avendano M A 1994 Randomised controlled trial of respiratory rehabilitation. Lancet 344: 1394–1397

Griffiths T L, Burr M L, Campbell I A et al 2000 Results at 1 year of outpatient multidisciplinary pulmonary rehabilitation: a randomised controlled trial. Lancet 29(355): 362–368

Guyatt G H, Berman L G, Townsend M et al 1987 A measure of quality of life for clinical trials in chronic lung disease. Thorax 42: 773–778

Guyatt G H, Townsend M, Keller J L, Singer J 1989 Should study subjects see their previous responses: data from a randomised control trial. Journal of Clinical Epidemiology 42: 913–920

Jones P W 1995 Issues concerning health-related quality of life in COPD. Chest S107: 1875–1935

Jones P W, Quirk F H, Baveystock C M, Littlejohns P 1992 A self-complete measure of health status for chronic airflow limitation: the St George's respiratory questionnaire. American Review of Respiratory Disease 145: 1321–1327

Lacasse Y, Wong E, Guyatt G H et al 1996 Meta-analysis of respiratory rehabilitation in chronic obstructive pulmonary disease. Lancet 348: 1115–1119

Lacasse Y, Guyatt G H, Goldstein R S 1997 The components of a respiratory rehabilitation programme: a systematic overview. Chest 111: 1077–1088

Leblane P, Bowie D M, Summers E et al 1986 Breathlessness and exercise in patients with cardiorespiratory disease. American Review of Respiratory Disease 133: 21–25

McGavin C, Gupta S, Lloyd E, McHardy G 1977 Physical rehabilitation for the chronic bronchitic: results of a controlled trial of exercises in the home. Thorax 32: 307–311

McSweeny A J, Grant I, Heaton R K et al 1982 Life quality of patients with chronic obstructive pulmonary disease. Archives of Internal Medicine 142(3): 473–478

Mahler D, Mackowiak J L 1995 Evaluation of the short form 36 item questionnaire to measure health related quality of life in patients with COPD. Chest 107: 1585–1589

Mejia R, Ward J, Lentine T, Mahler D 1999 Target dyspnoea ratings predict expected oxygen consumption as well as target heart rate values. American Journal of Respiratory and Critical Care Medicine 159: 1485–1489

Morgan M D L 1991 Experience of using the chronic respiratory disease questionnaire (CRDQ). Respiratory Medicine 85 (suppl B): 23–24

National Institutes of Health 1994 Workshop summary: pulmonary rehabilitation research. American Journal of Respiratory and Critical Care Medicine 149: 825–833

Nouri F M, Lincoln N B 1987 An extended activities of daily living scale for stroke patients. Clinical Rehabilitation 1: 301–305

Ries A L 1997 Pulmonary rehabilitation. Joint ACCP/AACVPR evidence-based guidelines. Chest 112: 1363–1396

Ries A L, Ellis B, Hawkins R W 1988 Upper extremity exercise training in COPD. Chest 93: 688–692

Ries A L, Kaplan R M, Limbery T M, Prewitt L M 1995 Effects of pulmonary rehabilitation on physiologic and psychosocial outcomes in patients with chronic obstructive pulmonary disease. Annals of Internal Medicine 122: 823–832

Singh S J, Morgan M D L, Scott S, Walters D, Hardman E 1992 Development of a shuttle walking test of disability in patients with chronic airways obstruction. Thorax 47: 1019–1024

Singh S J, Morgan M D, Hardman A E et al 1994 Comparison of oxygen uptake during a conventional treadmill test and shuttle walking test in chronic airflow limitation. European Respiratory Journal 7(11): 2016–2020

Sweer L Zwillich C W 1990 Dyspnoea in the patient with chronic obstructive pulmonary disease: etiology and management. Clinics in Chest Medicine 11(3): 417–445

Vale F, Readon J Z, Zuhallack R L 1993 The long-term benefits of outpatient pulmonary rehabilitation on exercise endurance and quality of life. Chest 103: 42–45

Ware J E, Sherbourne C D 1992 The MOS 36-item short-form health survey. Medical Care 30: 473–483

Wedzicha J A, Bestall J C, Garrod R et al 1998 Randomised controlled trial of pulmonary rehabilitation in severe chronic obstructive pulmonary disease patients, stratified with the MRC dyspnoea scale. European Respiratory Journal 12: 363–369

White R J, Rudkin S T, Ashley J et al 1997 Outpatient pulmonary rehabilitation in severe chronic obstructive pulmonary disease. Journal of the Royal College of Physicians 31: 541–545

Wijkstra P J, Ten Vergert E M, Van Altena R et al 1994a Reliability and validity of the chronic respiratory disease questionnaire (CRQ). Thorax 49: 465–467

Wijkstra P J, Van Altena R, Kran J et al 1994b Quality of life in patients with chronic obstructive pulmonary disease improves after rehabilitation at home. European Respiratory Journal 7: 369–373

Wijkstra P J, Postma D S, Koeter G H 1999 Which patient is a good candidate for rehabilitation? European Respiratory Journal. Madrid Abstract

World Health Organization 1980 International classification of impairments, disabilities and handicaps. World Health Organization, Geneva

Zigmond A S, Snaith R P 1983 The hospital anxiety and depression scale. Acta Psychiatrica Scandinavica 67: 361–370

12

End stage management of respiratory disease

Susan Madge   Glenda Esmond

One of the most important principles of medical care and treatment is human dignity. This principle is particularly relevant in the case of the terminally ill patient, whose treatment and care should not start from the medical axiom of preserving life at all costs but from the right of these patients to die with dignity (Kuuppelomaki 1993).

RECOGNIZING THE TERMINAL PHASE OF RESPIRATORY DISEASE

Management of the end stage of any chronic disease places great demands on the multidisciplinary team involved with the patient's care. With respiratory disease there is often no clear event that signifies the beginning of the terminal phase because of the gradual deterioration over many years. The team must be alert to the subtle changes in symptoms and psychosocial status that indicate declining health and the beginning of the terminal phase. These can include:

- no relief from breathlessness despite optimizing medical management
- an inability to get out of the house due to breathlessness despite pulmonary rehabilitation
- increasing number of hospital admissions
- limited improvement following admission for acute exacerbations
- patient voices concerns about dying
- expression of fear and anxiety and development of panic attacks.

The patient himself often recognizes a change in health as breathing becomes more laborious and mobility becomes compromised. The family however may not have become aware of these changes; indeed the patient may have taken care not to allow these changes to become obvious to family members in an effort to protect them. Breaking the news to the family therefore may come as a great shock and acknowledgement of the reality of the situation may often take some time. Time and privacy are important for the family and patient to allow them to come to terms with the changing state of the disease and the effect that it is having, both physically and emotionally.

DECISION MAKING

There are many decisions that have to be made by the patient and his family during this stage and the teams involved can be a source of both practical and psychosocial support to guide them through this often difficult period. Support however must be as unbiased as possible and patients and their families should be fully involved in the decision making processes. Sullivan et al (1996) and McNeely et al (1997) examined the influence of the physician in talking to patients and families about end stage choices and found that although physicians advocated a shared decision making approach, they were strongly influencing the deliberation process. Information was often presented in modified form in order to influence the decision that was being made by the patient or family. It is therefore essential that all members of the healthcare team are aware of the importance of providing the patient and his family with information that has not been modified, so that they can make informed choices based on the full facts. The skill is to have the ability to provide such information in a sensitive and supportive manner and to offer time, so that the patient and family can explore issues further.

AGGRESSIVE INTERVENTION VERSUS A PALLIATIVE MODE OF CARE

In respiratory care many treatments used in the aggressive treatment phase of the disease may continue once patients enter the terminal phase

Case study 12.1

Robert is 64 years of age and has smoked from the age of 22 years. He was diagnosed with chronic obstructive pulmonary disease 12 years ago. He is married and has two grown up sons. Deterioration has taken place over the past 2 months and currently Robert requires 2 litres of oxygen via nasal cannula 24 hours per day. Robert was admitted to hospital and after 3 weeks of treatment there was minimal improvement despite changing antibiotics and maximizing bronchodilation.

Robert's progress was discussed at a multidisciplinary meeting and following a review of medical notes and input from each discipline it was decided that Robert was entering the terminal phase of his chronic obstructive pulmonary disease. Previous discussion with the respiratory nurse specialist had allowed Robert to raise concerns regarding his anxiety about his family watching him die of breathlessness. All members of the team felt that Robert knew he was entering the terminal phase. It was agreed that a sensitive, open and honest discussion should take place and the issue of non-invasive ventilation and resuscitation status should be discussed. The team decided that as the respiratory nurse specialist had already had a discussion with Robert regarding breathlessness and dying, she would arrange a time to revisit these issues with him, and that the consultant would see him afterwards.

The team's assessment of Robert's insight into the severity of his disease was correct and the discussions with both the respiratory nurse specialist and the consultant physician were very positive. Robert asked for somebody to be with him when he told his sons, but felt that he did not need anybody with him when he told his wife as he was sure she already knew.

After being given all the facts, Robert decided that he would not be resuscitated if he had a cardiorespiratory arrest as he did not want to die in intensive care. He was aware that non-invasive ventilation was an option and would consider this if it was used to control breathlessness but would also want opioids to control his breathlessness when the time came. It was agreed that these issues would be revisited as and when either Robert or the team felt it appropriate.

This open discussion reduced Robert's fear and anxiety as he felt he no longer had to pretend that he was doing well. The team found it easier to care for Robert knowing they were not hiding anything from him and that a clear treatment plan could be made.

of their disease, for example oxygen to control hypoxaemia and antibiotics to reduce the volume of sputum. It is therefore not always obvious from the treatment regimen that the patient has entered the terminal phase and in need of palliation of symptoms. It is essential that there is a discussion regarding the change, otherwise the patient may be deprived of treatment for palliation of symptoms or may have unnecessary investigations such as taking of arterial blood gases. The decision to change from aggressive intervention to a palliative mode of care should be collaborative among patient, carers and healthcare professionals. If patients and their families are properly educated and supported it is possible for them to participate actively in 'life and death' decisions, including the use of ventilatory support (Gilgoff et al 1989, Meduri et al 1994, Piper et al 1992).

It must be acknowledged that treatment choices and the dilemma of aggressive management versus palliative care are difficult decisions for both the families and the healthcare professionals concerned. The pre-terminal and terminal stages must be handled with sensitivity and compassion together with sound judgement and involvement from the patient, the family and all members of the multidisciplinary team. Withdrawal of any aspect of active treatment, such as chemotherapy or intravenous antibiotics, has to be highly individualized and must follow careful discussion with the patient and family. Communication at this time is paramount and it is essential that the patient and the family receive sufficient information to enable them to make informed decisions about treatment and the possibility for flexibility of choice. These treatment decisions may include whether terminal care should be carried out in the home or in hospital, the options for respiratory support such as non-invasive ventilation, pain management and symptom control and the management of cardiorespiratory failure.

SYMPTOM CONTROL

Recognizing and managing symptoms during the terminal stages of illness relies on specialist assessment and the formulation of a clear and appropriate plan of care that is flexible enough to account for fluctuating needs. This assessment must be open to change, acknowledging the ongoing requirements of both the patient and the family. The symptoms that patients with end stage respiratory disease most commonly experience are:

- breathlessness
- anxiety, depression and panic
- pain
- inability to cope with lung secretions
- cough
- complications related to immobility
- haemoptysis
- stridor.

Symptom control is not just a matter of prescribing and administering analgesia or sedation. An holistic approach allows relief to be found in many ways, from changing position or relieving constipation to acknowledging fear and anxiety. The nurse responsible for assessing patient needs at this time must be aware of all the contributing factors and be in a position to discuss them with colleagues such as the physiotherapist, occupational therapist, dietitian, palliative care team, psychologist and medical staff.

Breathlessness

Breathlessness is the most overwhelming and distressing problem associated with end stage respiratory disease and successful alleviation may dramatically improve the physical and psychological status of the patient. Unfortunately, breathlessness can also be the most difficult symptom to manage and may often involve a variety of approaches that include:

- positioning
- psychosocial intervention
- oxygen therapy
- opioids.

Positioning

Some breathlessness may be alleviated by allowing the patient to find the most comfortable position in which to sit or lie and then obtain support from pillows and bed rests. A patient's favoured position may remain the same for days or change throughout the day, and careful discussion with the patient and the family will guide the nurse. It may be that the patient needs advice on an appropriate position or help to get into the position. Most patients

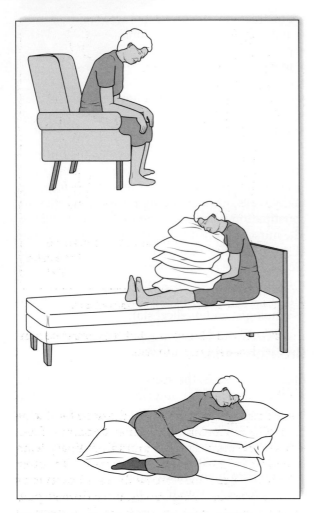

Figure 12.1 Positioning to alleviate breathlessness.

who are breathless need to sit upright and be well supported (Fig. 12.1).

Oxygen therapy

Patients with severe respiratory disease often commence oxygen therapy at home before the disease reaches the end stage. This will be provided through a variety of sources, from cylinders to concentrators, and is commonly delivered via nasal cannula or face mask, with or without humidification. The multidisciplinary team will decide, with the patient, the most appropriate method of delivery throughout the changing stages of the disease process.

Oxygen therapy will have been commenced to aid symptomatic relief of breathlessness by correcting hypoxaemia. Oxygen therapy in this situation will often be recommended for use as intermittent therapy during the day and continuously overnight. However, as the patient becomes more unwell their dependence on oxygen will increase such that by the time they are in the end stage of their disease they will be using it constantly, and in some cases will panic if it is withdrawn for any reason. Care must be taken to maintain appropriate oxygen levels in order to prevent introduction of new symptoms such as excessive drowsiness and headaches due to carbon dioxide retention. Sometimes, carbon dioxide narcosis can in itself result in symptomatic relief as the patient may become slightly drowsy. However, continuing rises in carbon dioxide levels can lead to confusion and severe headache. Maintaining a balance between monitoring arterial blood gases to ensure that new symptoms are not introduced and avoiding the invasive nature of taking arterial blood gases is important. A single arterial blood gas measurement taken while the patient is receiving the chosen percentage of oxygen is often sufficient.

Anecdotal reports indicate that occasionally some patients find using a fan to blow cool air in their direction or being near a wide open window very helpful, although they may not feel hot or be pyrexial. Patients report that the cool, moving air makes them feel that they can breathe more easily and that when the fan is turned off or all the windows in the room are closed they feel suffocated and start to panic. A similar response is sometimes found with the use of mask or nasal oxygen, where it is often the feeling of the oxygen flow that helps. This can be a problem when the required flow rate is low; entrainment of air into the delivery system may be helpful in this situation. Other useful agents in the management of breathlessness are nebulized bronchodilators such as salbutamol or terbutaline.

Opioids

As death approaches, the respiratory patient is likely to become increasingly breathless and the aim of treatment at this time is to control this distressing symptom. Opioids can alleviate breathlessness provided the dosage is titrated in the same way as when used for pain control (Davis 1998). To avoid respiratory depression, opioids should be introduced at low dosages, for example 2.5 mg morphine elixir 4 hourly and increasing following assessment of breathlessness and signs of respiratory depression. If opioids are not considered by the multidisciplinary team because of fear of respiratory depression, the patient may suffer unnecessarily.

Occasionally medication is necessary to relieve constipation, and laxatives or stool softeners may be administered, especially at the commencement of opioids. These issues may often cause embarrassment for the patient and the nurse

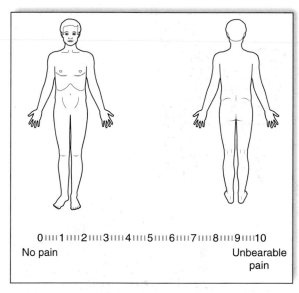

Figure 12.3   Pain chart – an assessment tool.

involved should be aware that they must be handled with sensitivity and tact.

Pain

Assessing the fear of pain and the need for it to be controlled can be one of the most important functions of the nurse and the multidisciplinary team in caring for the terminally ill patient. This must not always be assumed to be the case however as during some end stage respiratory disease pain may not be the primary problem. It is essential therefore to spend time talking carefully with the patient in order to identify the source and cause of the pain so that appropriate analgesia or other methods of pain relief may be offered. The concept of total pain (Saunders 1967) encompasses the following areas:

- physical
- emotional
- social
- spiritual.

Pain control needs to address all these areas if pain relief is to be achieved. Pain charts (Figs 12.2 and 12.3) are useful in measuring the patients' perceptions of their pain and in reassessing effectiveness of pain control.

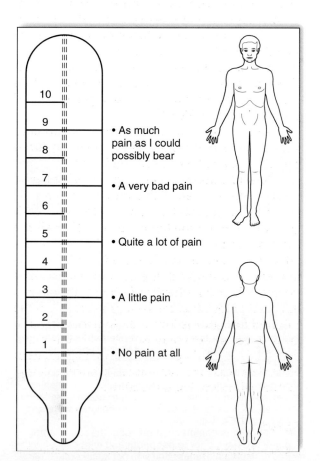

Figure 12.2   Pain chart – an assessment tool.

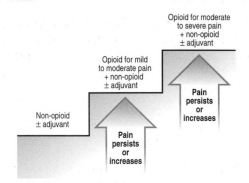

Figure 12.4 Analgesic ladder.

In respiratory disease pain is primarily centred around the chest and back, although the abdomen may also be involved due to coughing and the work of breathing. There may also be limb pain due to problems with immobility or referred pain. The World Health Organization's (1996) analgesic ladder (Fig. 12.4) can be a useful tool to guide the prescription of appropriate and adequate analgesia. Selecting the most appropriate analgesia, and the dosage and route of administration may sometimes require specialist expertise. Most hospitals, hospices and community teams have access to palliative care or pain teams and their advice should be sought whenever possible.

Lung secretions

End stage respiratory disease may often be accompanied by problems associated with viscous or copious lung secretions, which are a particular problem for patients with cystic fibrosis and bronchiectasis. Any interference with the ability to breathe can be terrifying and the management of lung secretions is fundamental in symptom control.

Both thick and copious lung secretions are optimally managed with a combination of inhaled medication and chest physiotherapy. Nebulized mucolytics such as normal (0.9%) or hypertonic (3–7%) saline and dornase alfa may help to thin the mucus, making it easier to expec-

torate. However, inadequate hydration also contributes to the dehydration of secretions, and fluid intake, whether oral, enteral or intravenous, should be closely monitored.

The constant build up of secretions in the lungs can be a frightening experience; patients describe struggling to breathe or feeling as though they are drowning. The importance of this problem and its management can therefore not be underestimated. Anticholinergic agents such as atropine or hyoscine may often be helpful in reducing the over production of lung secretions. Unfortunately, although it can cause distress, it may be necessary occasionally to administer oropharyngeal suction, especially during chest physiotherapy. The decision to perform suctioning must be weighed in relation to whether it will cause more or less distress than the secretions.

Case study 12.2

Wendy was a 48-year-old lady with bronchiectasis. She was in the terminal stages of her disease and had chosen to die in hospital where she had been receiving care for the past 14 years. She felt secure in the environment and felt she would benefit from the experience of the physiotherapist: her main concern was control of lung secretions as she became very breathless if she did not clear sputum from her lungs.

The plan of care, which Wendy was involved in creating, consisted of administering humidified oxygen therapy, as she found the coolness of the humidification comforting, intravenous antibiotics so that her sputum volume was minimized, intravenous fluids and modified physiotherapy.

Four days before her death she became more breathless due to sputum retention and was getting more anxious due to breathlessness. Wendy was therefore commenced on chlorpromazine to reduce anxiety, which had the desired effect, allowing her to have a good night's sleep. At this point the physiotherapist treating her knew that even the modified form of physiotherapy she was receiving would be likely to cause more distress than relief. Instead, the physiotherapist used the time to help make Wendy comfortable by means of positioning, and spent time listening to her talk about unrelated issues such as how successful her children were and how proud she was of them.

Wendy was commenced on subcutaneous diamorphine two days prior to her death and died peacefully, free from breathlessness and with her family around her.

There are many techniques for administering chest physiotherapy, which may be active or passive procedures. Each patient will use a technique tailored to his or her particular requirements and this may change as their condition changes. Patients with end stage respiratory illness may be used to carrying out daily physiotherapy in their homes as well as in hospital, and they may find that chest physiotherapy relieves their symptoms until the very late stages of the illness; however, consideration may be given to its withdrawal when there is no longer any physical or emotional benefit. The patient should be offered chest physiotherapy, often in a modified form, for example breathing control sitting in an upright position, rather than postural drainage and percussion. The patient should be allowed to decline physiotherapy in the terminal phase but wherever possible the time that would have been spent on it should be used to help with positioning to alleviate breathlessness or to provide psychological support.

Cough

Cough is a physiological reflex that protects the airways and lungs by clearing secretions and foreign matter. Cough can be an unpleasant symptom and is a particular problem in patients with lung cancer (Cowcher & Hanks 1990), although it can be a symptom that patients can experience in the end stage of any respiratory disease. The consequences of cough include:

- loss of sleep
- chest wall pain from muscular strain
- headaches
- rib fractures
- haemoptysis.

Cough can be described as productive or dry and the aim of management is to alleviate the unpleasant symptoms. The treatment options can include:

- cough suppressants (i.e. codeine linctus)
- mucolytics (i.e. nebulized saline)
- nebulized local anaesthetic
- antibiotics
- antimuscarinics (i.e. hyoscine).

Haemoptysis

In the terminal stage of lung disease haemoptysis can be fatal. Patients with the following problems are most likely to have a massive haemoptysis:

- lung cancer
- aspergilloma
- lung abscess
- bronchiectasis.

If the possibility of haemoptysis as a terminal event can be predicted in a patient, then the treatment plan should reflect this potential problem. The aim is to reduce awareness and fear, and a combination of an intravenous opioid and a benzodiazepine is usually required to do this (Davis 1998).

Stridor

Stridor can be described as an obstruction of the larynx or major airways resulting in a harsh inspiratory wheeze (Davis 1998). Corticosteroids can provide relief but in extreme cases the patient may require radiotherapy or insertion of a tracheal or bronchial stent to provide symptom relief.

Immobility

An inability to move effectively and painlessly has an immediate effect on independence and the feeling of being in control. Immobility may also cause serious problems with:

- pressure areas
- constipation
- muscle wasting
- personal hygiene.

These often intimate issues may be alleviated practically with the provision of a wheelchair and commode, a pressure relieving mattress or cushion, the maintenance of good hydration and diet, regular pressure area care, passive or active exercise and help with washing. Occupational therapists, in hospital or in the community, can be invaluable in assessing individual needs and providing equipment that will allow both patients and carers to manage daily life optimally.

PSYCHOSOCIAL SUPPORT

Patients with end stage respiratory disease commonly experience symptoms of:

- emotional distress
- depression
- anxiety
- panic.

These symptoms can cause increased breathlessness resulting in more distress (Fig. 12.5).

The level of advice and support offered to help patients understand what is happening to them has to be related to their level of understanding. With this in mind the aim of any intervention is to provide the patient with strategies to enhance:

- coping abilities
- symptom relief
- quality of life.

There can often be a conspiracy of silence surrounding patients, created by family and staff in a well meaning effort to protect them. This however leaves the patient with unanswered questions, unresolved fears and a feeling of isolation. Most patients wish to 'leave their house in order'. This may be through achieving certain dreams, leaving a will or belongings to their family and friends, or organizing their own

funeral. Some patients want to plan the terminal process themselves with a 'living will', an advance directive determining the use of ventilatory support or medication, and some simply want to prepare to say goodbye. To prevent patients' involvement in the terminal stages of their disease may therefore cause them more distress and reduce their ability to cope with the treatment demands placed upon them.

Some respiratory diseases, such as cystic fibrosis, are inherited and this may often cause guilt and frustration in parents and healthy siblings; whereas smoking related diseases such as lung cancer and chronic obstructive pulmonary disease (COPD) may generate fear and social stigmatization since society views smoking related diseases as self-inflicted. When a family begins to recognize the terminal stages of an illness a range of emotions can be experienced, including:

- anger
- guilt
- denial
- disappointment
- helplessness.

These emotions are displayed in a variety of ways and are often directed towards the professionals caring for the sick relative. Junior members of the multidisciplinary team may find this difficult to deal with and supervision is important in supporting colleagues at these times. Most family members become concerned about the nature of the terminal phase and demand a detailed description of the stages that will follow, with a time scale, even though this may be impossible to predict.

Counselling

Early counselling for both patients and their families is a way of preparing people for dealing with loss when it occurs. Early counselling will ideally have given those concerned time to think about the future and what will be involved. Inability to plan for the future and only being able to live one day at a time adds to the stress suffered by patients and families. Preparation helps everyone, particularly the patient, family and health-

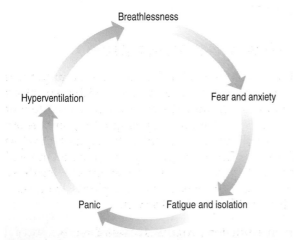

Figure 12.5   Cycle of breathlessness.

care professionals, to cope with difficult issues more thoughtfully and successfully. It is possible and even helpful to discuss issues regarding end stage management with patients over many years. Patients with cystic fibrosis, for example, who know that they have a significantly reduced life expectancy, are often prompted to discuss their feelings about dying when a peer dies.

The needs of the patient and their family are in a constant state of flux during the end stage of any illness and the nurse must be alert to the complexity and changing nature of each patient's care. By offering support and acknowledgement of their situation the nurse can help the family come to terms with and adapt to the changes (Bell & Shale 1993). The psychological distress suffered at this time by both the patient and the family means that the nurse becomes an advocate (Pursell 1994), enabling all involved to accept new ways of:

- coping
- recognizing denial
- respecting wishes
- making decisions about treatment
- discussing issues around dying.

There are often practical issues that the patient and family are concerned with, some of which they may feel inhibited about discussing with healthcare professionals. These can include:

- financial problems
- housing problems
- time off work to stay with the patient – whether at home or in hospital
- loss of wages or benefits when the patient dies
- funeral expenses.

Confidence in the team involved will allow these issues to be raised without embarrassment.

Anxiety, depression and panic

There are many ways to approach the psychological trauma of coping with the knowledge of approaching death. Offering basic reassurance and ensuring security play a major role in calming an anxious patient. This can be offered through talking to the family or carers, sharing information,

involving patients and families in decision making, or by providing distraction appropriate to the patient. Counselling in its many forms is often helpful. However, it must be remembered that each patient may require a different approach and it is the responsibility of the nurse and colleagues in the multidisciplinary team to ensure that the counselling being offered is appropriate for the patient.

The various complementary therapies are becoming more popular in practice today and are increasingly being provided in hospitals, hospices and patients' homes. Many patients find some types of complementary therapy, such as aromatherapy and reflexology, helpful on both an emotional and a physical level and find this either preferable to taking medication or a helpful addition to their treatment regimen. Practitioners are often willing to come to hospitals or visit private homes to treat individuals and there are recognized institutions which can recommend therapists able to fulfil this request.

It must be recognized, however, that medication continues to play an important role in relieving anxiety and at certain stages in the terminal process appropriate use of anxiolytics should be considered. Most commonly used are diazepam or chlorpromazine, which can be administered in a variety of ways, including orally, intravenously or rectally.

Symptom control is a fundamental right of a dying patient. Table 12.1 summarizes symptom control approaches used for respiratory patients.

LUNG TRANSPLANTATION

Lung transplantation has become an important therapeutic option for patients with respiratory failure and limited life expectancy. The advent of heart–lung, double lung, single lung and, more recently, living donor lobar transplantation has for some, however, greatly complicated the end stage of respiratory disease, especially for those with cystic fibrosis. Lung transplantation is usually considered when there is:

- an estimated prognosis of less than two years
- deteriorating chronic respiratory failure

- lung function below 30% of predicted values
- a seriously compromised quality of life.

Absolute contraindications to transplantation are decreasing. New techniques are being developed and advances in immunosuppressive agents and postoperative medical care have led to improving survival rates and quality of life. Obliterative bronchiolitis, however, continues to remain a serious problem (Madden & Geddes 1993). Despite advances, transplantation is not suitable for or desired by all patients and unfortunately, due to poor organ availability, will only be available to a small percentage of those who have been assessed as possible successful recipients.

Although there is much to discuss with patients who are thinking about transplantation as

Table 12.1   Symptom control – suggested approaches

Problem	Pharmaceutical management	Other measures

Breathlessness	• Morphine syrup (titrate and breakthrough)
	• Morphine sulphate tablets (maintenance)
	• IV/SC diamorphine (infusion if no oral route)
	• Nebulized morphine
	• Fentanyl patches (slow release)
	• Bronchodilators
	  – salbutamol
	  – terbutaline
		• Oxygen therapy
		• Fan
		• Positioning
		  – sitting over pillows
		  – high side lying

Viscous lung secretions	• Mucolytic agents
	  – nebulized saline
	  – dornase alpha
		• Adequate hydration
		  (oral/enteral/IV)
		• Humidification
		• Modified physiotherapy

Copious secretions	• Review mucolytics
	• Anticholinergic agents
	  – atropine
	  – hyoscine
		• Oropharyngeal suction if
		  necessary

Oedema	• Diuretics if symptoms troublesome	
Anxiety	• Diazepam (oral, PR, IV or infusion) • Chlorpromazine • Midazolam infusion	• Reassurance and security • Information and involvement • Distraction • Complementary therapies • Counselling
Mobility		• Wheelchair • Commode/urinal/bedpan • Pressure relieving mattress • Attention to pressure areas and personal hygiene
Loss of appetite/nausea	• Metoclopramide • Cyclizine • Prochlorperazine • Domperidone	• Avoid strong smells • Small amounts of food and drink
Constipation	• Laxatives and stool softeners • Senna, lactulose (consider starting with opioids)	• Hydration • Diet
Pain	• Identify and treat source with appropriate analgesia (non-steroidals, opioids)	• Involve palliative care team • Patient controlled analgesia • TENS

(From Cystic Fibrosis Nurse Specialist Group 2001 with permission of June Dyer (CF CNS Bristol))

an option for treatment, there are also some important issues to be considered:

- Patients and their families undergo considerable stress waiting, sometimes for years, for organs to become available, and this has an impact on the entire family and their day-to-day life which should not be underestimated.
- The positive aspects of waiting for organs on an active waiting list can sometimes blinker both healthcare professionals and families to alternative options for treatment. Careful consideration must be given to the risk of not recognizing the end and to the timely institution of palliative care when appropriate.

Case study 12.3

Rebecca was a 13-year-old with cystic fibrosis who had frequent courses of intravenous antibiotics, was on oxygen, wheelchair dependent and was no longer able to leave the house. Rebecca was therefore referred and assessed for a heart–lung transplant and began the long wait at home for organs to become available.

Rebecca's mother carried the pager with her wherever she went, and put it by her pillow at night. Family life became centred on the pager and this source of stress and anxiety 24 hours a day, 7 days a week caused relationship problems within the family. The cystic fibrosis team and the transplant team saw Rebecca and her family regularly, and were both concerned about how the family were coping and the problems that were starting to appear. Psychological intervention was recommended and the family started seeing a psychologist who was working with the cystic fibrosis team.

After 6 months both teams, in discussion with the family, decided to remove Rebecca from the transplant list for a break, despite her declining health. Almost immediately after coming off the list her parents reported feeling as though they had been holding their breaths for the last 6 months and now they could breathe again. Rebecca and her family decided that transplantation was no longer an option for them and that the wait was spoiling the time they had left together.

Rebecca died 3 months later in her local hospital with her family and friends beside her. Rebecca's parents reported that coming off the list was the best thing that they had done as it allowed them to relax and enjoy the rest of Rebecca's life. Both Rebecca's mother and her father said that being able to talk about death and make plans without the 'what if' anxiety hanging over them enabled the family to cope more successfully with the situation.

The option for transplantation has made decision making difficult for patients and their families and has often altered their attitudes towards effective terminal care. Delay in acknowledgement that the end stage has been reached and in 'letting go' of the goal of transplant so that the patient may die with dignity often causes unnecessary pain and suffering. The multidisciplinary team must be alert to these problems and support the patient and family in recognizing the appropriate options for care.

BEREAVEMENT

Bereavement begins when someone acknowledges that the person they care about is dying (Sheldon 1997). The grief process for family and friends may begin even before the patient with respiratory disease dies. The healthcare professional caring for the dying patient and their family should be aware not only of the possible five stages of grief (Kuebler-Ross 1970), but also that these stages may occur in any order and may be repeated:

- denial
- anger
- bargaining
- depression
- acceptance.

Recognition of grieving can help support the family and the dying patient. Donnellan (1999) suggests that simple support can be provided by being:

- aware
- there
- sensitive
- human
- ready
- patient.

When a person with respiratory disease dies, bereavement follow-up is often required. The members of the primary healthcare team are of prime importance at this time in providing such support, and therefore liaison between primary and secondary care is essential.

THE HEALTHCARE PROFESSIONALS

Working with the terminally ill will, to some greater or lesser degree, have a physical and psychological effect on the healthcare professionals caring for this group of patients. Due to the chronic nature of respiratory disease many of the multidisciplinary team will have known these patients for years and therefore death, particularly in younger patients, can have an impact on the team. Recognition of the need to provide support, supervision and guidance at all levels and to all disciplines may protect staff from the anguish suffered through being so closely involved with dying patients. Every member of the multidisciplinary team must be aware of the others, both emotionally and physically, to allow recognition and prevention of the stress and 'burnout' often described in staff working in these situations.

A strong multidisciplinary team allows a mutual respect for each other's welfare (Madge & Khair 2000). In caring for terminally ill patients and to be able to continue to do so usefully, staff must acknowledge their feelings and seek support, formally or informally, from appropriate sources. In situations where staff are routinely caring for dying patients, provision must be made for staff supervision on a formal level; informal arrangements may not be reliable, may be expensive or may be too much trouble to arrange.

When patients start to deteriorate the dilemma of what should or should not be done for the patient leads to two questions, 'When is enough enough?' and 'Who decides?' (Fratianne et al 1992). Management of these decisions has been reported to lead to stress within the professional team but this can be overcome through group involvement in the decision making, with the final decision then being presented to the family and patient as a team decision. Studies have shown that a decision made by the team removes from any one individual the responsibility of having to make a stressful decision, and the families experience a great deal of relief as they are not forced into making difficult decisions alone (Fratianne et al 1992, Konigova 1996).

Often the terminal stages of care can become extended and at times confusing; healthcare professionals report emotional exhaustion and a low feeling of personal accomplishment (van Servellen & Leake 1993). It has been found that agreed coping strategies employed by teams enable staff to cope with the continuing stressors of caring for the dying. Sutton (1993) suggests that continuing education, supervision by senior staff and smaller staff/patient ratios allow staff to manage their caseloads more successfully.

There can be no doubt that caring for dying patients, whatever their age, is complex and stressful. All the staff involved should acknowledge the support they can not only receive, but also offer each other by working within a multidisciplinary team. An holistic approach to the care of patients and their families allows each person to benefit from the rewarding and challenging experience that caring for the dying patient can bring.

CONCLUSION

The end stage of any respiratory disease need not be a painful or frightening experience for the patient. Clear clinical assessment, knowledge of all the available treatment options and involvement of all members of the multidisciplinary team will ensure that all patients will have an individualized plan of care appropriate to their changing needs.

REFERENCES

Bell S, Shale D 1993 Terminal care in cystic fibrosis. Palliative Care Today 2(4): 48–49

Cowcher K, Hanks G W 1990 Long term management of respiratory symptoms in advanced cancer. Journal of Pain and Symptom Management 5(5): 320–330

Cystic Fibrosis Nurse Specialist Group 2001 National consensus standards for the nursing management of cystic fibrosis. Cystic Fibrosis Trust, Bromley

Davis C L 1998 Breathlessness, cough and other respiratory problems. In: Fallon M, O'Neill B (eds) ABC of palliative care. British Medical Journal Publishing Group, London

Donnellan C 1999 Bereavement. Independence, Cambridge

Fratianne R B, Brandt C, Yurko L, Coffee T 1992 When is enough enough? Ethical dilemmas on the burn unit. Journal of Burn Care Rehabilitation 13(5): 600–604

Gilgoff I, Prentice W, Baydur A 1989 Patient and family participation in the management of respiratory failure in Duchenne's muscular dystrophy. Chest 95(3): 519–524

Konigova R 1996 Do-not-resuscitate orders and withheld or withdrawn treatment. Acta Chirurgiae Plasticae 38(2): 73–77

Kuebler-Ross E 1970 On death and dying. Tavistock, London

Kuuppelomaki M 1993 Ethical decision making on starting terminal care in different health-care units. Journal of Advanced Nursing 18: 276–280

McNeely P D, Hebert P C, Dales R E et al 1997 Deciding about mechanical ventilation in end-stage chronic obstructive pulmonary disease: how respirologists perceive their role. Canadian Medical Association Journal 156(2): 177–183

Madden B P, Geddes D M 1993 Which patients should receive lung transplants? Monaldi Archives for Chest Disease 48(4): 346–352

Madge S, Khair K 2000 Multidisciplinary teams in the United Kingdom: problems and solutions. Journal of Pediatric Nursing 15(2): 131–134

Meduri G U, Fox R C, Abou-Shala N et al 1994 Noninvasive mechanical ventilation via face mask in patients with acute respiratory failure who refused endotracheal intubation. Critical Care Medicine 22(10): 1584–1590

Piper A J, Parker S, Torzillo P J et al 1992 Nocturnal nasal IPPV stabilizes patients with cystic fibrosis and hypercapnic respiratory failure. Chest 102(3): 846–850

Pursell E 1994 Telling children about their impending death. British Journal of Nursing 3(3): 119–120

Saunders C M 1967 The management of terminal illness. Medicine Publications, London

Sheldon F 1997 Psychosocial palliative care: good practice in the care of the dying and bereaved. Stanley Thornes, Cheltenham

Sullivan K E, Hebert P C, Logan J et al 1996 What do physicians tell patients with end-stage COPD about intubation and mechanical ventilation? Chest 109(1): 258–264

Sutton G 1993 Entry to the burns team: stressors, support and coping strategies. Burns 19(4): 349–351

Van Servellen G, Leake B 1993 Burn-out in hospital nurses: a comparison of acquired immunodeficiency syndrome, oncology, general medicine and intensive care unit nurse samples. Professional Nurse 9(3): 169–177

13

Primary and secondary care interface

Linda M Mackay

CHAPTER CONTENTS

The care of the respiratory patient demands a multidisciplinary approach but this needs to be set within the wider context of general healthcare provision. Primary care is the setting where approximately 90% of all contacts between the public and the National Health Service (NHS) occur (Mant 1997). It has also been shown that about 80% of people consult their GP once a year and that this figure is greater for smokers (OPCS 1994). It is this group of smokers who are most likely to suffer impaired respiratory health. It is suggested that active participation in prevention and detection of early respiratory disease, and achievement of a correct diagnosis and treatment (British Thoracic Society 1997, Raw et al 1998) will improve the respiratory health of all.

Exploration of the primary and secondary care interface is essential if 'seamless care' is to be achieved. This is where the individual requiring health interventions can move between the different healthcare settings (Fig. 13.1) using an agreed management plan which enables continuity of care without constraining boundaries.

INFLUENCE OF GOVERNMENT POLICY ON HEALTHCARE

Healthcare in the United Kingdom (UK) today is primarily delivered through the NHS. The underlying service philosophy is to treat according to need, not ability to pay or membership of insurance schemes. This ideal is reiterated in the government consultation paper on quality *A first class service: quality in the new NHS* (Department

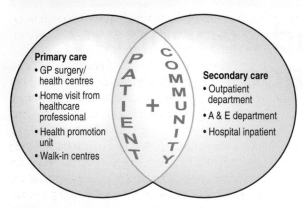

Figure 13.1   Healthcare settings.

of Health (DOH) 1998a). Prior to this, in 1990 the *NHS and community care act* (DOH 1990) introduced an internal market into the NHS, the ideology being to promote improved efficiency and more patient choice. Then followed *The patient's charter* (DOH 1991) which set rights and standards for care. *The health of the nation* (DOH 1992) White Paper set targets for disease prevention, then in 1996 a new system was introduced for dealing with NHS complaints. All this legislation affected those working within the NHS and the pace of change increased with the election of a

new government in 1997 which brought more changes in policies.

The NHS reforms in *The new NHS* (DOH 1997) are led by an altered ideology into what has been termed the 'third way'. This change in healthcare policy aims to enable more flexible working between health and social care agencies, thus facilitating interagency working and the formation of healthy alliances aimed at implementing a public health model for health. The English White Paper *Saving lives: our healthier nation* (DOH 1999a), part of the UK public health strategy, acknowledges that social and cultural factors are main determinants of health (Fig. 13.2). It establishes targets focused on health trends and potential risks but fails to set overall targets for reducing poverty and social inequalities.

INEQUALITIES IN HEALTH

The Black report (Black 1980) demonstrated that inequalities in health and healthcare existed but it was mainly ignored by the government of the day. More recently *The Acheson report* (Acheson 1998) again highlighted inequalities in health that have not gone away. The government's White Paper on

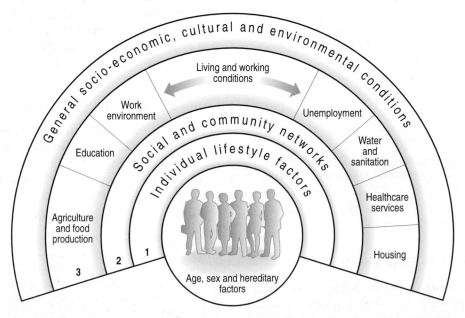

Figure 13.2   The main determinants of health (Acheson 1998). Crown copyright material is reproduced with the permission of the Controller of Her Majesty's Stationery Office.

public health, *Saving lives: our healthier nation* (DOH 1999a) confirms the findings of the Acheson inquiry and outlines a strategy to address lifestyles and life circumstances. One strand of this acknowledges evidence that people can improve their health if they take a lead in self-managing their chronic illness. This approach is supported by Bagnall & Heslop (1987) who demonstrated a relationship between chronic respiratory patients managing their health at home and improved respiratory health outcomes. The UK Public Health Association views this national health strategy as a step forward but points out that an NHS centred approach cannot by itself narrow the widening gap between rich and poor. The fact that the health inequalities gap exists and is widening raises the question of how health can be improved so that the difference is reduced. At the clinical level, action that is continuously directed at reducing inequalities is the only way that practitioners can develop and implement government policy. In reality this means:

- There needs to be an awareness of changes in policy through a personal and organizational commitment to continued professional development. For many this demands a major shift in culture with an appropriate mix of incentives and sanctions of behaviour. This is explored and explained in *Clinical governance: moving from rhetoric to reality* (NHS Executive North Thames 1998).
- Healthcare workers need to receive training and help to translate concepts such as clinical governance into practice. They need to address actively what is labelled the 'theory/practice gap' (Thompson 1995).
- It has to be acknowledged that conflicts of interest often exist. In the real world these have to be noted and, if it is not possible to resolve them, any risks that may be present must at least be minimized.

CLINICAL GOVERNANCE

'Clinical governance can be defined as a framework through which NHS organisations are accountable for continuously improving the quality of their services and safeguarding high standards of care by creating an environment in which excellence in clinical care will flourish' (DOH 1998a).

Clinical governance can be used as a tool to help healthcare professionals to achieve good quality care, but translating theory into practice is a challenge. By working together, questioning the evidence for their own practice, updating professional knowledge and skills, sharing their findings and addressing gaps or omissions in care delivery, healthcare professionals should be able to deliver better quality care for the population they serve (Fig. 13.3).

Implementation of clinical governance

Clinical governance can be implemented in several ways; one example that involves multidisciplinary teamwork is the shared governance or shared leadership model (Brooks et al 1998). This model can be used to facilitate communication, learning and breaking down barriers both between professional groups and between the primary and secondary healthcare settings. This model is based upon a network structure that offers opportunities for sharing ideas, information and resources, directed towards a common goal (Porter-O'Grady 1994). This model is in contrast to the traditional hierarchical and bureaucratic structure previously associated with healthcare delivery.

Professional self-regulation

Clinical governance is linked to professional self-regulation and lifelong learning. It also involves the patient and the public, as well as healthcare professionals. This ideal is embodied in government policy:

Professional and statutory bodies have a vital role in setting and promoting standards, but shifting the focus towards quality will also require practitioners to accept responsibility for developing and maintaining standards within their local NHS organisations. For this reason, the government will require every NHS Trust to embrace the concept of 'clinical governance' so that quality is at the core, both of their responsibilities as organisations and of each of their staff as individual professionals   (DOH 1997)

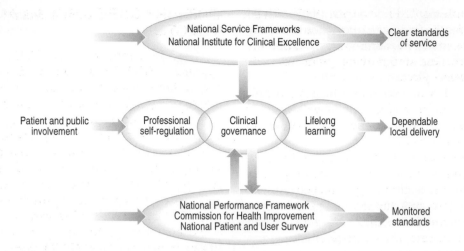

Figure 13.3 Clinical governance: what the quality framework means for patients (NHS Executive 1998). Crown copyright material is reproduced with the permission of the Controller of Her Majesty's Stationery Office.

Clinical risk management

Quality care requires team members to coordinate their work towards agreed goals; achievement of teamwork requires members to communicate effectively and should involve the local population. For practitioners delivering care, there are choices to be made about what is the most appropriate care for an individual or group, and how to deliver the care. Will it need other practitioners' input? Inevitably there is a chance that the care provided may not produce the desired outcome or may be less than optimal, so it is necessary to learn from such situations and try to reduce the likelihood of less than optimal care being given. In the past the NHS culture has been one of blame, which has not encouraged learning from less than optimal practice, so the idea of risk management is new to many practitioners. It has been defined thus:

risk management is a means of reducing the risks of adverse events occurring in organisations by systematically assessing, reviewing and then seeking ways to prevent their occurrence. The problem is that health care is, by its very nature, a risky business and only a proportion of adverse incidents are avoidable.
(NHS Executive North Thames 1998)

All healthcare workers can give examples of poor communication or poor teamwork that may have contributed to less than ideal patient care.

At a national level the National Institute for Clinical Excellence exists to promote clinical and cost-effective care. It will be the responsibility of all healthcare workers to implement health improvement plans (HImP) and standards that will be monitored. Therefore we will have a duty to identify occurrences of conflict or poor care, to learn from mistakes and to set out strategies to address these difficulties. This may mean managing or limiting the risks involved.

Quality

As the government translates into practice the proposals outlined in *A first class service* (DOH 1998a), a framework is evolving called *The NHS performance assessment framework* (DOH 1999b).

Box 13.1 The six areas of the performance assessment framework

- Health improvement
- Fair access to services
- Effective delivery of appropriate healthcare
- Efficiency
- The patient and carer experience
- The health outcomes of NHS care

This was implemented from April 1999, with six areas of underpinning activity, to assess current performance, improve performance and account locally for progress in improving quality and efficiency of local services.

All these areas are set within the government strategic human resources agenda, explained in *Working together – securing a quality workforce for the NHS* (DOH 1998e).

Translation of the concept of what clinical governance actually means for healthcare professionals who are delivering interventions at clinical level demands that the clinicians address the issue of quality in healthcare. At the organizational level it means that strategic plans should be shaped by the wider HImP for a population.

HEALTH IMPROVEMENT PLAN (HImP)

At the organizational level any strategic plan needs to be shaped by the wider HImP for a population. The innovations of Health Action Zones (HAZ) and Sure Start have been introduced in an attempt to reduce inequalities in health.

Health Action Zones are areas where there are particularly high levels of illness and the target is to improve health faster in these areas than among the rest of the population. Government funding has been set aside for this and a collaborative bid is made by health service managers, social service directors, clinicians, local business people, community group leaders and voluntary bodies for their area, in order to achieve a reduction in inequalities. The other government initiative to tackle social exclusion is Sure Start, a parenting initiative designed to promote the health and educational development of pre-school children. This is of relevance to respiratory health because there is some evidence that intrauterine and childhood factors play a part in determining adult respiratory disease (Barker 1993). Present policy involves setting up primary care groups (PCG) and primary care trusts (PCT) to implement HImPs for local populations. PCGs and PCTs are therefore central structures in the commissioning of healthcare for a population and set health within a public health framework.

PRIMARY CARE GROUPS AND TRUSTS

The White Paper *The new NHS: modern and dependable* (DOH 1997) outlined new arrangements for service provision from March 1999. These changes involved commissioning services through the introduction of long term service agreements and more effective arrangements for specialist services. Central to the success of these changes was the introduction of primary care groups (PCGs). Each group has a single budget reflecting the size of the population served, usually 100 000 people. PCGs can develop from a basic level through to the top level of freestanding primary care trust (PCT) status, when they have responsibility for providing community health services as well as hospital care.

Statute demands that each PCG must have between four and seven GPs, one or two community nurses, one social services officer, one lay member, one health authority non-executive member and one PCG chief officer (ex-officio (non voting) member). However, little reference is made to other colleagues such as professions allied to medicine (PAMs). Sackman (1999) refers to a survey that demonstrated that most PCGs have two nurses and seven GPs, and that there are several models being used based on the bottom-up, developmental approach, with power shared between members to represent the local community interests rather than the professionals' agenda. To be truly representative, PCGs

---

Box 13.2 Spectrum of primary care group development (4 levels)

1. Minimum support from the Health Authority which acts in an advisory capacity to commission care for its population.
2. Formally, as part of the Health Authority, take devolved responsibility for managing the budget for its population.
3. Become a freestanding body accountable to the Health Authority for commissioning.
4. Become an established freestanding body (Trust status) accountable to the Health Authority for commissioning care and with additional responsibility for the provision of community health services for its population.

must include lay members and build bridges with social services and other local authority departments. All team members need to gain an understanding of the contribution they and members of the other disciplines can make in order to develop a shared and agreed perception of what the PCG or PCT role is.

The PCG or PCT needs to become a reference group for the community it serves and needs to collect evidence about the population's perception of health. To achieve this it is necessary to call upon experts to provide input on specific health issues, such as smoking cessation or asthma care, across the primary and secondary care interface. The four principles of health visiting (CETHV 1977) provide a useful framework for determining a population's health needs (Fig. 13.4).

Using this framework would be one way in which the public could work in partnership with professionals to influence health outcomes. An example of how a respiratory nurse could influence the PCG or PCT in relation to respiratory health is outlined in Case study 13.1.

Case study 13.1

A respiratory nurse specialist was part of the clinical effectiveness reference group of the local PCG. She raised the topic of the respiratory health of both the resident and the working populations of the area. The respiratory nurse was invited to give a 10-minute presentation on the relevance of the government's White Paper Smoking kills (DOH 1998d), which clearly outlines a more committed public health approach to respiratory care. This document attempts to offer a 'joined-up' approach to the promotion of respiratory health by suggesting an advertising ban on tobacco promotion and the curtailment of sponsorship of sports events, as well as offering prescriptions for nicotine replacement therapy to individuals. This area of health had been identified in the local authority health improvement plan (HImP) and so the PCG was expected to include it on its agenda for its population. The PCG agreed to gather evidence about local respiratory morbidity and mortality, with a view to making a business case to bid for government funds for smoking cessation work.

This illustrates how the respiratory nurse raised awareness of the importance of respiratory health at a community population level, thus linking government policy to action planning at the HImP and PCG level.

If healthcare professionals are implementing the public health approach, then they will be strategically influencing respiratory care by linking with PCGs and implementing their strategic plans at HImP or Health Action Zone (HAZ) level.

PUBLIC HEALTH FRAMEWORK

The government is aware of the complexity of the situation and is approaching public welfare by advocating that 'joined-up' problems need 'joined-up' solutions and a public health framework to help achieve this. If a public health approach is to shape healthcare delivery, members of the population need to be involved as partners; therefore service provision will be influenced by factors such as the population's characteristics. Some examples of how this might happen are:

- Ethnicity may influence how information and care are given and received. For example, newly arrived immigrants with cultural and communication difficulties need to be sensitively helped to be partners in their care.
- Age – an older population, which includes chronic respiratory patients, may find learning more difficult due to factors such as failing sight and/or hearing.
- Educational needs – literacy may be a consideration as respiratory disease affects social classes 4 and 5, who may be educationally disadvantaged.
- Carers' needs – what are these? The literature identifies that their needs include more information and greater communication with the multidisciplinary team. Carer here is defined as the person related to or living with the patient.

Partnership approach to care

In September 1998 the government produced a discussion document, *Partnership in action* (DOH 1998b), which addressed this agenda and created new opportunities for joint working between health and social services. This is an ambitious development and it is helpful to examine how teamwork within the NHS has fared before try-

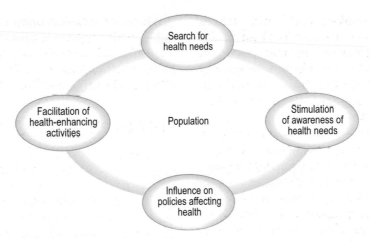

Figure 13.4   Framework for determining a population's health needs.

ing to approach teamwork between the two organizations of health and social services. Success for this new agenda will require more teamwork, often with a single agency taking the lead in care provision. Healthcare needs to be flexible and creative to meet the needs of the population often labelled as 'socially excluded'. For example, those with no fixed abode, or who have different cultural or health beliefs, will need a different route of access to the NHS for their healthcare than the more conventional route through the GP. This can be illustrated by Case study 13.2 about a refugee who develops pulmonary tuberculosis.

Seamless respiratory care

Many chronic respiratory patients become caught between the boundaries of health and social services. Whether meeting hygiene needs is a social or a health issue will be a familiar question to readers; another example is the scenario of repeated admissions, or lack of funding for the respiratory patient to be maintained at home, often because the level of home help support is reduced too quickly. This contributes to patients failing to cope and being readmitted. With a more proactive approach that allowed more flexibility for increased social support early in any deterioration, patients might cope better with difficulties and recover at home,

Case study 13.2

The refugee arrived in England with his cousin, after his home country became a war zone. He could not speak any English and, after 6 weeks, settled in London with a 'friend of a friend'. The rented accommodation was cold and damp, and the one room was shared with another refugee. After 3 months he developed a cough which worsened over several weeks, and he began to lose weight. He did not understand how to access a GP or other healthcare services. One day when he was out shopping he collapsed in the street and was taken to hospital by ambulance. Due to his presenting symptoms, cough, emaciated appearance and a suspicious chest X-ray, he was put into a side room, as an infection control measure. A sputum specimen was obtained and an interpreter was contacted. The interpreter was able to ascertain details of his social background and health problems and to explain to him that TB was the most likely diagnosis. Then, with the help of the multidisciplinary team, the patient was involved in the plan of care. He was admitted to a negative pressure side room and the consultant for communicable disease control (CCDC) was advised of the situation. The diagnosis of infectious TB was confirmed the next day, with the sputum smear positive for acid alkaline fast bacillus (AAFB). He remained an inpatient for 3 weeks until he was responding to treatment and considered non-infectious. His general health was also improving, and he began to put on weight. Whilst he was an inpatient, the social worker (attached to the local social services asylum seekers team) was able to help him to address his other health and social needs (e.g. registration with a GP, contact with the housing department and a link with a community worker).

thus avoiding an admission. The British Thoracic Society COPD guidelines (1997) identify that the level of support available at home is a consideration when deciding whether to admit or treat at home. There is a need for professionals to understand care needs and become advocates for patients and carers. Heslop (1995, 1997) identified that the respiratory nurse is in an ideal position to act as an advocate for patients and carers through supporting the psychosocial aspects of coping with breathlessness at home. The WHO framework of impairment, disability and handicap (WHO 1980), can be used to advocate such support in relation to breathlessness (Fig. 13.5).

Role of the respiratory nurse in providing seamless care

The challenge is, how can the respiratory nurse facilitate the communication of background

details such as home conditions to the acute situation of the Accident and Emergency department? Primary and secondary care have a longer history of working together for respiratory patients than do many other specialities (Holmes & Macfarlane 1999). However, there is no room for complacency. The importance of seamless care and the need to promote it between primary

Case study 13.3

Ada, a 69-year-old smoker, suffers from chronic obstructive pulmonary disease (COPD). She has visited her GP as she has become more breathless over the past few days and is coughing and producing light green sputum. Her GP refers her to the acute respiratory assessment service based at the local hospital.

Assessment

- Lives with husband and has daughter who visits twice weekly.
- Pulse oximetry on air at rest: SaO_2 89%.
- Arterial blood gases on air: pH 7.37; PaO_2 7.1 kPa; $PaCO_2$ 5.8 kPa.
- Arterial blood gases on oxygen: pH 7.37; PaO_2 10.5 kPa; $PaCO_2$ 5.6 kPa.
- Blood pressure: 130/85; Pulse: 96/min.
- Slight ankle oedema.
- Wheeze and crackles present.

Following assessment it was decided that Ada was suitable to be managed at home with the support of the respiratory nurse specialist. An oxygen concentrator was arranged and delivered the same day so that Ada could receive oxygen at 2 L/min via nasal cannula, thereby correcting her hypoxaemia. She was prescribed oral antibiotics and a course of oral steroids. She was given advice on how to use the oxygen and on the importance of smoking cessation, in particular of not smoking while using oxygen. She was discharged home without needing admission. The respiratory nurse specialist visited the next day to assess Ada in her own home, to ensure the treatment was understood, and to offer support with her smoking cessation action plan.

Over the next week Ada improved, with her SaO_2 returning to 94% on air. The respiratory nurse specialist referred Ada for an occupational therapy assessment, as it had been identified that Ada was unable to have a bath because there was no rail and she was frightened of falling. Advice on smoking cessation was given. Following three home visits by the respiratory nurse specialist over a 10 day period, Ada no longer required oxygen therapy as her SaO_2 was above 92%. Ada was discharged from the ARAS and her care was returned to her GP. A full summary of Ada's care while under the ARAS was faxed to the GP.

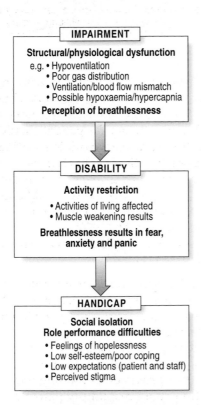

Figure 13.5 The concepts of impairment, disability and handicap in relation to breathlessness.

Table 13.1 Theoretical summary of differences between groups and teams

Characteristic	Group	Team
Definition	Number of people or persons near together or belonging or being classed together	A side of players such as a football team
Size	Unlimited	Max 12
Focus	Task	People
Communication structure	Commands downwards and reports upwards	Upwards, downwards and laterally
Members	Task may have 'thrown' them together because of their job description, may not be interconnected in any other way	Mix of personalities with overall vision and corporate objectives to guide them to achieving outcome(s)
Members' roles	May be designated by status alone	Awareness of others' roles, a mixture of personalities creating balance that enables roles to be matched (not exclusively by profession or status) by functional requirements. Sympathetic to others' roles and encouragement to develop special interests
Leadership (Argyle 1973)	Autocratic style	Facilitative style, mainly democratic but in a crisis can change to autocratic. Team members enabled to take the lead when appropriate
Learning style	Style varies with the individual but also the organizational preference or philosophy will be an influence. For healthcare workers all need to show evidence of 'lifelong learning'.	

and secondary care assumes a higher priority than in the past, and this has led to innovations in respiratory care delivery. For example, some patients will require care from both settings simultaneously, and this has been achieved by schemes such as 'hospital at home' and the acute respiratory assessment service (ARAS) (Flanagan et al 1999) and the acute chest triage rapid intervention team (ACTRIT) (Callaghan 1999). In such schemes the contribution that nursing, and in particular respiratory nursing, can make to help bridge the primary and secondary care interface is clear. Such ventures will involve an element of clinical risk but these complex issues can be addressed within the frameworks of clinical governance and performance assessment.

Multidisciplinary teamworking

At a strategic level, government policy encourages interagency and interorganizational working which crosses the settings of primary and secondary care. Care across settings must there-fore involve multidisciplinary working with statutory and voluntary groups. The care required by the patient will influence who is involved, but in theory the patient should be the focus of the team. Teamwork is a difficult concept, with each individual having his or her own perception of what a team is, one definition being: 'A group of people who make different contributions towards the achievement of a common goal' (Gilmore et al 1974).

In promoting multidisciplinary teamwork it is important to identify where:

- Duplication occurs and consider how to minimize this. (Is it always a bad thing?)
- Gaps in care can occur, and try to identify and address these.
- Resources could be used more effectively. This may involve referral to other agencies or provision of training and education about respiratory patients' needs to other professionals or the public.

The interpersonal relationships and use of individual skills will be governed and influenced by the objectives for achieving the goal. Generally a team differs from a group, in that teams are led and groups are managed. The team members primarily determine authority, control and role, whereas in groups a different echelon of management in the organization determines these characteristics (Table 13.1).

Many groups and teams lie in between the two poles and move position to be in different places at different times. Bales (1950) and Tuckman (1965) generated a lot of interest in and research into group dynamics (Box 13.3).

More recently, interest in healthcare teams has built upon this work and developed our understanding of teams (Belbin 1981, 1993). Pearson & Spencer (1995) point out that the idea that if a team is working well it is therefore more effective is based largely on anecdotal evidence. They write about pointers to effective primary care teamwork and have produced four major indicators of team effectiveness, as well as suggestions for their practical measurement (Box 13.4).

Field & West (1995) identified that effective teamwork is difficult to achieve but through identifying good practice the following can be used to achieve success:

- Facilitators – enable practices to identify the need for team building, provide support activities and start-up help where needed.
- Meetings – some are vital to developing team work and it is important to have the necessary skills to organize and run effective meetings.
- Training – greater emphasis is required to provide this for all members, to cultivate team members' potential, improve skills and increase the confidence of all members to participate.

Many of these practices have been referred to earlier in this chapter and support government policy to promote lifelong learning. Clearly healthcare professionals need to optimize their effectiveness in communicating with others and to be aware of how much they may be influenced by others. This is not something new but was acknowledged by Ley in 1977: '. . . it is no longer reasonable to claim that concern with the communications side of health care is merely an optional extra'.

A lot has been written about teamwork in primary care, mainly in general practice, but little has been written about how the acute setting and the community can work together as a team. Perhaps it is more realistic to aim at collaboration. Effective collaboration demands good

---

Box 13.3 Tuckman's (1965) five phases that groups pass through

1. **Forming**: start of group's life, testing of ideas, start of trust between members, leader sets tone demonstrating acceptance of differences.
2. **Storming**: members express ideas and opinions, conflict and disagreement can occur, openness and honesty without destruction is encouraged.
3. **Norming**: 'norms' for behaviour emerge as members interact and learn to accept their differences (strengths and weaknesses), the mix of people (Belbin 1981, 1993) achieves cooperation and ways of achieving the group outcomes (tasks), leader needs to identify potentially damaging norms.
4. **Performing**: members work in harmony, work flexibly to achieve tasks and enjoy working together to solve problems.
5. **Mourning**: when members leave or the group ends its life there is a sense of sadness but also of achievement.

Box 13.4 Effective and successful teams

Indicators of team effectiveness:
- agreed aims, goals, objectives
- effective communication – this requires all disciplines to use the same vocabulary (Pietroni 1992)
- patients receiving the best possible care
- individual roles defined and understood

Conditions for successful team work:
- conscious and continuous efforts to integrate both the nursing team and the primary healthcare team as a whole
- the inclusion of induction courses, team meetings and in-service courses
- provision for learning about other professions, both in training and in service
- a minimization of status differences between team members, each being encouraged to develop special interests

(Pearson & Spencer 1995)

communication and the decision making skills of individual team members. In reality, because team members are busy, finding the necessary time to make and develop collaborative working relationships is often difficult. However, with the focus now on quality and the use of the clinical governance tool, perhaps practitioners will be able to justify time set aside for collaboration and teamwork.

Communication

All members of the multidisciplinary team need to place high priority on developing effective communication channels and working in partnership with patients and carers.

There are many definitions of communication. Krech et al (1962) define it as: 'The interchange of meanings between people, primarily accomplished through the use of conventional symbols.' Hinchliff's (1979) definition is: 'A process by which people influence one another by transmitting and receiving ideas, opinions, feelings and attitudes, usually involving the use of language. Whether what is received is the same as what is transmitted therefore depends on a common perception of the meanings of the language or symbols used.'

Communication has two important components, the non-verbal and the verbal (Porritt 1990).

The combination of both components gives human beings a greater variety of expressions than any other animal. The quality of the communication and therefore of the interaction is dependent upon the networks used for the process. In fact the message transmitted may not be the message that is received. Mackay (1996a,b) found Gillespie & Yarbrough's (1984) communication model useful when considering nursing practice involving chronic respiratory patients (Fig. 13.6). This model and its theory afford a dynamic conceptual framework (in this case healthcare) in which change may occur. The model presents the communication event within a framework, allowing for a particular change in one part to influence the whole system, including an outcome of acceptance or rejection of the message. Awareness of these interactions should ensure that the message that is sent goes through the most effective channel and potential barriers are minimized.

When communicating with patients and their carers it is essential to consider their health beliefs and their experience of illness, as well as to examine one's own professional health beliefs. If they differ, both can affect communication and the differences can become barriers (Mackay 1993). The translation of good communication into practice, together with the use of appropriate channels, should minimize barriers and help create accurate

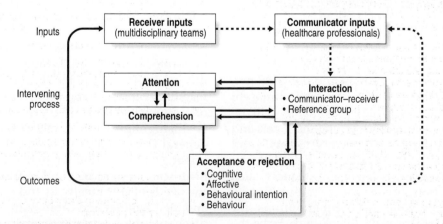

Figure 13.6 Communicating: a conceptual framework of the dynamic process. Adapted from Gillespie & Yarbrough 1984. Reprinted with permission from the Society for Nutrition Education. A conceptual model for communicating nutrition, Gillespie A and Yarbrough P, *Journal of Nutrition Education*, 16(4):169, 1984.

perceptions of the contribution each multidisciplinary team member can make to healthcare. Achievement of this will depend upon local care group settings, geographical circumstances, the care required, and team composition. Consideration of the practical communication options available to healthcare providers is needed, for example measures such as:

- regular team meetings, and/or network meetings
- effective use of information technology – the telephone, fax, databases
- quality written information in letters or patient/client-held notes.

All these need consideration when choosing the most effective channel for a given situation. However, receipt of the intended message can also be influenced by the perceptions of those involved. When considering communication, there are also ethical issues to be addressed such as confidentiality, what information is collected, how it is stored, by whom, for what purpose, and how it is shared between healthcare professionals. There should be agreement on these issues between all parties involved in health, including the patient. Non-direct patient care activity, such as letter writing, may be as important as direct care but is often perceived as less important.

Information technology

With the pace of change in new information technology (IT) there is an increasing number of options open to the multidisciplinary team, such as video conferencing, e-mail and the NHS net, even Telemedicine (Panahi & Shahtahmasebi 1999). The options actually available will be influenced by resources for IT, staffing levels and mix and the interface between NHS trusts and purchasing authorities, all of which have an influence upon any existing health alliances, such as Health Action Zones. The geography of an area can dictate what are feasible options; for example in a rural area the telephone may be the only option if a team meeting would involve hours of travelling. This differential access to services is one of the problems identified in the

government document *A first class service: quality in the new NHS* (DOH 1998a). Government policy is to address and minimize such problems by working in partnership with professionals and patients. The need to use information technology is acknowledged in *Modernising health and social services: national priorities guidance* (DOH 1998c). Sharing of information contained within databases is being explored and guidance will be issued (NHS Executive HSC 1998/098).

Discharge planning

The complex issues surrounding communication, as well as the pressure to use acute services in the most cost-effective way, mean patients are discharged sooner back into the community, reducing time available to organize care. Dennis et al (1996) state: 'As the length of hospitalisations decreases, there is less time to implement a comprehensive discharge plan that includes meeting patients' learning needs for home self care.'

Discharge planning is a process that helps the patient progress along the continuum from the hospital setting back into the community, be that home or more suitable accommodation, for example sheltered housing, or into a community rehabilitation setting before eventually going home. It should be a multidisciplinary task and the respiratory nurse may have an important role not only in coordinating care but also in aiding assessment of the patient's healthcare needs and potential for rehabilitation. This role is highly important as many healthcare professionals have little understanding of the chronic nature of some respiratory diseases and therefore lack awareness of pulmonary rehabilitation. Nolan & Nolan (1997) highlighted the fact that rehabilitation in general is receiving renewed interest and that nursing has a contribution to make in helping the healthcare system respond more adequately to the needs of chronically ill and disabled people and their families and carers. Any assessment for discharge to a different care setting should involve the patient as a partner, but some individuals may want to adopt a more passive role in their own care (Martin 1999). Care must focus on the patients and their carers and the ultimate aim should be good safe discharge (BTS 1997).

RESPIRATORY NURSE SPECIALIST

The unique contribution of nursing to healthcare underpins the development of respiratory specialist nursing. The changes are best summed up as evolutionary because they continue to be shaped by factors from both outside and inside nursing. As with any evolutionary process there exists conflict of interest, which can be used creatively. The metaphor of a cube is used by Marks-Moran (1997; Fig. 13.7) to express the many facets of nursing, including the 'opposites' of: art and science; theory and practice; thinking and doing; knowledge and action. The faces of a cube are not all visible at once (at least one face remains hidden when it is looked at) but they are interconnected because all are needed to form the cube. If the skills of the generalist nurse and those of the specialist are placed on opposite cube faces then it is possible to see how nursing responds to the needs of respiratory patients in a variety of ways: for example through the generalist nurse with an interest in respiratory care, such as a district nurse or a ward based nurse; through the nurse who specializes in all respiratory diseases; and also through the nurse with an even more specialist role, focusing on a specific respiratory disease such as asthma, cystic fibrosis, COPD or tuberculosis.

Liaison role of the respiratory nurse specialist

The respiratory nurse specialist has an important liaison role between primary and secondary care and is therefore in an ideal position to contribute to healthcare by undertaking a central coordinating function (Fig. 13.7; Case study 13.4) through the activities of discharge planning and collaborative interagency working.

The majority of contacts between the public and the NHS occur in the community setting, therefore it is important to explore the value of contact in the home for respiratory patients. The value of such an approach with chronic respiratory patients was shown by the early research of Cockcroft et al

(1987) and more recently by Flanagan et al (1999). Cockcroft et al showed that home visits by a respiratory nurse specialist may have contributed to better survival rates in chronic respiratory patients. One explanation for this is that these chronic respiratory patients were taught to seek help, rather than to ignore signs of deterioration. Heslop & Bagnall (1988) used a nursing model framework to help assess and plan care. They addressed the patients' and carers' agendas and included teaching about physical health, knowledge of medicines and identification of psychological and social issues. Flanagan et al (1999) demonstrated high patient satisfaction with this type of service. This approach to care delivery by the respiratory nurse is endorsed in the COPD guidelines (BTS 1997).

By bridging the gap in both directions between primary and secondary care, the respiratory nurse specialist can see patients in both settings. This can be achieved by home visiting, empowering patients to self-manage, acting as an advocate when the patient is unable to address concerns related to health, and being involved in discharge planning. In undertaking these activities the nurse is improving the flow of information about the patient or group of patients. In particular, if the nurse has visited in the home then he or she can help set realistic goals for rehabilitation.

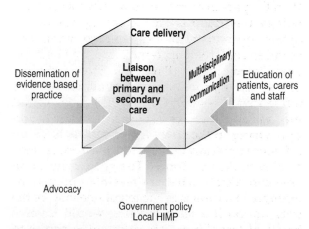

Figure 13.7 Coordinating function of the respiratory nurse. Adapted from Marks-Moran 1997.

Case study 13.4

James (68 years) was admitted to hospital with an ex-acerbation of COPD. Whilst an inpatient he made a slow recovery, but was obviously frailer than when seen at home by the respiratory nurse specialist. The discharge plan was to send him home with a nebulizer (which he learned how to use in hospital), the district nurse was fully briefed about discharge and management of the equipment, and a package of care was arranged. This consisted of a carer calling morning, lunch time and evening, and provision of meals on wheels.

After James' discharge the respiratory nurse specialist visited him at home and found that he was very anxious about how he would cope when his level of social support was reduced to once a day. The respiratory nurse specialist liaised about these real concerns with social services, the GP and the district nurse. James was to be reassessed by the social services home care organizer and the medical and nursing colleagues agreed that the minimum he required was an early morning and an evening call. The district nurse continued to call weekly.

The respiratory nurse specialist visited the following month to find that James was less confident about managing his care and was using more cylinders of oxygen although his SaO_2 was stable at 93%. His anxieties centred on how much he felt 'unable to cope' despite trying to remain independent; this was now worse in the evenings. It also appeared that he had a disagreement with one of his carers, who he said had given him the feeling that he 'should be coping better by now'. Despite these concerns being addressed, it was clear that James had lost his desire to, as he put it, 'battle for independence'. Again the respiratory nurse specialist shared findings with the GP, who was willing to support a case for increased support at home. However, before any action could be taken James was readmitted with another exacerbation. This time, when the respiratory nurse specialist saw him on the ward, James was adamant that he wanted to go into residential care in an area 50 miles away because this was near to his niece. His request was documented in the nursing and medical notes and his named nurse on the ward arranged for a social worker to advise him on the options and begin an assessment.

In reality, finding suitable, acceptable placements for chronic respiratory patients is a challenge. It seems that other agencies do not always understand or appreciate the problems of breathlessness, the unpredictability of the course of the disease and how stigmatized patients can feel (Williams 1993).

THE FUTURE

Quality respiratory care must be evidence-based and involve multidisciplinary audit, not just medical audit – valuable though that is. Health and social care agencies are beginning to embrace the concept of total quality improvement (TQI), which places emphasis on the customer. This approach to care delivery sits comfortably with shared clinical governance and clinical effectiveness (Alexander et al 1994), which were discussed earlier.

The key factors in improving respiratory health are:

- Preventive work, which could also be labelled primary prevention (e.g. smoking cessation).
- Rehabilitation – secondary and tertiary prevention.
- Palliative care (WHO 1990 states the aims of palliative care).
- Information technology (to help deliver care).
- Leadership – with the advent of nurse consultant posts (DOH 1999c) it will be interesting to see if such posts are created for respiratory care, thus developing a career structure for the respiratory nurse.
- Implementation of a public health model where patients are partners and carers are given more voice (Nolan & Philip 1999).

'Hope' is not just a concept for our patients to hold onto (Kylma & Vehvilainen-Julkunen 1997) but is relevant to healthcare professionals, as we all adjust to changes in the evolution of how healthcare is provided. It has to be accepted that change is not easy but affects us all. For respiratory nurses it is important that we are clear about nursing's unique contribution to respiratory care. Books such as this help develop thinking not just about the science but also about the art of nursing, especially respiratory nursing.

REFERENCES

Acheson D 1998 Report of the independent inquiry into inequalities in health (The Acheson Report). The Stationery Office, London

Alexander M K, Bourgeois A, Goodman L R 1994 Total quality improvement: bridging the gap between education and service. In: Strickland O L, Fishman D J (eds) Nursing issues in the 1990s. Delmar, Albany, NY, pp 280–289

Argyle M 1973 Social interaction. Tavistock, London

Bagnall P, Heslop A 1987 Chronic respiratory disease: educating patients at home. Professional Nurse 2(9): 293–296

Bales R F 1950 Interaction process analysis. Addison-Wesley, Cambridge, Mass

Barker D J P 1993 Fetal and infant origins of adult disease. British Medical Association, London

Belbin R M 1981 Management teams. Heinemann, London

Belbin R M 1993 Team roles at work Heinemann/Butterworth, London

The Black Report 1980 Inequalities in health. HMSO, London

British Thoracic Society 1997 Guidelines for the management of COPD. Thorax 52 (suppl 5): S1–S28

Brooks F, Mitchell M, Pugh J 1998 Shared governance as a way to involve staff in decision-making. Nursing Times 94(46): 56–57

Callaghan S 1999 ACTRIT: Acute Chest Triage Rapid Intervention Team. Accident and Emergency Nursing 7(1): 42–46

Cockcroft A, Bagnall P, Heslop A et al 1987 Controlled trial of respiratory health worker visiting patients with chronic respiratory disability. British Medical Journal 294: 225–228

Council for the Education and Training of Health Visitors (CETHV) 1977 An investigation into the principles of health visiting. CETHV, London

Dennis L I, Blue C L, Stahl S M et al 1996 The relationship between hospital readmissions of Medicare beneficiaries with chronic illness and home care nursing interventions. Home Healthcare Nurse 14(4): 303–309

Department of Health 1990 The national health service and community care act. HMSO, London

Department of Health 1991 The patient's charter. HMSO, London

Department of Health 1992 The health of the nation. A strategy for health for England. HMSO, London

Department of Health 1997 The new NHS: modern and dependable. The Stationery Office, London

Department of Health 1998a A first class service: quality in the new NHS. The Stationery Office, London

Department of Health 1998b Partnership in action. New opportunities for joint working between health and social services. A discussion document. The Stationery Office, London

Department of Health 1998c Modernising health and social services: national priorities guidance. The Stationery Office, London

Department of Health 1998d Smoking kills: a White Paper on tobacco. Cm 4177. The Stationery Office, London

Department of Health 1998e Working together – securing a quality workforce for the NHS. The Stationery Office, London

Department of Health 1999a Saving lives: our healthier nation. The Stationery Office, London

Department of Health 1999b The NHS performance assessment framework. The Stationery Office, London

Department of Health 1999c Making a difference: strengthening the nursing, midwifery and health visiting contribution to health and healthcare. The Stationery Office, London

Field R, West M 1995 Teamwork in primary health care. 2. Perspectives from practices. Journal of Interprofessional Care 9(2): 123–130

Flanagan U M, Irwin A, Dagg K 1999 An acute respiratory assessment service. Professional Nurse 14(12): 839–842

Gillespie A H, Yarbrough P 1984 A conceptual model for communicating nutrition. Journal of Nutrition Education 16(4): 168–172

Gilmore M, Bruce N, Hunt M 1974 The work of the nursing team in general practice. CETHV, London

Heslop A 1995 A study to explore the impact of disabling breathlessness and the influence of a carer in patients with chronic airflow limitation. MSc dissertation in Nursing Studies. West London Institute of Higher Education (a college of Brunel University)

Heslop A 1997 The role of the respiratory nurse and home care. In: Morgan M, Singh S (eds) Practical pulmonary rehabilitation. Chapman & Hall Medical, London

Heslop A P, Bagnall P 1988 A study to evaluate the intervention of a nurse visiting patients with disabling chest disease in the community. Journal of Advanced Nursing 13: 71–77

Hinchliff S M 1979 Teaching clinical nursing. Churchill Livingstone, Edinburgh, p 245

Holmes W F, Macfarlane J 1999 Introduction. Issues at the interface between primary and secondary care in the management of common respiratory disease. Thorax 54: 538–539

Krech D, Crutchfield R S, Ballachey E L 1962 Individuals in society. A textbook of social psychology. International Student Edition. McGraw-Hill, New York, p 307

Kylma J, Vehvilainen-Julkunen K 1997 Hope in nursing research: a meta-analysis of the ontological and epistemological foundations of research on hope. Journal of Advanced Nursing 25(2): 364–371

Ley P 1977 Communicating with the patient. In: Coleman J C (ed) Introductory psychology. A textbook for health students. Routledge & Kegan Paul, London, ch 12

Mackay L 1993 Evaluation is the key to success. A nurse-led tuberculosis contact tracing service. Professional Nurse 9(3): 176–180

Mackay L 1996a Nutritional status and chronic obstructive pulmonary disease. Nursing Standard 10(39): 38–42

Mackay L 1996b Health education and COPD rehabilitation: a study. Nursing Standard 10(40): 34–39

Mant D 1997 Research and development in primary care. National Working Group Report, NHSE, Leeds

Marks-Moran D 1997 Reconstructing nursing: beyond art and science. Baillière Tindall, Edinburgh

Martin N J 1999 Commentary on Thorne and Paterson's review: research on chronic illness. Evidence Based Nursing 2(1): 32

NHS Executive 1998 Clinical governance: quality in the new NHS. The Stationery Office, London

NHS Executive HSC 1998 Implementing the recommendations of the Caldicott report. Consultation paper on 'Caldicott Guardians' and the NHS strategic tracing service. Health service circular 1998/098. DOH, London

NHS Executive North Thames 1998 Clinical governance: moving from rhetoric to reality. DOH, London

Nolan M, Nolan J 1997 Rehabilitation: realizing the potential nursing contribution. British Journal of Nursing 6(20): 1176–1180

Nolan M, Philip I 1999 COPE: towards a comprehensive assessment of caregiver need. British Journal of Nursing 8(20): 1364–1372

OPCS 1994 General household survey. HMSO, London

Panahi G R, Shahtahmasebi S 1999 The implications of telemedicine for nursing. Professional Nurse 14(12): 835–838

Pearson P, Spencer J 1995 Pointers to effective teamwork: exploring primary care. Journal of Interprofessional Care 9(2): 131–138

Pietroni P 1992 Towards reflective practice – the languages of health and social care. Journal of Interprofessional Care 6(1): 7–16

Porritt L 1990 Communication: the basis of interaction. In: Interaction strategies: an introduction for health professionals, 2nd edn. Churchill Livingstone, London, ch 1

Porter-O'Grady T 1994 Whole systems shared governance: creating seamless organisation. Nursing Economics 12(4): 187–195

Raw M, McNeill A, West R 1998 Smoking cessation guidelines for health professionals. Thorax 53 (suppl 5, part 1): S1–S19

Sackman T 1999 CPHVA PCG board members' network. Community Practitioner 72(7): 220–222

Thompson N 1995 Theory and practice in health and social welfare. Open University Press, Buckingham

Tuckman B W 1965 Developmental sequence in small groups. Psychology Bulletin 63: 384–399

Williams S J 1993 Chronic respiratory illness. Routledge, London

World Health Organization 1980 International classification of impairment, disability and handicap. WHO, Geneva

World Health Organization 1990 Cancer pain relief and palliative care. Technical Report Series 804. WHO, Geneva

Index